I0797401

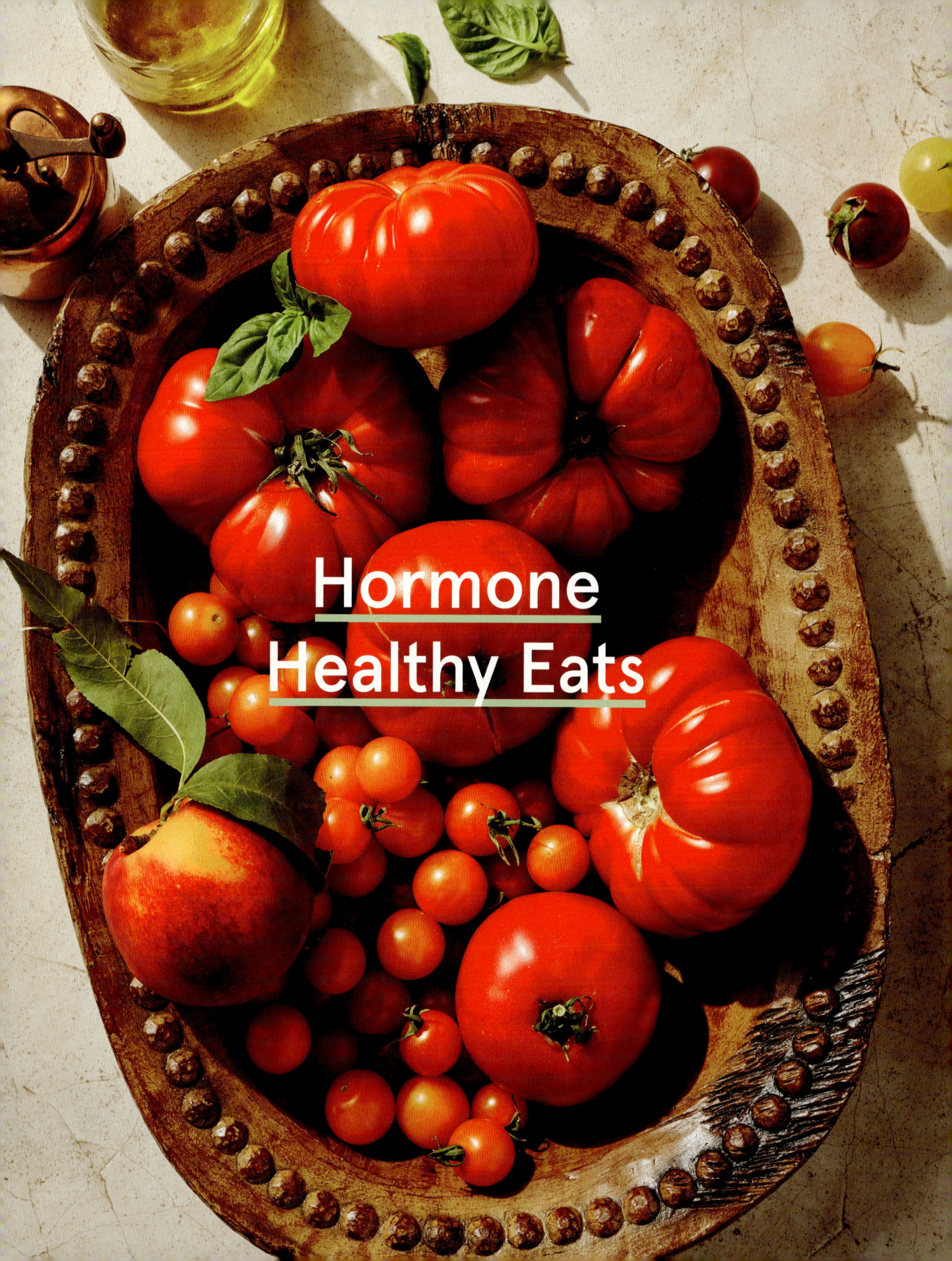

Hormone Healthy Eats

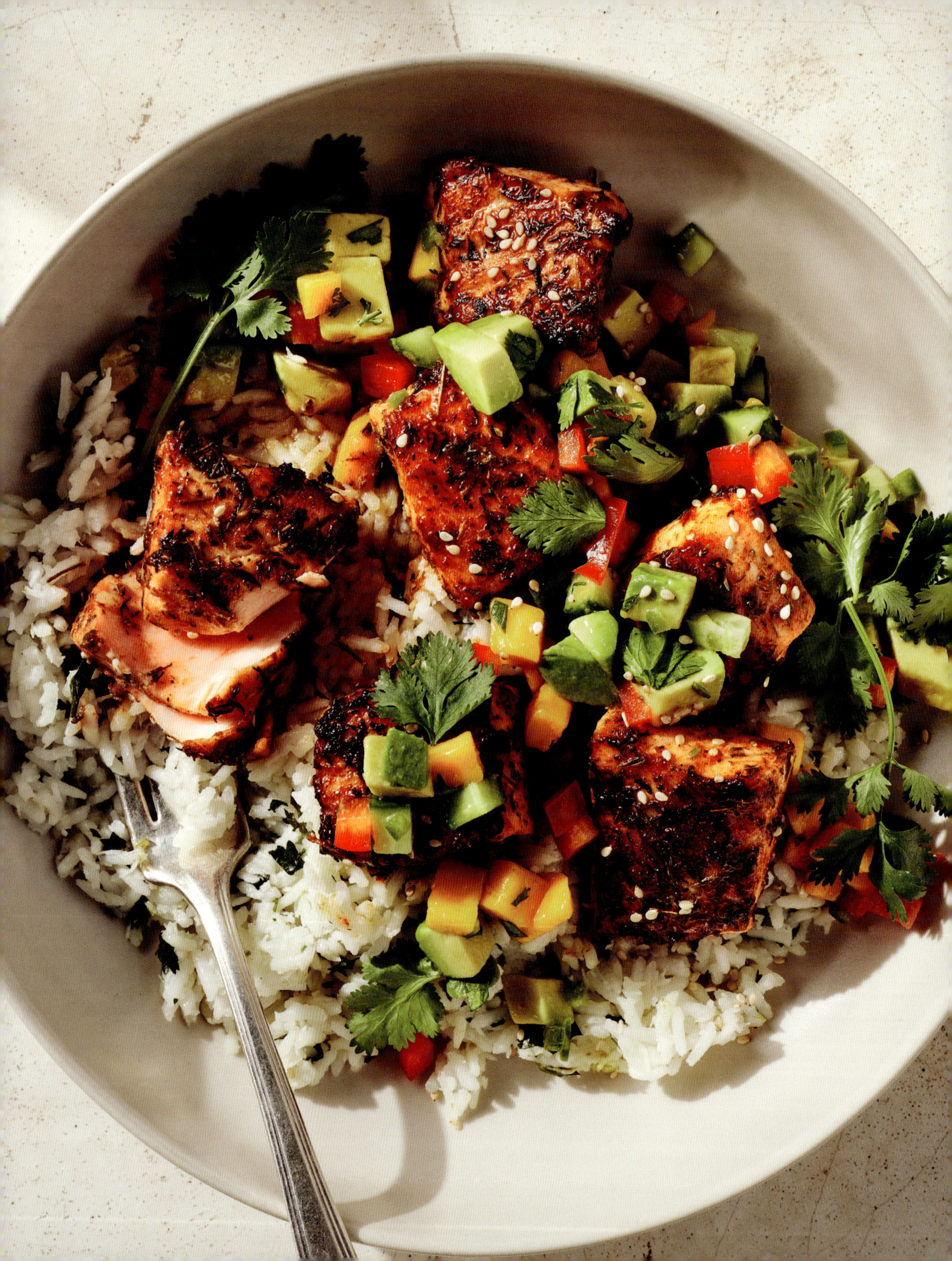

Hormone Healthy Eats

100 Recipes to Balance Your Hormones, Support Your Cycle, and Feel Your Absolute Best

LAUREN CHAMBERS

Photographs by Eva Kolenko

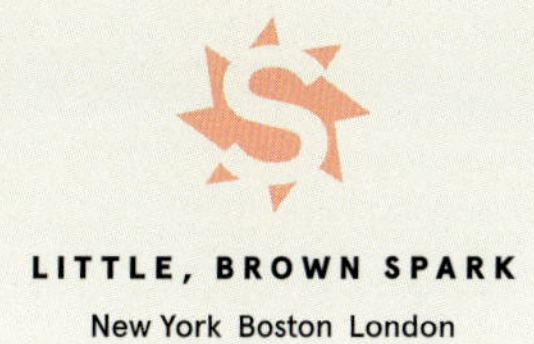

LITTLE, BROWN SPARK

New York Boston London

The information in this book is provided for educational purposes only and is not intended to diagnose, treat, cure, or prevent any condition or disease. This book is not intended as a substitute for consultation with a licensed practitioner. Please consult with your own physician or healthcare specialist regarding the suggestions and recommendations made in this book.

Little, Brown Spark
Hachette Book Group, 1290 Avenue of the Americas, New York, NY 10104
littlebrownspark.com

First Edition: February 2026

Little, Brown Spark is an imprint of Little, Brown and Company, a division of Hachette Book Group, Inc. The Little, Brown Spark name and logo are trademarks of Hachette Book Group, Inc.

Photography by Eva Kolenko
Styling by Emily Caneer, Genesis Vallejo, and Allison Fellion
Text illustrations by Leigh Savage
Book design by Laura Palese

ISBN 9780316577885
LCCN 2025941562

10 9 8 7 6 5 4 3 2 1

1010

Printed in China

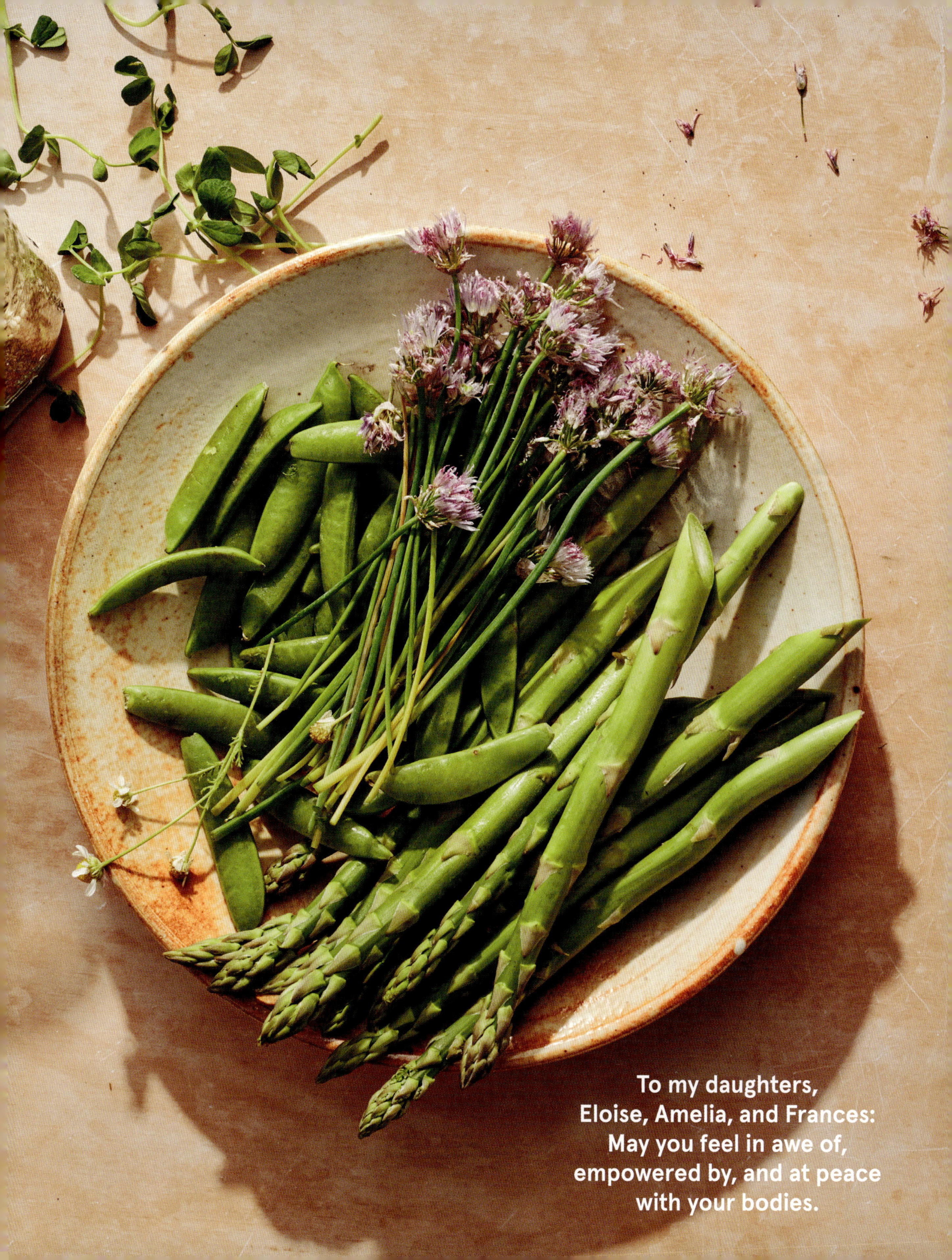

To my daughters,
Eloise, Amelia, and Frances:
May you feel in awe of,
empowered by, and at peace
with your bodies.

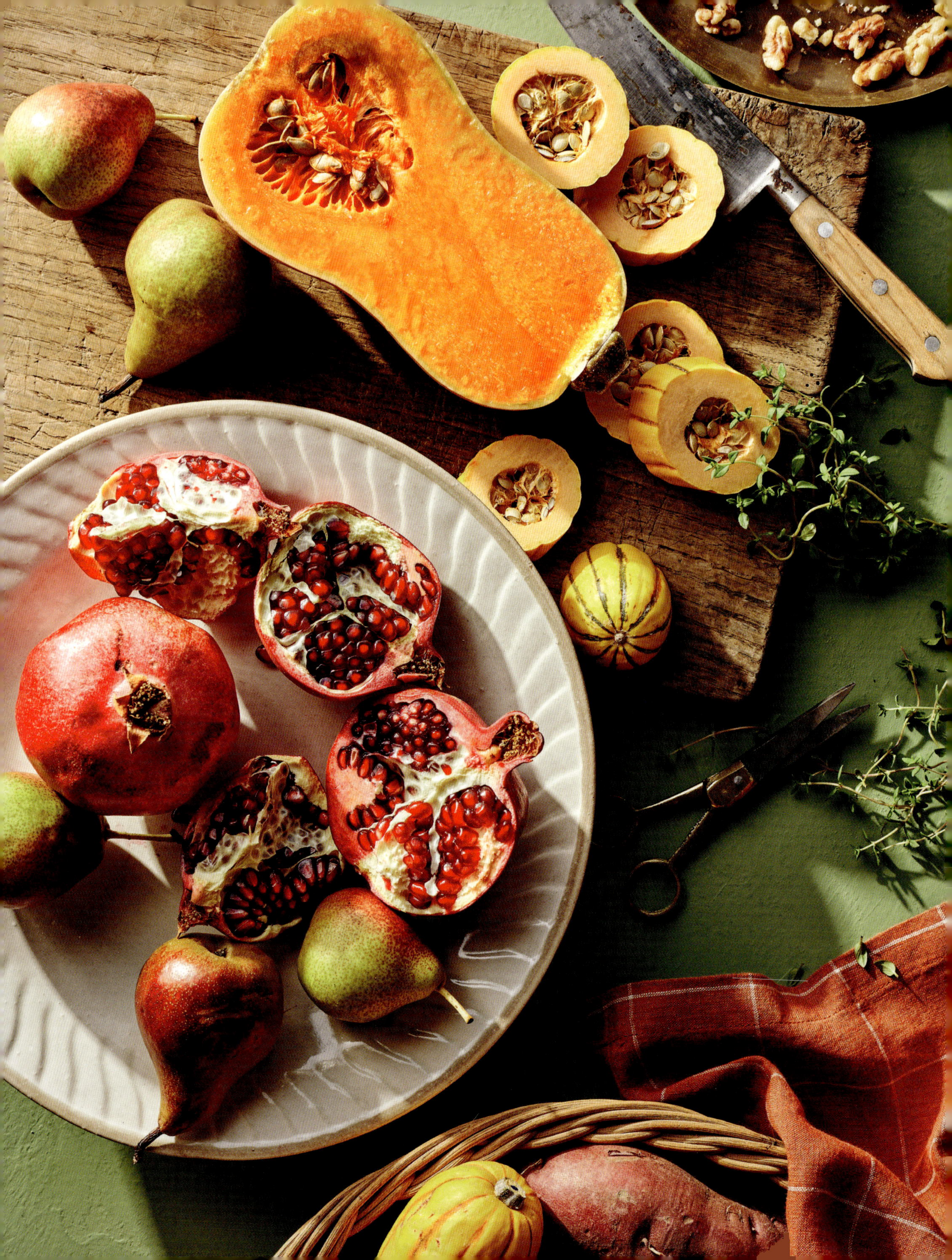

Contents

INTRODUCTION

For over a decade I struggled with symptoms of hormonal imbalance, including heavy, painful, and irregular periods; mood swings; acne; depression; anxiety; digestive issues; hair loss/thinning; and stubborn weight gain around my midsection. I was resigned to the fact that this was all just a "normal" part of being a woman with a period every month—until I went back to school specifically to study women's hormone health.

I'd always loved food, but I also grew up in the 1990s, when low-calorie and fat-free foods were all the rage, and spent much of my adolescence and 20s following a plethora of fad diets (Atkins, anyone?!) and consuming ultra-processed foods like Lean Cuisine, fat-free Jell-O with Cool Whip, and Kashi GoLean Crunch in an effort to keep up with the wafer-thin magazine models and sorority girls I envied in college.

And I did manage to stay skinny, at the cost of my health and happiness. First, I lost my period for two years, which at the time I considered a badge of honor: No PMS or period to deal with for one to two weeks every month? Amazing. But then, as a result, more symptoms cropped up, ranging from uncomfortable digestive issues (irritable bowel syndrome [IBS] and small intestinal bacterial overgrowth [SIBO]) to insomnia to mood swings to crippling anxiety.

But I kept on. And the more I white-knuckled it through each day, never feeling fully satiated or nourished, the worse my hormonal imbalance symptoms became. Of course, I had no idea the two were related at that time, so the more I struggled, the more I punished and deprived myself, pushing myself to train for grueling marathons and eating the same "safe" foods day in and day out (baked chicken breast, low-calorie protein bars, etc.) to regain some sort of control.

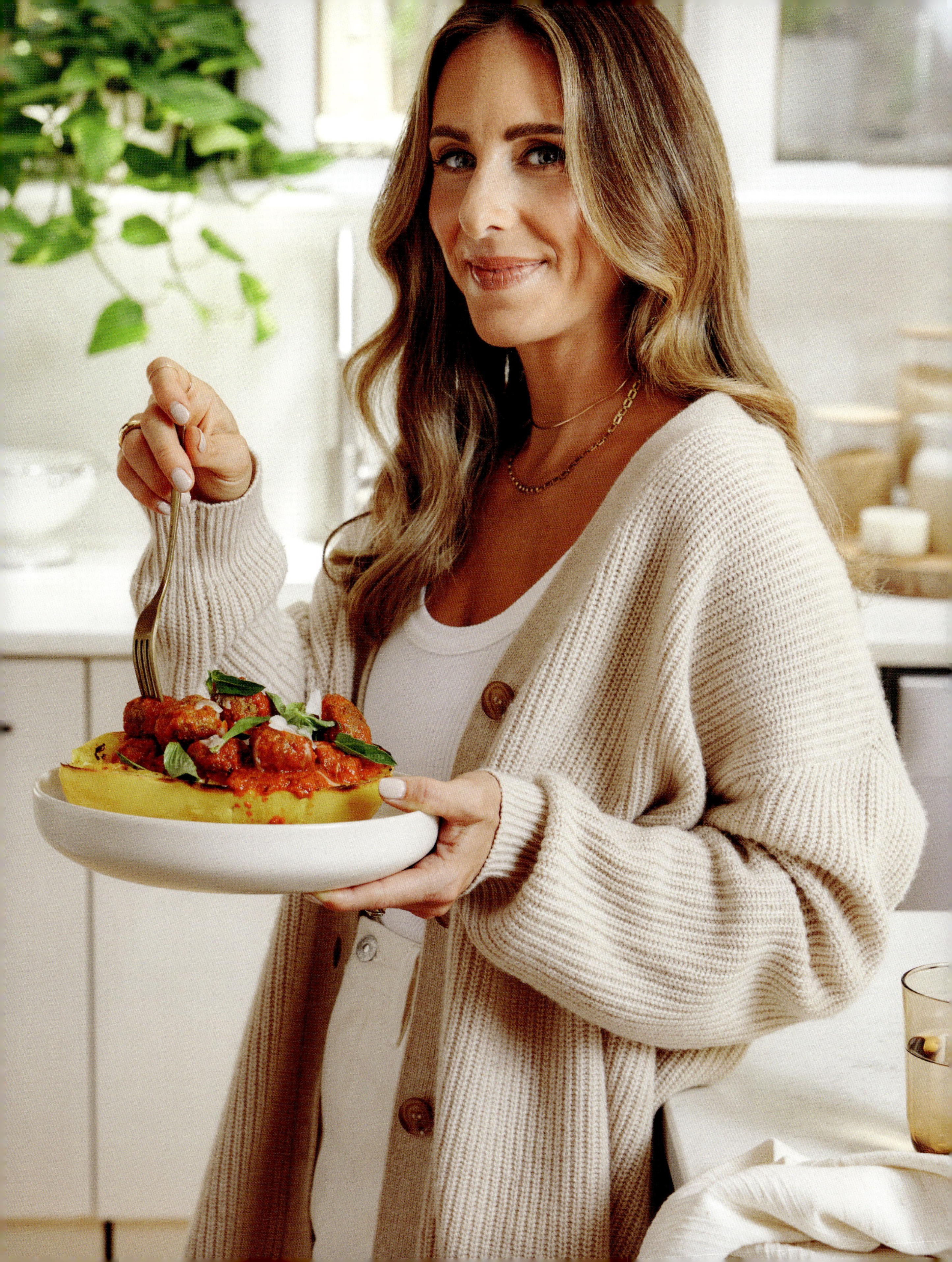

At the Institute for Integrative Nutrition, I learned that while these uncomfortable symptoms are incredibly common, with 90 percent of menstruating women in the United States reporting they experience some sort of period pain or symptom each month, they aren't, in fact, normal. Rather, they are your body's way of telling you that your hormones are out of balance and need support.

I also learned that undernourishment (i.e., not eating enough or regularly, restricting food groups or certain nutrients, skipping meals, fasting, stress around foods, etc.) is one of the leading culprits of hormonal imbalances. Food is to our hormones what gas is to a car, driving our cells, giving us energy and the fuel our hormones need to function and do their jobs effectively, which in turn regulates our metabolism, weight, appetite, overall appearance, and so much more.

After getting my accreditation in hormone health, I began integrating my new knowledge into my daily life, especially as it related to my complex relationship with food.

For the first time in decades, instead of focusing on calorie counting, deprivation, restriction, and only eating a specific list of foods deemed "safe" or "healthy," I started adding a wide variety of nutrient-rich foods to my meals, experimenting with rotating ingredients, and creating delicious recipes to support each phase of my menstrual cycle.

The results were surprising, in the best possible way:

- I began having consistent, dependable menstrual cycles for the first time ever, and all of my symptoms gradually diminished over time.
- I no longer needed Midol, a hot water bottle, and oversized sweatpants to accommodate the bloat and cramping I had previously experienced in the days leading up to and during my period.
- As my mood stabilized, the fighting with my husband during "that time of the month" began to naturally subside.

- I was also able to say goodbye to my zit cream and my Proactiv subscription once and for all.
- My bouts of fatigue, intense sugar cravings, and erratic sleep behavior were eventually replaced with even energy throughout the day, a healthy appetite, and deep, restful sleep at night.
- My hair became thick and full, my SIBO and IBS symptoms dissipated, and I began to get compliments on my "glowing skin."
- Last but certainly not least, when it came time to try to get pregnant, I was able to conceive naturally (three times, with three girls!), something I wasn't sure I'd ever be able to achieve due to my previously erratic cycles.

Before I learned how to balance my hormones, primarily through nourishing foods and recipes, I had no idea feeling this good was possible, especially without making major sacrifices. But I am living proof that balanced hormones are the key and can be achieved simply through eating *more* delicious food and integrating easy action steps into a daily routine.

I had discovered the secret sauce, and I want to share it with as many women as possible, making sure no female out there has to ever suffer or "just deal with" her uncomfortable symptoms again. So, ten years ago I opened my private practice, So Fresh N So Green, and dedicated my time to providing women with delicious recipes, simple tips, and natural remedies to help them optimize their hormones, health, and lives.

And after years of empowering women to nourish and take care of their bodies, but with the drive and determination to scale and help many more women than a 1:1 practice allows, I am so excited to share *Hormone Healthy Eats,* a cookbook designed to help you balance your hormones through food to live your best, most vibrant life.

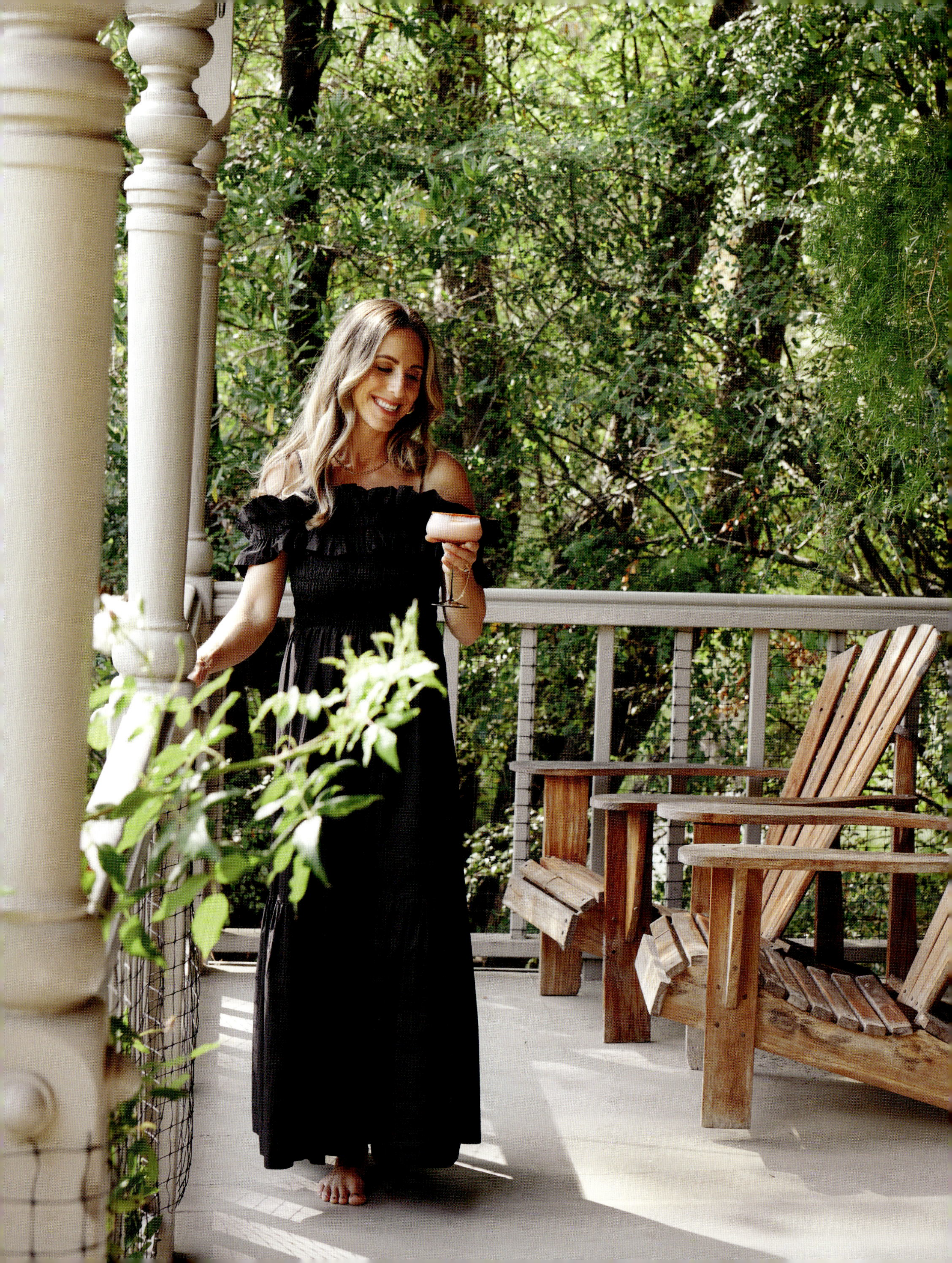

PART ONE

How Your Hormones and Menstrual Cycle Work

HORMONES 101

Our hormones, and periods, aren't out to get us—rather they exist to empower us. Their functionality isn't just designed to keep us alive, it's to help us *thrive*.

IF YOU'RE A WOMAN in your reproductive years, defined as being from your first period until menopause, roughly 30 to 40 years, your hormones dictate almost every aspect of your life:

- Appearance
- Energy
- Confidence
- Mood
- Metabolism
- Sex drive
- Cravings
- Weight
- Sleep
- Focus
- Digestion
- Memory
- Stress levels
- Ability to conceive and carry a healthy baby to term
- And let's not forget: your period

With so much influence over how we look, feel, act, eat, and think every day, from our first period to our last, the lack of education most of us have received about hormones is mind-blowing. Instead, the cumulative message many of us were taught via the media, school, healthcare providers, and peers was that our hormones (and periods) were something unfortunate to simply be dealt with every month. The uncomfortable and downright debilitating symptoms we experienced were, and still are, dismissed as normal, conditioning us to become victims of our own bodies, rather than being empowered by them.

While this attitude is incredibly unfortunate and even damaging, especially for those of us who have been struggling with symptoms of hormonal imbalance for years, the amazing news is that we carry the ability to change the status quo.

Our hormones, and periods, aren't out to get us—rather they exist to empower us. Their functionality isn't just designed to keep us alive, it's to help us *thrive*. And when they're supported, balanced, nourished, and attended to, they'll do everything they can to help us look and feel our best. They'll enable us to tap into the unique skills that only women in our reproductive years have access to: going out and living our best, most vibrant lives and feeling capable, powerful, and inspiring as women unhindered by health problems, hormonal imbalances, or body issues and positively impacting everyone in our orbit as a result.

So no, our hormones themselves aren't the problem. The problems are a lack of education around hormones combined with modern lifestyle factors that unwittingly throw them into chaos, particularly as related to mixed messaging around diet culture, "healthy" eating habits, and a plethora of "wellness" trends.

This is a huge reason why I created *Hormone Healthy Eats,* a guide to empower women to flip the script society has dealt us by utilizing nourishing recipes and supportive foods and lifestyle habits—helping us become the co-creators of our health, hormones, body, and life.

The first steps in this journey are education and awareness, beginning with an overview of the major hormones and the roles they play in our bodies. This will ultimately help you understand what's really behind symptoms you're experiencing—as well as how to reduce or reverse them in the long run.

OVERVIEW OF THE ENDOCRINE SYSTEM AND MAJOR FEMALE HORMONES

The Endocrine System

The endocrine system is a complex network of glands and organs. As humans, we simply could not survive without our endocrine system, which includes our:

- Brain (most notably the hypothalamus, pineal gland, and pituitary gland)
- Thyroid
- Parathyroid
- Thymus gland
- Adrenal glands
- Pancreas
- Ovaries (in women) and testes (in men)

This extremely sophisticated system uses hormones as chemical messengers to provide signals to various organs and tissues in your body to control and coordinate super important functions such as your:

- Metabolism
- Energy production
- Blood pressure
- Blood sugar
- Body temperature
- Growth and development
- Fluid and electrolyte balance
- Sexual function
- Reproduction and fertility
- Sleep/wake cycle
- Response to injury, stress, and mood

So yeah, pretty important stuff, right?

Major Female Hormones

While there are over fifty hormones identified in the human body, let's look at some of the major players and how they specifically interact with our bodies.

ESTROGEN

Produced by the ovaries, this proliferative (growth-promoting) hormone is involved in our reproductive system and menstrual cycle, as well as regulating cholesterol levels, the urinary tract, heart and blood vessels, bones, breast health, skin, hair, mucous membranes, pelvic muscles, and brain health and function.

WHEN IN BALANCE: Estrogen helps us feel happy, energetic, outgoing, and confident.

PROGESTERONE

Also produced by our ovaries, this steroid hormone plays a key part in female reproduction and a healthy menstrual cycle. It's best known for its role in preparing the endometrial lining to thicken to potentially house a fertilized egg after ovulation. It also helps to maintain a healthy pregnancy, reduce stress and anxiety, regulate mood, behavior, and cognitive function, stimulate weight gain and appetite, maintain fat tissue, and keep estrogen levels in check.

WHEN IN BALANCE: Progesterone helps us feel cool, calm, and collected.

TESTOSTERONE

The primary function of testosterone, produced in our ovaries, is to maintain our reproductive tissues along with growth and development, bone mass, and sex drive.

WHEN IN BALANCE: Testosterone makes us feel confident, bold, and sexy. However, when it is high it can lead to male-like characteristics, including acne, facial hair, and infrequent periods, often associated with polycystic ovarian syndrome, or PCOS for short.

The Female Endocrine System and Its Hormones

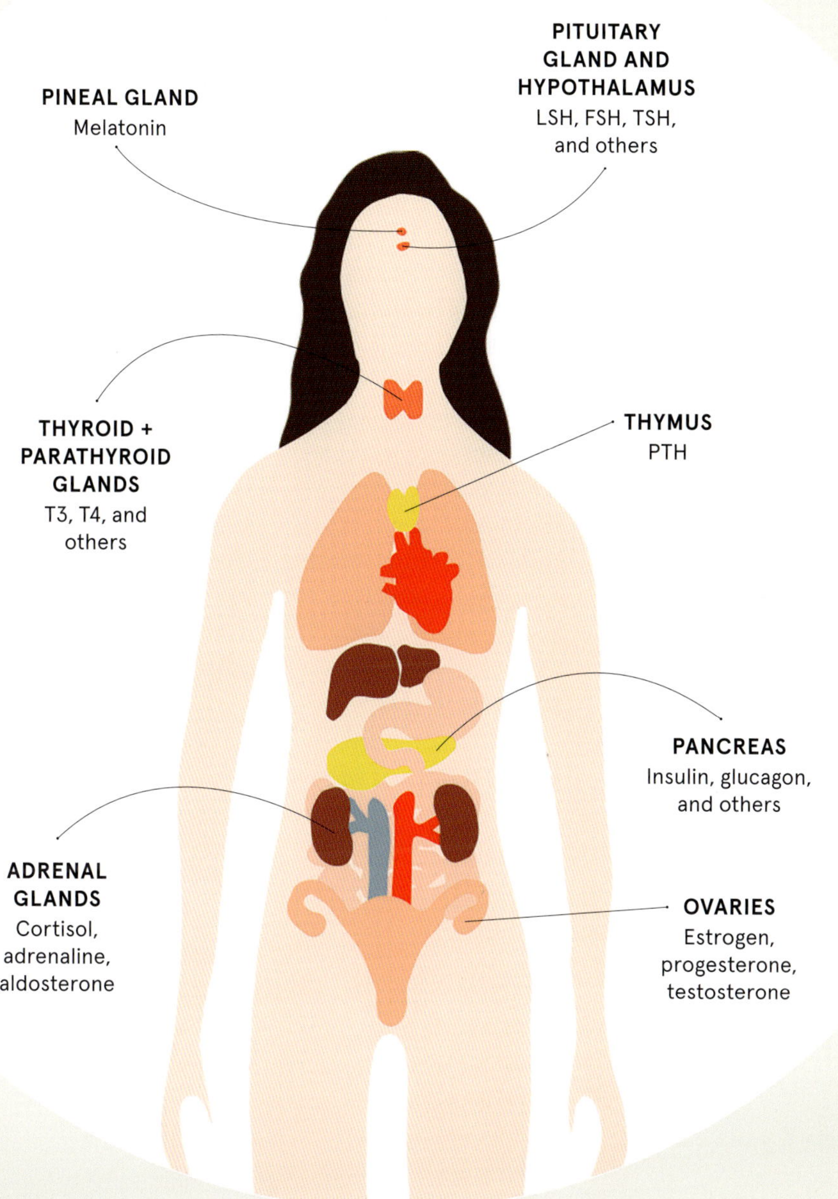

ESTROGEN
A proliferative (growth-promoting) hormone involved in your reproductive system and menstrual cycle.

TESTOSTERONE
Maintains our reproductive tissues along with growth and development.

INSULIN
Helps maintain your blood sugar levels.

LSH + FSH
Stimulate follicular growth and ovulation.

PROGESTERONE
Plays a key part in reproductive health and menstrual cycle. Thickens the uterine lining and keeps estrogen in check.

THYROID HORMONES
Regulate metabolism, heart function, digestion, muscle control, brain development, and bone maintenance.

CORTISOL
Regulates the body's response to stress.

MELATONIN
Regulates the sleep/wake cycle.

THYROID HORMONES

The thyroid hormones T3 (active form) and T4 (inactive form) are produced by the thyroid gland, which is shaped like a butterfly and sits at the base of your neck, right above the collarbone. T3's main job is to regulate metabolism by converting the food consumed into usable energy. It also regulates heart function, digestion, muscle control, brain development, and bone maintenance.

WHEN IN BALANCE: T3 helps us maintain a healthy weight, prevent brain fog, optimize digestion, and keep us feeling happy.

CORTISOL

Cortisol is released by the adrenal glands, the triangular organs that sit above your kidneys, and is essential in regulating our body's response to stress. It also helps control the body's use of fat, carbohydrates, and protein. Cortisol tends to get a bad rap, but without adequate production, we would die, as it also regulates blood pressure and blood sugar, and suppresses inflammation.

WHEN IN BALANCE: Cortisol releases cyclically, rising and peaking within the first 30 minutes we're awake and then slowly declining throughout the day and night, helping us stay alert and regulating our sleep/wake cycle.

INSULIN

Produced by your pancreas, which is not only a part of the endocrine system but the digestive system as well, insulin is responsible for releasing digestive enzymes that help to deliver glucose (which is what the meal you just ate turns into) from your bloodstream into the cells, where it is stored and used as energy. This helps to maintain blood sugar levels, which, just like hormones, need to be kept Goldilocks-style: not too little, not too much, just right. The pancreas also produces glucagon, which breaks down glucose stored in muscles and tissue to increase blood sugar.

WHEN IN BALANCE: Insulin enables us to effortlessly maintain a healthy weight, muscle mass, and energy levels, and rarely experience cravings.

As you can see, hormones are a really big deal and a part of a complex system that impacts our bodies in so many important ways. Our endocrine system and hormones are so interconnected with a variety of important roles and functions within the body that when one hormone is out of balance it likely impacts the rest of the system in a myriad of ways, which we then experience as uncomfortable, embarrassing, and painful hormonal imbalance symptoms.

COMMON HORMONE DISRUPTORS

When I step back and think about it, it's kind of crazy that 80 to 90 percent of menstruating women report experiencing symptoms related to PMS and underlying hormonal imbalances.[1]

What's at the root of all of these symptoms? Why do women seem to be hit so hard?

The short answer: Modern-day obstacles such as exposure to toxins and chemicals, processed foods, diet culture, and stress, just to name a few, are to blame. As you'll soon learn, many of these disruptors were only introduced within the last century, and were most often designed out of convenience and with good intentions but, as we're now learning, have disastrous effects on our hormones and endocrine system.

Let's cover some of the more common hormone disruptors so that you can start to identify whether they may be contributing to your specific symptoms and, I hope, resolve them effectively.

Toxin Exposure

While our bodies were originally designed to detoxify naturally, today we're exposed to a variety of toxins that didn't even exist in our environment one hundred years ago. *In fact, over 80,000 chemicals are in use today in the United States alone!*[2] And the research is showing that toxic chemicals are taking a dramatic toll on our hormone health, with 1 in 10 women within their reproductive years being diagnosed with PCOS,[3] 1 in 8 women developing a thyroid disorder within her lifetime,[4] and 1 in 6 couples worldwide struggling with infertility.[5]

Most of these toxins wreak havoc on the endocrine system by disrupting its normal function. They act like copycats, mimicking hormones normally produced in the body, which causes major confusion and a disruption in the feedback system. Often our bodies then stop making these hormones naturally, leading to...you guessed it, a hormonal imbalance.

Processed and Conventional Foods

While we're on the topic of toxins, let's touch on the hormone-disrupting chemicals found in many processed and conventionally grown foods, including plants sprayed with pesticides and animal proteins injected with hormones, antibiotics, and chemicals. While not all, many processed foods (think chips, candy, baked goods, cereals, dressings, canned goods, etc.) as well as conventionally grown fruits, vegetables, and animal proteins contain endocrine-disrupting chemicals that have been found to be the culprit in not only hormone imbalances (especially impacting the thyroid, adrenals, and reproductive organs) but also heart disease, metabolic syndrome, and obesity. We'll go over these later in more detail, but I always encourage clients to start by reading every single ingredient label before purchasing foods, even those marketed as "healthy." If it contains a long list of ingredients you don't recognize or can't pronounce, chances are it's going to negatively impact your hormones and health as a result.

Chronic Stress

We do need stress hormones to survive, and a little bit can often be a good thing, keeping us alert in high-risk situations or supplying us with a boost of energy during an intense workout. But chronic stress depletes our bodies of micronutrients needed to make hormones. Not only that, chronic stress instructs our adrenals to consistently pump out cortisol, keeping our bodies in a constant state of fight-or-flight. These elevated cortisol levels tell our ovaries to decrease estrogen and progesterone production, as the body must prioritize a stress response over other functions (because it thinks it must do so to survive). This means our body diverts resources from things not important in a life-or-death situation—including ovulation and a healthy menstrual cycle—so chronic stress is seen as a key culprit in many hormonal imbalances and fertility challenges.

Diet Culture

While we're still thinking about stress, it's worth noting that diet culture has had a profound impact on female hormones. Most diets, workout regimens,

> "HORMONES ARE A PART OF A COMPLEX SYSTEM THAT IMPACTS OUR BODIES IN SO MANY IMPORTANT WAYS.

and "wellness plans" that target women are only scientifically backed by research done on men. This is because females were often considered too difficult or risky to include in health research due to fluctuating reproductive hormones. It was not even required that women be included in clinical trials until 1993, thanks to the NIH Revitalization Act. Because men only have one biological rhythm (their circadian rhythm) and women have two (circadian and infradian; see page 24), most things impact us very differently, especially when it comes to food and exercise. Specifically, when women in their reproductive years restrict food or calories, fast or eat infrequently, or engage in extreme exercise and dieting, it completely backfires on our hormones, driving up stress hormone production and inflammation, messing with our menstrual cycle, slowing down our metabolism (increasing fat storage as a result), and disrupting our gut microbiome, which is directly linked to our hormones.

Hormonal Birth Control and Medications

Birth control, antibiotics, antidepressants, and other common drugs like aspirin and ibuprofen (also known as NSAIDs) can disrupt the balance of bacteria in your digestive tract, an essential factor in menstrual cycle health and fertility (as the metabolism of estrogen happens in your gut).[6]

Recent research also shows that synthetic birth control shrinks your vulvar tissues (including your clitoris)[7] and can reduce your ovarian volume (aka shrink your ovaries) by almost 50 percent.[8] Not only that, but it's been shown to disrupt a variety of metabolic processes that affect nutrient absorption (necessary for healthy hormone function),[9] and puts you at an increased risk for developing autoimmune and inflammatory diseases, such as Crohn's and ulcerative colitis.[10]

Gut Health Issues

All of the disruptors mentioned above can lead to gut health issues, and many hormone imbalances begin in the gut. This is because our gut is inextricably involved in hormone production and processes, ranging from thyroid hormone conversion to metabolizing and eliminating estrogen from the body. It also absorbs nutrients from our food to synthesize hormones, supports the elimination of toxins and chemicals that can lead to hormone imbalances, and houses 70 to 80 percent of our immune system, which if disrupted or inflamed can lead to autoimmune and hormone imbalance conditions. Keep in mind that if you're experiencing any sort of digestive issue (including diarrhea, bloating, constipation, food sensitivities, or acne) it's most likely in tandem with a hormonal imbalance.

Dysregulated Blood Sugar

These days there are many modern obstacles and habits (processed foods, added sugars, skipping meals, intense workouts, caffeine and alcohol consumption, sleep issues, chronic stress) that disrupt blood sugar, often driving up insulin production in the body, which is linked to hormonal imbalances and conditions such as PMS, polycystic ovary syndrome (PCOS), premenstrual dysphoric disorder (PMDD), low thyroid, and gestational diabetes. Too much insulin production can also cause a woman's ovaries to produce more testosterone (preventing ovulation) or convert too much testosterone to estrogen, leading to estrogen dominance.

Alcohol, Caffeine, and Drugs

Don't get me wrong, I love a latte or spicy marg as much as the next person, but I would be remiss if I didn't bring up the negative impact these beverages, as well as drugs, can have on our hormones.

First, let's touch on alcohol, which has been shown to alter and impair the functions of hormone-releasing glands, including the hypothalamus and pituitary in the brain (altering brain function). It's also linked to a natural (and rather dramatic!) rise in estrogen, often leading to estrogen dominance over time, with each alcoholic beverage increasing estrogen levels by 5 percent, and four or more drinks per day increasing them by over 60 percent.[11] Moderate alcohol consumption has also been linked to decreased progesterone levels, increased testosterone levels, and a suppression of thyroid production.[12] It's a known circadian disruptor and changes the composition and function of your gut microbiome, often leading to the gut dysbiosis linked to many hormone imbalances. It's also considered an anti-nutrient, meaning it's not only void of nutrients, but uses up critical ones, like B vitamins, in the detoxification process. It could be a culprit behind your symptoms if regularly consumed.

Moving on to caffeine, studies have shown that it increases cortisol and insulin secretion—which is why we often get a sudden jolt of energy after consuming a cup. However, that chronic cortisol and insulin output can often lead to dysregulated blood sugar and hormonal imbalances, such as adrenal dysfunction and estrogen dominance. Additionally, caffeine is an anti-nutrient that depletes the minerals and vitamins necessary for optimal hormone balance.

When referring to drugs, I mean SSRIs and antidepressants, marijuana, some anti-seizure drugs, opioids, beta blockers, and anti-anxiety medications. All of these have numerous effects on our bodies and can cause endocrine abnormalities via different mechanisms, including altering hormone production, transport, binding, and signaling. This can result in your experiencing symptoms ranging from a decrease in libido and ability to achieve orgasm, to fertility challenges and impaired pregnancies, to a decrease in metabolism and increase in weight.

Pregnancy and Birth

As you can imagine, or may have already experienced, your body and hormones go through a ton of changes during pregnancy, birth, and the postpartum period. These vast fluctuations can result in symptoms ranging from initial baby blues and night sweats to decreased libido and increased emotional reactivity, as well as to hair loss, stubborn weight loss, anxiety, insomnia, and fatigue. Many times, these symptoms resolve themselves over the first six months postpartum. However, more and more women report ongoing symptoms and difficulty balancing hormones after birth, often due to nutrient deficiencies, lack of sleep, increased stress, and the toll having a new baby can take on their physical and mental health. Many hormonal imbalances can be traced back to pregnancy and birth and may go on for years until they are properly diagnosed and treated.

Medical Conditions

Pre-existing medical conditions, including diabetes, vascular disease, MTHFR gene mutation, and other gene mutations, are often linked to hormonal imbalances.

This information is intended to help you pinpoint any habits, exposures, or experiences that might be leading to your symptoms and hormonal imbalances. The better you get at identifying these root causes and triggers, the more aware you become, thereby making your own informed, conscious decisions to help your hormones achieve balance and your symptoms to go *byeeee*!

ALIGNING WITH YOUR MENSTRUAL CYCLE

If you're a woman in your reproductive years—from when you get your first period up until menopause—you experience two biological cycles, whereas men and prepubescent girls or postmenopausal women have only one.

WHILE HORMONES ARE COMPLEX, the mechanisms that drive them are often not. In fact, with hormone balance, it's really all about getting back to the basics. Sure, there are nuances, pricey products, and specific micro habits every individual could potentially benefit from, but even these practices are built around a few key principles of hormone balance, including:

- **ALIGNING** with your menstrual cycle
- **BALANCING** your blood sugar
- **SUPPORTING** your gut and detox pathways
- **REDUCING** stress and **BUILDING** stress resilience

Focusing on these principles consistently will have the most profound, sustainable impact on your hormones and health, which should also simplify your lifestyle in a myriad of ways and alleviate any stress or overwhelm around what you "should" or "should not" be doing.

All of the recipes in this cookbook are designed to support each principle, through offering a wide variety of functional nutrients that work to keep blood sugar stable, optimize gut and liver health, and reduce inflammation. However, how and when you consume these meals is also important, based on what phase of your menstrual cycle you're in. Because this is such a key concept of the book and will truly empower you to reap all of the benefits, let's dive into it further.

For over a decade—beginning as a senior in high school and all through my 20s—I was a chronic dieter who was obsessed with my weight and, consequently, what I ate. Some days I felt okay, but many felt like such a struggle, white-knuckling it in between the Lean Cuisines and Luna Bars that did nothing to satisfy my hunger while pushing myself through grueling CrossFit workouts and marathon training 6 to 7 days a week.

Eventually, the lack of nutrients combined with the stress I put on my body caused my hormones to take a major nosedive, which brought on symptoms ranging from hair loss, acne, bloat, and weight gain to missing my period (for two years!) and eventually resuming menstruation, but with extremely heavy and painful periods.

It wasn't until I learned about my menstrual cycle and how to support my hormonal fluctuations during each phase that my health, symptoms, and life *really* changed, which is why I'm *so* excited to share this knowledge with you.

For me, it was incredibly empowering to learn that as women in our reproductive years, our hormones aren't static (like men's) but rather fluctuate throughout a 28-day (give or take) menstrual cycle. Once I honored those shifts with a variety of nutrients, workouts, and lifestyle habits, literally everything in my life became so much easier.

For the first time since high school, I felt like my life was in a state of flow instead of always having to force things (portion sizes, low-calorie foods, intense workouts, productivity, creativity, etc.). I felt fluid, effortlessly moving from one phase to the next. I realized I didn't have to try so hard, and the less I forced things and the more I listened to my body, the better it responded, and as a result, my symptoms naturally diminished over time.

I truly want that for you, and I believe it begins with an understanding of your two biological rhythms—circadian and infradian.

CIRCADIAN AND INFRADIAN RHYTHMS

If you're a woman in your reproductive years—the time frame from when you get your first period up until menopause—then you experience two biological cycles, whereas men and prepubescent girls or post-menopausal women have only one.

The first biological cycle you experience is your circadian rhythm, a 24-hour biological cycle that is regulated by body temperature, daylight and its absence, and the earth's rotation on its axis. This cycle happens daily, and it's also often known as your sleep/wake cycle, as it helps you feel alert during the day and sleep at night. All men and women experience this cycle.

As a woman in your reproductive years, the second biological cycle you experience is called your infradian rhythm, which refers to monthly or annual cycles. Your menstrual cycle is a prime example of an infradian rhythm, as it happens monthly on average, about 28 days. Men, prepubescent girls, and postmenopausal women do not experience this cycle.

This second biological rhythm, also known as your menstrual cycle, consists of four different phases—menstrual, follicular, ovulatory, and luteal. Each phase is defined by distinct hormonal fluctuations that deeply influence your brain, metabolism, microbiome, immune system, stress response system, and reproductive system. Pretty big deal, right?

You've probably already noticed or felt these influences but may not have understood what exactly was behind them. For example, I used to get absolutely ravenous the week before my period and often ended up bingeing on carbs and sweets. I would fault myself for this, like I was weak or had no willpower, when really, I was just in my luteal phase and my metabolic rate had sped up, requiring an uptake of approximately 300 more calories per day.

I also remember times during my cycle when I looked in the mirror and thought I looked really good. My hair would seem shinier, my skin would glow, and I felt lighter, more toned, and less bloated. I'd feel much more inclined to be social and especially in the mood to date. Looking back, I was most likely ovulating, and the increase in hormones like estrogen and testosterone was improving my appearance, energy, and libido as a primal mechanism to attract a mate and reproduce—fascinating, right?

But alas, I did not know that at the time, and then it'd be the week before my period and I'd look and feel different and think there was something wrong with me, so I'd work out harder and cut more calories and feel worse as a result. It became an unrelenting cycle.

You may or may not relate to my personal experience, but if you're here I'm guessing you've felt the effects of the hormonal shifts of your menstrual cycle, especially if something is off balance, which is when all of those common but not normal symptoms tend to crop up.

But once you're able to understand, honor, and support the ebb and flow of your menstrual cycle—your second biological clock—it no longer is a burden; rather it is an empowering and beautiful thing. Your symptoms will naturally dissipate, and you'll feel good in your body—not just when you're about to ovulate but *all month long*.

> "
>
> **ONCE YOU'RE ABLE TO UNDERSTAND, HONOR, AND SUPPORT THE EBB AND FLOW OF YOUR MENSTRUAL CYCLE, IT NO LONGER IS A BURDEN, AND RATHER AN EMPOWERING AND BEAUTIFUL THING.**

THE FOUR PHASES OF YOUR MENSTRUAL CYCLE

To support your hormones, it's imperative to understand what's going on at a hormonal and biological level during the four phases of your menstrual cycle. My hope is that after reading this chapter you'll no longer feel like a victim of your period and menstrual cycle and instead feel incredibly in awe and empowered by it.

Phase One

THE MENSTRUAL PHASE

Let's begin with Phase One of your menstrual cycle, menstruation, also known as your inner winter phase.

WHAT IT IS

Menstruation begins the first day of your period and lasts anywhere from 3 to 7 days, when a quick drop in estrogen and progesterone triggers the shedding of the endometrium and you begin to bleed. This drop happens when your body gets the signal an embryo has not been implanted in the uterus—aka you're not pregnant—and therefore the cushy lining it prepared for an embryo is no longer needed, and it breaks down as a result.

All of your sex hormones are at their lowest levels during this phase, and with them your energy. Your body is also working extra hard and losing nutrients with the loss of blood, making this an essential phase to rest and replenish, similar to the essence of the winter season.

Biologically, these hormonal fluctuations impact your brain and body in various ways, including:

- **BRAIN:** The decline in hormonal levels creates the greatest communication between your two brain hemispheres, the left analytical side and the right feeling side. This means you are best able to synthesize how you feel while also considering the facts, making it a good time for strategizing, analyzing, and reflecting.

- **IMMUNE SYSTEM:** As sex hormone concentrations decrease, your immune system downshifts and becomes less active, so your body won't attack a fertilized egg in case you're pregnant. But it also means if your hormones are imbalanced, you're more susceptible to feeling run-down or getting a cold.

- **METABOLISM:** With both estrogen and progesterone low, your metabolism and appetite are steady and stable at this point, making it important to eat nourishing foods regularly and often.

- **GUT MICROBIOME:** Leading up to your period, your body releases prostaglandins, which force your uterine muscles to contract, thereby promoting the shedding of your uterine lining. These muscle contractions can also impact your intestine and bowels, causing more frequent, loose stools (aka period poop).

- **STRESS RESPONSE:** Your stress response and resting cortisol rate are most likely still heightened at the start of your period, which is nature's way of helping you protect a fertilized egg in the event you're pregnant, but start to decline as your uterine lining sheds and continue dropping throughout your follicular phase.

WHAT ALL OF THIS MEANS FOR YOU

These hormonal and biological shifts very much align with the winter season. Energy is low and you're feeling ready to hunker down and hibernate, much like how we feel during the dark, short, and cold days of winter. It's not a time you often feel like going out, being social, engaging in intense physical activities, or getting it on—but rather getting on your warmest pj's, making hot cocoa, and getting cozy on the couch. It's totally normal to feel this way during menstruation, as well as experience some muscle contractions or minor cramping and physical sensations. What is not normal is experiencing painful or debilitating symptoms such as intense cramping, heavy bleeding or blood clots, extreme fatigue, depression, anxiety, bloat, etc. These symptoms indicate you're dealing with one or more hormonal imbalances.

Phase Two

THE FOLLICULAR PHASE

Moving on to Phase Two, your follicular phase, also symbolic of your inner spring phase.

WHAT IT IS

This phase begins the first day after your period ends, typically lasting 7 to 10 days. Your brain releases follicle stimulating hormone (FSH), triggering the growth of follicles in the ovaries to prepare for ovulation. Your estrogen levels also start to ramp up to thicken your uterine lining to prepare for possible egg implantation, while increasing testosterone levels begin to stimulate your libido.

As this happens, you'll begin to experience a boost in energy, mood, and cognitive skills (especially when it comes to complex processing tasks). You'll start to feel more confident, powerful, bolder, and willing to take risks.

Biologically, these hormonal fluctuations impact your brain and body in various ways, including:

- **BRAIN:** Increasing estrogen levels lead to a boost in synaptic connections within the hippocampus, which can increase mental sharpness, creativity, and communication skills. Estrogen also enhances the release of serotonin, your happiness neurotransmitter, helping you feel more social, verbal, and outgoing.
- **IMMUNE SYSTEM:** As estrogen levels rise, your immune system is on high alert and ready to attack to protect your body and promote optimal fertility. This means you're less likely to feel fatigued or get sick.
- **METABOLISM:** As estrogen rises it naturally slows your metabolism and suppresses your appetite, conserving nutrients in preparation for a potential pregnancy. This means you'll often feel better eating lighter, but still nutrient-rich, foods.
- **GUT MICROBIOME:** When hormones are in balance, you typically don't experience many digestive symptoms during this phase. However, if out of balance, issues like constipation and slower GI transit time can arise, increasing problems with estrogen metabolism and often leading to estrogen dominance.
- **STRESS RESPONSE:** If hormones are balanced, resting cortisol levels are lower during this period, making it an ideal time to ramp up productivity at work or increase exercise intensity.

WHAT ALL OF THIS MEANS FOR YOU

Just like spring, you're feeling ready to emerge from hibernation and re-enter the social scene. Your energy, mood, and cognitive skills are increasing, getting you in the mood to move your body, get outside, connect with others, start to work on new projects, and get plans in motion. Your rising confidence and libido also mean you're willing to try new things and get into the dating scene. Basically, the sun's coming out, flowers are in bloom, and you're feeling it (and yourself). However, if you're dealing with symptoms including low energy and libido, acne, digestive issues, etc., it indicates there are most likely underlying hormonal imbalances at play.

Phase Three

THE OVULATORY PHASE

From the follicular phase, we transition into ovulation, also known as your inner summer phase:

WHAT IT IS

Ovulation typically occurs somewhere between days 12 and 17 of your menstrual cycle and is short, usually lasting only 2 or 3 days. Right before ovulation, you get a surge of luteinizing hormone (LH), which causes the dominant follicle to burst open and release an egg into the fallopian tube. The egg will be viable for roughly 12 to 24 hours, and if it's not fertilized by sperm (which can live up to 5 days in the female body), it will disintegrate.

Hormonally, levels of estrogen and testosterone are at their peak during this phase, helping you feel magnetic, energetic, outgoing, confident, and sexy while optimizing your creativity and communication skills. Your libido is running high, to naturally get you in the mood during your fertile window and attract a mate with genetic potential.

Biologically, these hormonal fluctuations impact your brain and body in various ways, including:

- **BRAIN:** Skyrocketing estrogen levels continue to enhance synaptic connections within the hippocampus, meaning your mental sharpness, creativity, and communication skills are at their peak. It's a great time for connecting with others, dating, being social, giving presentations, interviewing for a job, or working on a creative project.

- **IMMUNE SYSTEM:** Your immune system continues to be on high alert and ready to attack to protect your body and ensure you ovulate. This means you're less likely to feel fatigued or get sick.

- **METABOLISM:** Your metabolism slows, and appetite is suppressed as primally your body's trying to shift the focus from foraging to finding a mate. While you still need to eat nutrient-dense foods regularly, you may find yourself feeling satisfied with smaller portions and gravitating toward lighter and fresher "summer" foods.

- **GUT MICROBIOME:** High levels of estrogen can sometimes cause water retention and bloat, which should be minimal during this time. However, if you have a hormonal imbalance such as estrogen dominance, it can be very noticeable and uncomfortable.

- **STRESS RESPONSE:** If hormones are balanced, resting cortisol is lower at this phase. But if you have high cortisol or are dealing with an increase in stress nearing the ovulatory phase, it can delay or even prevent ovulation, as your body doesn't want to promote pregnancy during periods of heavy stress.

WHAT ALL OF THIS MEANS FOR YOU

It's summer vacation and you're at your peak—glowing, looking and feeling amazing, ready to see and be seen. You're focusing on having a good time and connecting with others (especially a significant other) while also feeling super productive and creative. Basically everything is firing on all cylinders. Despite all that amazingness, if you're struggling with hormonal imbalances, you may find yourself dealing with bloat, cramps, spotting, constipation, breakouts, or even pain—also known as mittelschmerz—during this phase.

> "
> IT'S SUMMER VACATION AND YOU'RE AT YOUR PEAK—GLOWING, LOOKING AND FEELING AMAZING, READY TO SEE AND BE SEEN.

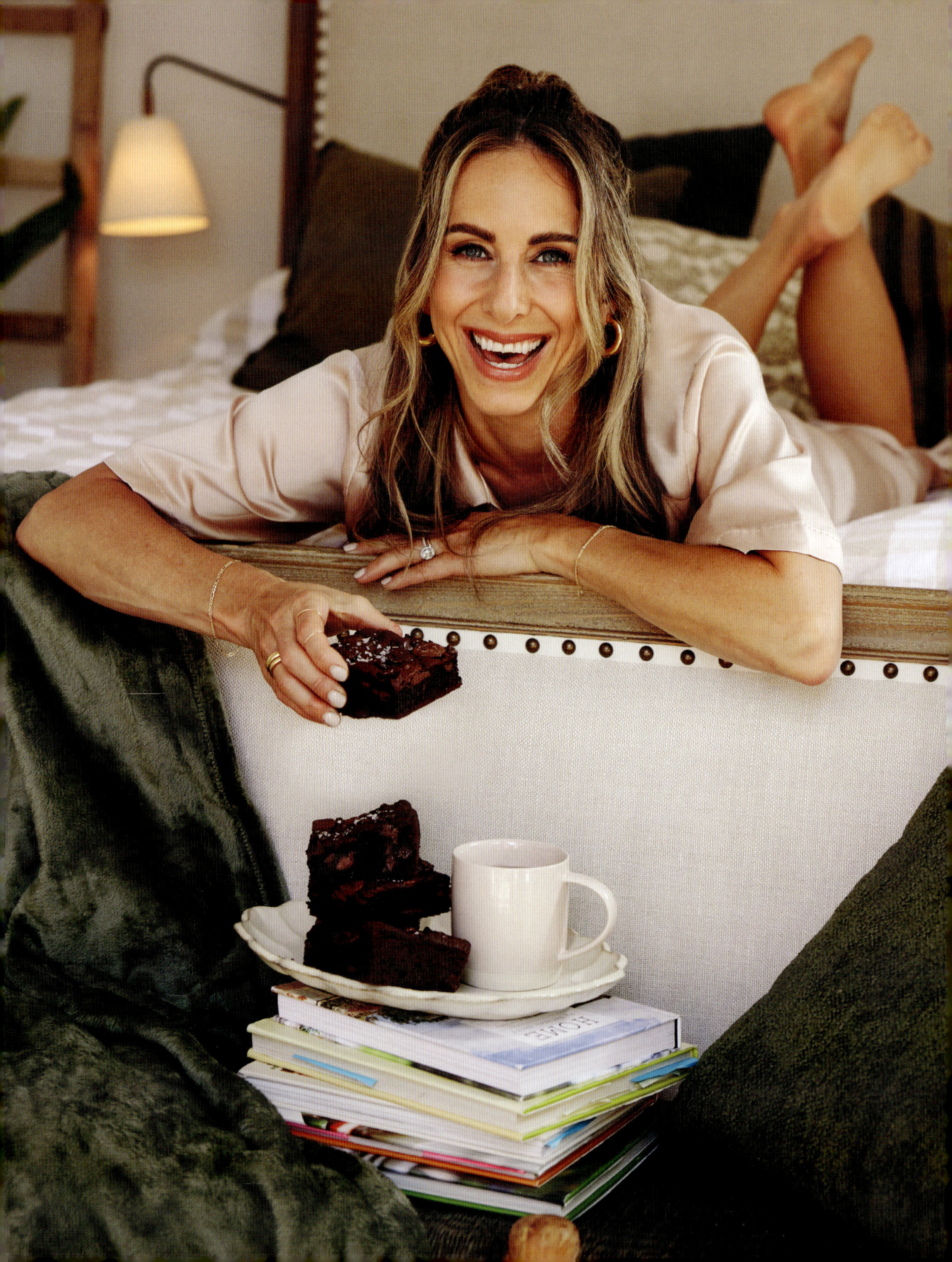
HOME

Phase Four

THE LUTEAL PHASE

Last, but not least, we enter the luteal phase, also known as your inner fall:

WHAT IT IS

The luteal phase typically lasts 12 to 14 days and occurs immediately after ovulation, making up the entirety of the second half of your menstrual cycle. Hormonally, estrogen, testosterone, and LH begin their decline while progesterone rises to stimulate the growth of the uterine lining in preparation for a potential pregnancy (if you're not pregnant it will shed during the menstrual phase).

During the first half of the luteal phase, you're still typically riding high off the feel-good effects of ovulation. However, as progesterone production increases, you'll find yourself starting to wind down, with a strong attention to detail and desire to complete tasks and get things done—much like the transition from summer to fall.

Biologically, these hormonal fluctuations impact your brain and body in various ways, including:

- **BRAIN:** Your brain chemistry is optimized for task and detail orientation, as well as bringing projects to completion. Progesterone stimulates the GABA receptor in the brain, which helps you feel relaxed and calm. Thus, if you find yourself experiencing PMS symptoms like anxiety, moodiness, or trouble sleeping, it may be attributed to low progesterone.

- **IMMUNE SYSTEM:** As hormone concentrations decrease, your immune system downshifts to protect a potentially fertilized egg (instead of attacking it as a foreign invader). This makes you more susceptible to illness and fatigue, especially if you're already dealing with a hormone imbalance.

- **METABOLISM:** During your luteal phase, your metabolism and appetite increase as your body is preparing to meet the nutrient demands of pregnancy in the event an egg has been fertilized. Energy expenditure jumps anywhere from 8 to 16 percent, requiring an average intake of 200 to 300 additional calories per day. This is why it's especially important to eat nourishing foods regularly and often, as restricting calories could backfire on your metabolism and turn on fat storage.

- **GUT MICROBIOME:** Progesterone can slow digestion and GI transit time, which means food moves more slowly through your intestine, resulting in bloating and constipation. This makes it an especially important time to ramp up fiber and water intake to keep things moving, as well as eat warm, well-cooked foods that are easier to break down.

- **STRESS RESPONSE:** Our resting cortisol rate increases and stress response is heightened during this phase, as nature's way of helping you protect a fertilized egg in the event you're pregnant.

WHAT ALL OF THIS MEANS FOR YOU

Just like the beginning of fall, you're still feeling your summer self while also craving a sense of routine and stability (not to mention a clean, organized space to create it in). And just as the fall days grow shorter, darker, and colder, you'll want to lean into soft sweaters, warm soups, and all things cozy the second half of your luteal phase. While this can be such a beautiful phase, it's often the worst for those dealing with hormonal imbalances, as PMS symptoms such as bloat, cramping, intense cravings, breast tenderness, moodiness, anxiety, and sleep issues tend to rear their ugly heads.

Now that you've learned about the four phases/seasons of your cycle and how they impact you on a physical and emotional level, use the cheat sheet on page 31 to help start syncing your meals, movement, and mindset accordingly. These habits work to support your hormonal fluctuations, alleviate symptoms, and maximize how you feel during your entire cycle.

HOW TO TRACK YOUR MENSTRUAL CYCLE

At this point you might be thinking, *Okay, well, this is all interesting and cool stuff, but what if I don't even know what phase I'm in or how to figure it out?* So that's why I'm going to give you the tools to effectively track your cycle.

Phase One

MENSTRUAL PHASE

If you have no idea what phase you're in, make a note of the day your next period starts (when you first use a tampon, menstrual cup, etc.). This is day 1 of your *entire* cycle, and it typically lasts anywhere from 3 to 7 days.

Phase Two

FOLLICULAR PHASE

Technically, the first half of your cycle (when your period begins through ovulation) is considered the follicular phase. However, most professionals (including myself) further break down the menstrual cycle into four distinct phases based on hormonal fluctuations.

Thus, on the day your period ends (the day you stop bleeding) you have officially entered your follicular phase. This phase typically lasts 7 to 10 days.

Phase Three

OVULATORY PHASE

Detecting when you're ovulating can be tricky because every menstruator ovulates on a different day of their cycle.

A few ways to effectively track and confirm ovulation include:

- Check your cervical fluid, which becomes wet and stretchy, similar to egg whites.
- Track your basal body temperature, which rises slightly after ovulation.
- Observe your cervical position and texture (soft and high).
- Watch for a natural increase in libido, mood, and energy.
- Test with an LH strip, which detects the surge in luteinizing hormone that occurs prior to ovulation. (*Please note,* this does **not** confirm ovulation, but only predicts when it may occur.)

While ovulation typically lasts only 24 hours, you will feel the hormonal effects leading up to and after it for several days.

Phase Four

LUTEAL PHASE

You only enter your luteal phase upon completion of ovulation.

Things you might notice as you transition into this phase include:

- A change in cervical fluid from wet, stretchy, and slippery to thick and dry
- A low and closed cervical position
- A decline in energy and mood
- A gravitational pull inward
- PMS symptoms such as breast tenderness, cramping, mood swings, breakouts, headaches, bloat (remember, these are common but *not* normal)

This phase typically lasts 12 to 14 days, up until your next period. On day 1 of your period the entire cycle begins again.

Menstrual Cycle Cheat Sheet

	MENSTRUAL	FOLLICULAR	OVULATORY	LUTEAL
SEASON	Winter	Spring	Summer	Fall
DURATION	First day of period until period ends, typically days 1 to 7	Day period ends until ovulation, typically days 7 to 14	Egg released from ovary, typically days 14 to 17	After ovulation until period begins, typically days 17 to 28
WHAT'S HAPPENING	Sex hormones drop, triggering uterine lining to shed	Estrogen, testosterone, and FSH rise, triggering growth of follicles (will mature into an egg) and uterine lining (for potential egg implantation)	LH surges, triggering ovaries to release an egg; estrogen and testosterone at their peak	Estrogen and testosterone decline, progesterone rises, stimulating the growth of the uterine lining to prepare for egg implantation (if not pregnant it will shed in the next menstrual phase)
HOW YOU'LL FEEL	Low energy, hibernation mode, analytical, intuitive	Energized, creative, bold, confident	Sexy, social, verbal, powerful	Productive (at first), detail-oriented, withdrawn, in your feelings
MEAL FOCUS	Mineral-rich, warm, slow-cooked foods	Fresh, vibrant, fiber-rich, gut-friendly foods	Raw, cooling foods like salads, smoothies, fresh fruits, veggies	Cozy carbs, warm soups, stews, casseroles
MOVEMENT FOCUS	Slow, gentle, restorative movement	Ramp up the intensity, increase cardio	Full-on HIIT mode	Shift to strength- and flexibility-based movement
MINDSET FOCUS	Rest, replenish, low-key cozy	Plan and start new projects, try new things	Get social, go on dates, see and be seen	Complete tasks, set boundaries, self-care regimens
HERBS	Chamomile, ginger	Peppermint, nettle, oat straw	Dandelion root, nettle, hibiscus	Red raspberry leaf, ginger, cinnamon

MIA MENSTRUAL CYCLE SUPPORT

So...how do you track and support your cycle if you're not even having a period?

There can be many reasons why your period is absent (including chronic stress or illness, under-nourishment, conditions such as PCOS, etc.), but I know this is an especially frustrating experience for many of my clients who come off hormonal birth control, as most of them are hoping to return to regular cycles quickly in the hopes of getting pregnant. Unfortunately, because of the effects hormonal birth control can have on hormones, my clients find it can take months, sometimes even years, for their period to return and cycles to normalize, not to mention that they get hit with a ton of hormonal imbalance side effects that have gone under the radar for years. Usually, these have never been treated or resolved, leading to major discomfort, frustration, and sometimes pain.

While I don't have the ability to wave a magic wand and make it all better, I can do the next best thing and provide you with recipes and tips to help you support your hormones and get your cycle back on track, whether it's missing due to birth control, postpartum, nursing, or a condition such as amenorrhea.

Before we get into these in the next chapter, let's cover the parameters of what a healthy, optimal period and menstrual cycle looks like, so you can correctly identify when yours is back on track.

Optimal Menstrual Cycle and Period Parameters

- **CYCLE LENGTH:** Your menstrual cycle should be regular and consistent for you every month, typically lasting between 26 and 34 days, give or take, without spotting in between.

- **PERIOD COLOR:** Your period blood should be a deep red cranberry color from start to finish.

- **PERIOD LENGTH:** Your period should last anywhere from 3 to 7 days.

- **PERIOD CONSISTENCY:** You should have a strong flow without any clots or extremely heavy bleeding (i.e., bleeding through your menstrual care products in less than 1 to 2 hours).

- **PHYSICAL SENSATIONS:** You may feel slight sensations, contractions, or warmth from your pelvic region, but you shouldn't experience any kind of pain that makes you reach for drugs or hot water bottles, or interferes with your daily routine.

On the other hand, these are the signs of underlying hormonal imbalances:

- Your cycle is typically less than 25 days or longer than 35 days.
- Your cycle is irregular (i.e., skips a month or you never know when your next period will come).
- Your cycle is completely MIA.
- You experience symptoms such as regular spotting in between periods, dark or light period blood, periods that last less than 3 days or longer than 7 days, or extremely heavy or painful periods.

All these signs point to hormonal imbalance and do not meet the parameters of a healthy, optimal period and menstrual cycle.

A Note on Perimenopause and Menopause

Depending on where you are in life, perimenopause may or may not be on your mind. For many years it seemed to me something I didn't really need to think about or plan for, but the more I've learned (and the older *and wiser* I get), the more I understand that supporting and nourishing our hormones now is imperative for a smooth transition into perimenopause and beyond.

This is because perimenopause—defined as the period when your body starts making the natural transition to menopause, ultimately marking the end of your menstrual cycle and reproductive years—represents a decline in reproductive hormone production, most notably estrogen and progesterone.

As you've previously learned, these hormones are responsible for *a lot* of functions and feelings.

ESTROGEN: Estrogen regulates cholesterol levels, the urinary tract, heart and blood vessels, bones, breast health, skin, hair, mucous membranes, pelvic muscles, and brain health and function.

When in balance, estrogen helps us feel happy, energetic, outgoing, and confident.

PROGESTERONE: Progesterone helps to reduce stress and anxiety; regulate mood, behavior, and cognitive function; stimulate weight gain and appetite; and maintain fat tissue and keep estrogen levels in check.

When in balance, progesterone helps us feel cool, calm, and collected.

As these hormone levels naturally lower, you can imagine the types of symptoms one might experience (night sweats, weight gain, anxiety, brain fog, mood swings, depression), especially if you're entering this phase in a depleted state with your hormones already out of whack.

Remember, we rely on our ovaries to produce estrogen and progesterone throughout our reproductive years, but this slowly declines as we enter perimenopause, until production halts at menopause. When this happens, our adrenal glands take over, producing smaller amounts of estrogen and progesterone, which are important to help mitigate uncomfortable symptoms.

I want to help you avoid approaching this phase in a state of burnout, as I was on the path to doing myself prior to my education: I was taxing my adrenal glands from *years* of undernourishment, chronic stress, ignoring my body's cues, and constantly pushing myself to keep up with the never-ending demands of a very linear, masculine society. If I had kept going at that pace, my adrenal energy reserves would have depleted, and I would have had nothing to pull from to support myself during this transition. Cue the symptoms, felt at an even deeper, more intense level.

Using this book as a guide *now* is going to help you pave the way for perimenopause by restoring and replenishing your nutrient reserves.

When you focus on restoring and replenishing, you support your natural hormonal rhythms and help your body ovulate and have a healthy period each month, which is crucial for progesterone production and keeping estrogen levels in check. This helps to mitigate symptoms now so that you're not experiencing them at a magnified level in the future. It also places far less demand on your adrenal glands, so that you can transition into perimenopause with a robust reserve tank, instead of running on empty.

BOTTOM LINE: How you show up for your hormones during your reproductive years will set the tone for your future. Take this opportunity to tune in to your body and give it what it needs by following the key hormone-balancing principles outlined in this book. (Or, if you're already in perimenopause, take these steps now to mitigate symptoms immediately.)

THE HORMONE HEALTHY EATS PHILOSOPHY

Women in their reproductive years have a higher need for vitamins and minerals than men or prepubescent girls and postmenopausal women due to the amount of energy it takes to orchestrate ovulation and a healthy menstrual cycle, not to mention pregnancy, childbirth, and lactation.

IF YOU'VE READ the introduction to this book, you already know I have my own long, drawn-out saga with dieting, which only left me feeling depleted, neurotic, kind of sad, *very* hungry, and dealing with a plethora of hormonal imbalance symptoms to boot (heavy periods, mood swings, breakouts, thinning hair, bloating, etc.).

While every person is on their own journey, and I don't intend to shame anyone following a diet or trend, I do want to address the fact that most mainstream diets don't consider our unique female biology and what *actually* works for women during the reproductive years.

Most studies done on the benefits of mainstream diets, exercise programs, or wellness trends are conducted on men—in fact, women were not even included in clinical research and trials until a law passed in 1993 mandating it! This discrimination was not only based on gender bias but was also in large part due to the concern over having to account for women's fluctuating hormone levels and reproductive cycles. Gender-biased research has had serious repercussions for women's health, and we are still trying to make up for it.

What the research conducted in the past few decades on normally cycling women shows is that an average of 2,600 to 2,700 calories per day needs to be consumed for the basal metabolic rate to function optimally,[1] with varying needs based on activity and stress levels as well as hormonal fluctuations during the menstrual cycle.

Undereating (defined as an intake of 1,500 calories or less per day) is a very well-researched cause of hormonal disruption,[2] with a calorie deficit below daily requirements disrupting the menstrual cycle in a matter of months leading to a decrease in both estrogen and progesterone production and a shortened luteal phase (making it especially difficult for those trying to conceive).[3]

Falling under the umbrella of undereating, skipping meals also proves problematic for women in their reproductive years, specifically breakfast, which is linked to irregular cycles and an increase in period pain (also known as dysmenorrhea). In my practice, I saw a large portion of my female clients skipping breakfast or substituting coffee for breakfast in an effort to intermittent fast and lose weight, which ended up suppressing their thyroid function, decreasing their metabolic rate, and ultimately leading to more fat storage (not to mention mood swings, intense cravings, dysregulated blood sugar, and increased risk of miscarriage).

And it's not just restricting calories that negatively impacts our fertility, menstrual cycle, and overall hormonal health, but omitting food groups as well. One study following women on a raw-food vegan diet found that 30 percent of the women had amenorrhea, or the absence of a menstrual cycle altogether, because they didn't have sufficient micronutrients to support ovulation and hormone production.[4] Another found that women with hypothalamic amenorrhea have low levels of IGF-1, an insulin growth factor needed to regulate tissue repair, bone health, and reproductive function, due to low protein intake.[5] Yet another study conducted on over 18,000 women found those with a low saturated fat intake (less than 10 percent) had the highest rate of ovulatory infertility, while those with the highest saturated fat intake (12 to 14 percent of total calories) had the most optimal ovulatory function and regulated menstrual cycles.[6]

The research shows not only that most mainstream diets have a vastly different effect on men vs. menstruating women, but also that there's another huge fundamental problem with the diet industry to consider: This industry relies on consumerism (through the continual purchase of medications, supplements, books, foods, etc.) to make money. If you succeed in achieving your weight loss goals and no longer need what they're selling, profits decline. Thus, the industry has designed these programs to help you achieve short-term success, so that when you eventually "fall off the wagon" you return to their goods or services. They rely on you as a repeat customer. Your loss is their gain, over and over again. Diets are designed for you to fail, and nobody likes to feel like a failure; this cycle leaves most women in a worse spot than when they began.

Ultimately, if the goal is to balance hormones in order to live a symptom-free and higher-quality life—one where we can maintain an effortless, healthy weight we feel really good at—we have to stop turning to diet culture and its overarching mentality of restrictive punishment or deprivation, and instead focus on what the research reiterates time and time again: We need to be eating an abundance of nutrient-dense food to support our unique biology and hormonal rhythms.

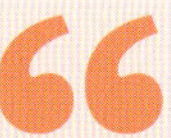

WE NEED TO BE EATING AN ABUNDANCE OF NUTRIENT-DENSE FOOD TO SUPPORT OUR UNIQUE BIOLOGY AND HORMONAL RHYTHMS.

FOUR PILLARS OF EATING FOR HORMONE BALANCE

Now that we've covered what eating for hormone health does *not* include—restriction, dieting, or anything stressful or negative surrounding our food choices—let's talk about what it does include, centering on four pillars.

Align Foods with Your Menstrual Cycle

As you learned in the previous section, your hormones follow a pattern with four distinct hormone fluctuations throughout each cycle. These fluctuations impact your female physiology in a myriad of ways and require a variety of macro- and micronutrients. Rotating a wide variety of nutrient-dense foods tailored to the phase of your cycle is one of the best hormone-balancing tools you have at your disposal.

While we cover this in depth in each chapter (with 25 delicious recipes per phase to help you truly enjoy this core concept), I do want to take a moment to encourage you if this is new or feels overwhelming. Here's a few tips I share with my clients:

START SMALL

If you're overwhelmed, just start with one thing. Maybe it's focusing on switching up one meal per day (breakfast, lunch, or dinner) or trying one new fruit or veggie for each phase. Whatever you do, don't stress yourself out. This should feel fun, aligned, and in flow with where you are at in your cycle.

THINK OF EACH PHASE AS A SEASON

Your menstrual cycle phases align perfectly with the four seasons we experience every year. Winter is symbolic of your period (low and inward energy, warm, nourishing foods, rest), spring with your follicular phase (new beginnings, making plans, fresh foods), summer with ovulation (a time to see and be seen, indulge in pleasures, lots of seasonal, ripe produce), and fall with your luteal phase (tying up loose ends, getting organized and cozy, preparing for the upcoming winter season). When you think of it this way it feels very natural and intuitive.

CHECK IN WITH HOW YOU FEEL

Once you begin to truly listen to what your appetite, energy levels, and body are telling you, you'll most likely find you naturally crave foods aligned with where you are in your cycle. For example, during your luteal phase your metabolic needs shift, causing you to naturally crave more carbohydrates to supply your cells with fuel. Leaning in to this signal by adding more complex carbohydrates (like apples and sweet potatoes) or eating more hearty meals supports your metabolism, helping to negate cravings, balance blood sugar, and reduce PMS symptoms.

Eat for Blood Sugar Balance

Eating for blood sugar balance is a non-negotiable when it comes to supporting your hormones and has been proven helpful for maintaining a healthy body composition and consistent energy levels, as well as being linked to lower overall inflammation and a reduction in menstrual cycle irregularities and PMS. Research has shown that elevated blood sugar levels due to a high intake of refined grains and sugar exacerbate PMS symptoms[7] and interfere with fertility[8] as they influence one of the main regulators of the menstrual cycle, the hypothalamic-pituitary-ovarian axis. They also lead to insulin resistance, which has a direct effect on ovarian hormone production.

While it's important to crowd out unrefined and processed carbohydrates with real, nutrient-dense whole foods to support blood sugar balance and overall hormone health, science has shown us there are also plenty of small, almost effortless tweaks we can make to our diets that make a big difference overall. Personally, I found a huge sense of freedom when I focused on eating in a way that supports optimal blood sugar balance, as it allowed me to experience so much joy and pleasure with food (without restriction!), while still feeling satiated and energized afterward.

Here are a few effective blood sugar balancing tips to get you started.

MAKE SURE EVERY MEAL AND SNACK CONTAINS AN OPTIMAL BALANCE OF PROTEIN, FAT, AND FIBER

If I could emphasize a pillar of eating for blood sugar and hormone balance, it would be the intentionality of including a high-quality source of protein, fat, and fiber at every meal or snack. First and foremost, these three macronutrients need to be consumed for hormones to synthesize, produce, and function optimally. Specifically, we need:

- **PROTEIN:** An essential structural component of *all* hormones, which means you must consume sufficient protein to make enough hormones.[9] High-quality protein sources include grass-fed meat, organ meat, poultry, wild-caught seafood, pasture-raised eggs, lentils and beans, and some sources of dairy such as cottage cheese, ricotta cheese, and Greek yogurt. Refer to page 43 for more information and recommended portion sizes.

- **FAT:** Dietary fat and cholesterol are considered essential "building materials" that help make steroid hormones, including your sex hormones—estrogen, testosterone, and progesterone. However, not all fat is created equal, and when I refer to high-quality fat, I am referring to essential fatty acids found in wild-caught fish, eggs, nuts, and seeds, as well as monounsaturated fats found in avocado, olives, and olive oil, and short-chain fatty acids found in grass-fed butter and ghee. See page 44 for more information.

- **FIBER (DERIVED FROM COMPLEX CARBOHYDRATES):** Despite the dietary dogma surrounding carbohydrates, they are an essential part of hormone production, as they help fuel our cells and drive the engines in the body that produce hormones. Complex carbs rich in fiber include all fruits and vegetables, as well as beans, lentils, quinoa, millet, oats, rice, corn, etc. See page 46 for more details.

So, not only are these three macronutrients vital building blocks of hormones, but when eaten together during meals and snacks they create a powerhouse combo that keeps your blood sugar from spiking or crashing and stimulates cholecystokinin (also known as CCK), a major hormone regulator that signals satiation. Basically, what this means is that every time you consume a meal or snack with this combo, it helps you feel steady, satisfied, and energized afterward, reduces cravings, and prolongs satiation between meals—meaning you don't need to rely on snacks or caffeine as often to get you through the day.

TRY SWITCHING THE ORDER OF FOODS AT MEALS

You can eat the exact same meal but balance your blood sugar simply by switching the order in which you consume certain foods. Specifically, when you eat fiber first (such as a salad, veggies, etc.) followed by a protein and fat (steak with butter) and any starches or sugars last (pasta, bread, or chocolate cake), it creates a lower, slower glucose rise than if you were to eat foods in a different (or opposite) order (i.e., bread/pasta first, steak second, veggies last). This is because fiber breaks down slowly in your digestive tract, creating a slow glucose rise, while starches are quickly converted into glucose, leading to a glucose spike. When you eat fiber first, it slows down the speed at which you digest starches, so glucose trickles into the bloodstream more slowly than if you had eaten the same foods in reverse order. Pretty cool, huh? This hack may not always work (for example, if you're eating a sandwich), but if you find yourself out at a restaurant or making a meal with multiple sides at home, it's fairly simple and intuitive to follow.

START WITH A SAVORY BREAKFAST

Okay, not gonna lie: ya girl *loves* a sweet breakfast. However, scientific studies show that eating a savory breakfast rich in protein, fiber, and fat (as well as low in starches and sugar)—such as an egg scramble with avocado, greens, and smoked salmon—not only helps curb a glucose spike at breakfast, but sets the tone for how your blood sugar responds the rest of the day.[10] This is because upon waking our blood sugar is typically very low, or in a fasting state, after not eating all night. When we eat a sweet or carb-heavy breakfast first thing (like pastries, cereal, doughnuts, etc.), the glucose enters our bloodstream quickly, leading to a massive spike, triggering a rush of insulin to remove the excess glucose, and culminating in a subsequent crash, increased fat storage, decreased energy, and intense cravings throughout the entire rest of the day. While I still like to enjoy my "sweeter" options that follow the protein, fat, and fiber formula, I must admit I almost always feel great after enjoying a savory breakfast, and I make sure to consume one if I need extra energy or to be on point for the day.

OPT FOR DESSERT AFTER A MEAL INSTEAD OF A SWEET SNACK BETWEEN MEALS

Eating a stand-alone dessert or sweet snack (such as a midday cookie or even a bowl of fruit) converts quickly into glucose, leading to a spike and crash that disrupt blood sugar and hormone balance. If you're craving something sweet, save it for a "dessert" after a meal rich in protein, fat, and fiber. This takes advantage of your body being in a "postprandial state," which is when it's still metabolizing what you've previously eaten, slowing the rate at which the sugar and starches convert to glucose in your digestive tract, curbing a spike, and helping to keep blood sugar stable.

AIM TO EAT A BALANCED MEAL OR SNACK EVERY 3 TO 5 HOURS

While every person is different and I always encourage you to listen to your body and hunger cues, multiple studies show that skipping meals, eating less than your caloric needs, and intermittent fasting negatively impact the hormones and blood sugar of women in the reproductive years. Aiming to eat nutrient-dense meals or snacks every 3 to 5 hours works to keep blood sugar balanced and hormones in a relaxed, optimal state.

EAT IN A CALM, RELAXED ENVIRONMENT

Speaking of being relaxed, when possible it's important to consume your meals in a calm, unrushed, and undistracted environment. Doing so helps your body slip into its parasympathetic nervous system, aka its rest and digest mode, so you can properly digest your meal and optimally absorb and assimilate nutrients in your digestive tract, working to keep blood sugar stable. Eating in a hurried, stressed, or distracted environment signals your body to stay in its sympathetic state—aka its stress state—leading to a higher glucose spike.

DRINK CAFFEINE, ALCOHOL, AND SUGARY BEVERAGES WITH OR AFTER MEALS

A common question that comes up with clients is whether they need to give up caffeine or alcohol, and truthfully, it all depends on your unique situation. My first tip before you give it up cold turkey (which can be a barrier to improvement since many women, including myself, simply refuse to give up their daily cup of coffee) is to consume it with or after a nutrient-dense meal that is rich in protein, fat, and fiber. Just as with a dessert or sweet treat, the fiber, protein, and fat slow the rate at which a sugary beverage enters your bloodstream, helping to curb a glucose spike. I never recommend drinking caffeine or alcohol on an empty stomach, especially first thing in the morning.

FOCUS ON MEAL DENSITY

Another great blood sugar–balancing hack is to anchor lighter meals with denser ones. These meals all typically contain a similar amount of calories and macronutrients (protein, fat, and fiber) but digest, assimilate, absorb, and hit the bloodstream very differently, impacting how nourished you feel as a result. For example, how you feel after you drink a smoothie with protein powder, nut butter, banana, and greens (light) will probably be much different than how you feel after sitting down with a knife and fork to eat a steak cooked with butter, potatoes, and a salad (dense). I encourage aiming for a combination of both light and dense meals throughout each day, especially emphasizing dense meals if you feel like you're doing *all of the things* and still feel starving or undernourished.

Eat for Optimal Gut and Liver Health

While our bodies do a pretty amazing job of detoxifying on their own, supporting this process through optimizing the health of our gut microbiome and pathways of elimination is crucial for healthy hormones due to the constant bombardment of toxins we experience in our modern world.

Let's jump into my top nutrition and lifestyle tips that will support your gut microbiome and detoxification pathways naturally:

CONSUME LIVER-SUPPORTIVE FOODS

Nutrients derived from the foods we eat (such as glutathione, vitamins B and C, selenium, and certain amino acids) are needed for your liver to break down toxins during its two-phase detoxification process. Foods rich in these nutrients include raw carrots, beets, dandelion greens, cruciferous vegetables, broccoli sprouts, citrus (especially lemon), chlorophyll (found in leafy greens), onions, garlic, and turmeric.

Additionally, it's important to consume enough high-quality animal protein, such as grass-fed red meat and poultry, wild-caught seafood, organ meats, eggs, and gelatin found in bone broth, as they provide your liver with sulfur-containing amino acids such as taurine, cysteine, glycine, and choline, specifically needed for phase-two liver detoxification. While you can find small amounts of some of these amino acids in plant-based sources, they are much more abundant and bioavailable in animal proteins, meaning they're more easily used and assimilated by the body. While every person is different and I'm not here to tell you to abandon your religious or cultural beliefs, if you're struggling with symptoms related to an overburdened liver (including fatigue, disrupted sleep—especially between the hours of 2 to 4 a.m.—acne or other skin conditions, blood sugar disorders, nutrient malabsorption, indigestion and acid reflux, chronic infections, asthma or allergies, and PMS) and do not consume animal protein, this could be an area to further pay attention to.

EAT A VARIETY OF NUTRIENT-DENSE WHOLE FOODS

A diet rich in nutrient-dense whole foods featuring protein, fat, and fiber, as well as vitamins and minerals, ensures you're providing your body with the raw materials it needs to produce healthy hormones, as well as optimizing digestion, regulating blood sugar, boosting good gut bacteria, and effectively eliminating toxins. Following the meal structure and making the recipes in this cookbook based on where you are in your cycle is one of the best ways to begin incorporating this practice. So if you've already started doing this, congrats, you're well on your way!

EAT FOR THE DIFFERENT PHASES OF YOUR CYCLE

Speaking of aligning with your menstrual cycle, consuming a variety of foods based on where you are in your cycle not only supports different hormone fluctuations by meeting specific nutrient needs but also maximizes your gut health. This is primarily because your gut microbiome thrives off diversity, and rotating different foods and cooking methods during each phase ensures your gut doesn't get too overexposed to any particular food that may be causing an inflammatory response.

INCORPORATE PREBIOTIC- AND PROBIOTIC-RICH FOODS

You may have heard of probiotics, which are a type of beneficial bacteria found within the gut microbiome. These microorganisms play a central role in health and are involved in both immune function and digestion. (Remember, 70 to 80 percent of our immune system is housed in the gut!) Historically people were able to consume plenty of probiotics from food grown in nutrient-rich soil and fermented foods, but harmful agricultural practices (including the use of pesticides) and decreased diet quality have caused our food supply to be significantly lower in probiotics than before. Even worse, conventional meat and dairy products contain antibiotics that kill off the good bacteria in our gut, leading to an unbalanced gut microbiome and directly affecting our hormones as a result. Fortunately, there are many probiotic-rich foods you can consume to provide your gut with these essential microorganisms, such as kefir, sauerkraut, kimchi, Greek yogurt, apple cider vinegar, miso, raw sheep and goat cheeses, pickles, and brine-cured olives.

Lesser known, but still equally important, is the incorporation of prebiotics into your diet, which are used as a food source for the probiotics and other healthy bacteria to feed off of to proliferate and thrive (i.e., you need enough prebiotic bacteria to have healthy probiotic bacteria, otherwise they won't survive!). Prebiotic-rich foods include cooked onion and asparagus, green or unripe bananas, chicory root, artichokes, dandelion greens, oats, and resistant starches such as sweet potatoes or squash that have been cooked and then cooled.

EAT PLENTY OF FIBER-RICH FOODS

Fiber is a vital part of the detoxification process, as it binds to the toxins filtered by your liver and safely eliminates them via your intestinal tract. Optimal sources of fiber include artichokes, cruciferous vegetables, starchy root vegetables, pears and apples, quinoa, gluten-free oats, beans and lentils, seeds, nuts, and avocado. Refer to page 46 for more specifics.

OPT FOR ORGANIC, REAL WHOLE FOODS WHEN POSSIBLE

I get that life is different for each of us and we don't always have time, access, or money to hit up the local organic farmers' market or make a home-cooked meal from scratch. But opting for animal proteins and produce sourced from local or organic farms you can trust, as well as limiting weird chemicals or ingredients found in many packaged or processed foods, will go a *long* way in supporting your liver and hormonal health. (Remember, we're exposed to an abundance of toxins via pesticides, herbicides, added hormones, antibiotics, dyes, and preservatives through conventional and processed foods.) If you're operating on a budget, check out the Environmental Working Group's Clean Fifteen and Dirty Dozen (see ewg.org) for produce contamination guidelines. If organic isn't an option, try soaking fresh produce in a mixture of 1 teaspoon baking soda per 2 cups of water for 15 minutes to help remove pesticides, or choosing fruits and veggies that have been flash frozen, which preserves their nutrients.

Eat to Support and Soothe Your Nervous System

What foods we consume and how have a huge effect on our stress levels, either contributing to stress and inflammation within the body or combating them. Let's cover the ways you can do so specifically with your eating habits.

AVOID INFLAMMATORY FOODS

As you know by now, I'm a big fan of adding things vs. taking them away (more abundance, less restriction), but if you truly want to maximize your gut, liver, and overall hormone health, it is important to avoid inflammatory triggers (listed in detail on pages 50–53). Please keep in mind this is also bio-individual to each person, and based on your unique genetic makeup, background, blood type, and current state of health. You may be able to digest certain foods like gluten or dairy that can be highly inflammatory or triggering to others (such as those with lactose intolerance or an autoimmune condition like Hashimoto's or celiac disease). Stick to foods with a minimal amount of ingredients on the label (as well as ones you recognize and can pronounce), along with organic produce, grass-fed and pasture-raised animal products, and wild-caught seafood when possible.

EAT IN A CALM, RELAXED ENVIRONMENT

Eating in a calm, undistracted state allows your body to tap into its parasympathetic nervous system (also known as rest and digest mode) and properly absorb the nutrients you're consuming. When you eat on the go, in a distracted environment, or in a stressed-out state, your body has to divert energy away from digestion in response to a potential "threat" and stays in its sympathetic state (also known as fight-or-flight mode).

The sympathetic nervous system diverts blood flow to other organs, interfering with regular contractions of the muscles along the digestive tract, and decreases secretions needed for proper digestion. These changes in the digestive system lead to poor nutrient absorption, a slower transit time, and irritation of the large intestine, which contributes to symptoms ranging from indigestion to constipation, diarrhea, cramping, and bloating.

Bottom line: It's not just what you eat, but also *how* you eat it. I encourage clients to try to start with a commitment to enjoy at least *one* meal (dinner often seems to work best) sitting down at a table, eating a meal on a plate with no distractions (i.e., phone, TV, etc.). Allow yourself to relax and fully enjoy.

EAT FOR PLEASURE

Finding joy, pleasure, and gratitude in preparing and eating meals is an underrated pillar of eating for health and happiness. When we approach food in this way it's so much easier to make long-term, sustainable changes for real results. It's not "following a diet," it's a lifestyle.

It's so important to figure out what you like, have the capacity for, and feels right for you. You're much more likely to follow through with cooking a

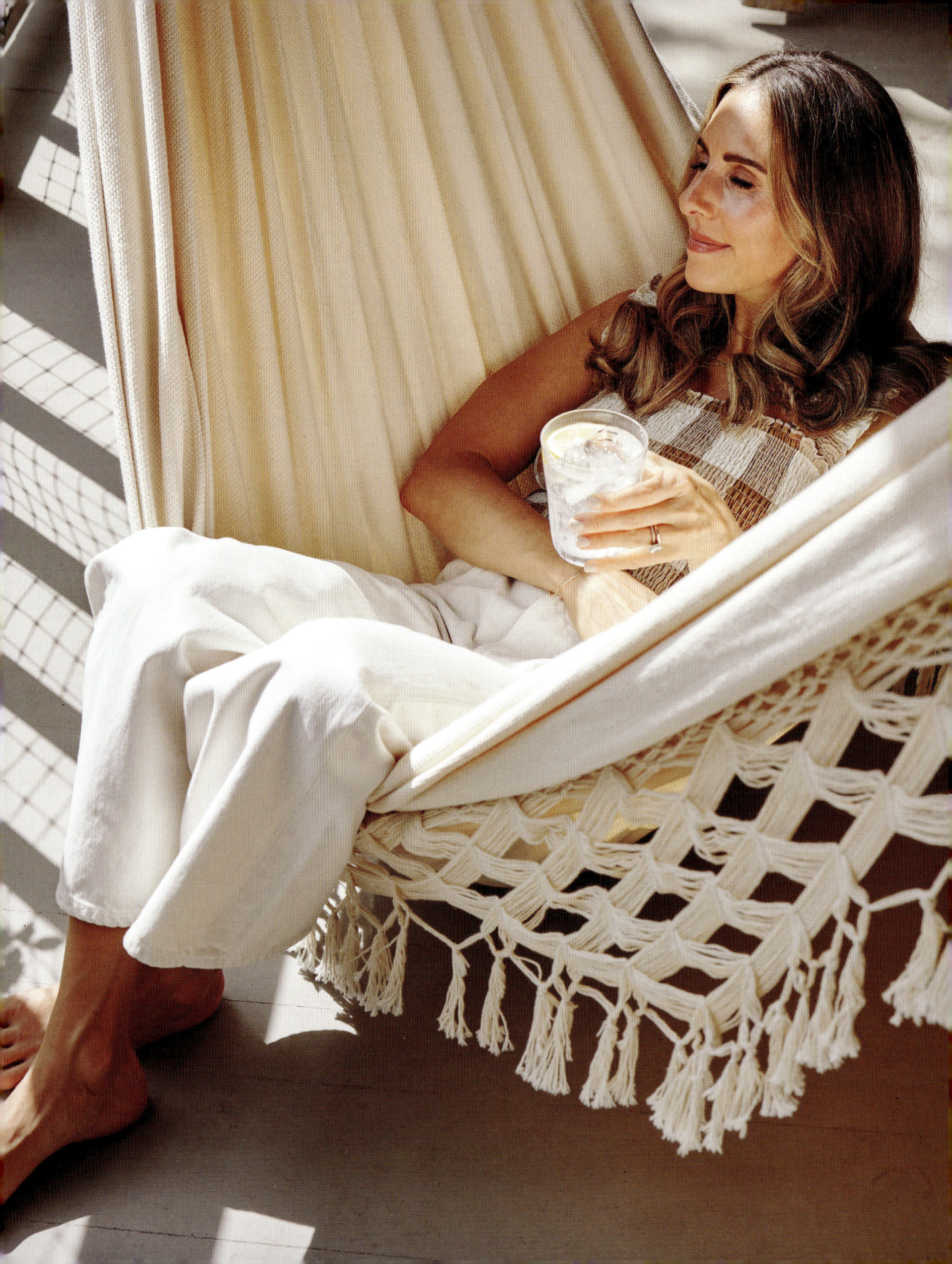

meal if it sounds appetizing and you feel comfortable cooking it vs. throwing in the towel and going with takeout or processed foods.

Eat food that brings you joy, in a way that also helps you feel your best (i.e., exactly what this cookbook is designed to do) and you'll not only find yourself feeling so much more nourished and satisfied, but also living a more fun, fulfilling, and beautiful life...and isn't that kind of the point?

ADOPT AN "ADD IN" VS. "TAKE AWAY" MENTALITY

Speaking of eating food in a way that brings you joy, swapping out the diet culture's take-away mentality for eating an abundance of nutrient-dense foods is a simple but profoundly impactful mindset shift. Instead of thinking of all the foods you need to eliminate at each meal or snack to "be healthy," try thinking of foods you can add to your plate that will fuel your hormones, thereby positively affecting your metabolism, energy, libido, skin and hair health, fertility, menstrual cycle, and overall health.

For example, is there a way to add more protein to your breakfast by scrambling your eggs with cottage cheese? Or to add more fiber to your burger by adding avocado and a side of sweet potato? Or maybe add more fat to your salad by drizzling it with extra virgin olive oil, or more minerals to your parfait by sprinkling it with nuts and seeds? This perspective is so much more enjoyable than thinking about taking away foods we love, and this is key for reducing stress and building sustainable eating habits.

Incorporating practices from each of these pillars will help you build a strong foundation for your hormones to thrive, but at the end of the day you've got to tailor it all to your unique preferences, lifestyle, and needs.

If something just doesn't work for you (timewise, taste-wise, budget-wise, etc.), it's highly unlikely that you'll follow through with doing it. And if you don't take consistent action, you won't get results.

Not only that, but every single person on this planet has their own unique genetic makeup, preference, lifestyle, and overall state of health. So what works well for one person may not work well for another. Please take this into account when approaching recipes and eating suggestions in this cookbook, as well as any other nutrition advice floating around out there.

You know your body best, and if something doesn't feel right or work well for you, honor it above all else.

BENEFICIAL FOODS FOR HORMONE HEALTH

Now that we've covered the basic tenets of a hormone-healthy eating mentality, let's dive into the food specifics. All of the food in this section has been scientifically proven to have a positive effect on your hormones, either directly or indirectly via a contributing mechanism such as improved gut health, liver function, or insulin sensitivity. That being said, I want to emphasize how different each person is, and therefore not all of these foods may work well for you. Take this into account as you read this section, noting which foods you'd be excited to try or incorporate into more of your meals moving forward (you can easily find them throughout the recipes in this book!).

Macronutrients

A macronutrient provides the body and cells with energy and is needed in large amounts (typically measured in grams). There are three major macronutrients—protein, fat, and carbohydrates (what I refer to here as fiber)—and all of them need to be consumed to achieve optimal hormone balance.

PROTEIN

Protein is an essential structural component of all hormones, meaning you must consume sufficient protein to make enough hormones.

Protein is made up of smaller components called amino acids, which help to make muscles, tendons, organs, skin, enzymes, neurotransmitters, and various molecules that do everything from foster metabolic health, fertility, and protection during pregnancy to ensure proper immune and cognitive function as well as regulate your menstrual cycle and blood sugar.

Animal studies have shown that too little protein can prevent or delay ovulation by suppressing the release of luteinizing hormone, which is the hormone that triggers ovulation.[11] If ovulation does occur on a low-protein diet, studies show, egg quality can be negatively impacted.[12] Furthermore, low protein intake can impair estrogen signaling, throwing off your entire menstrual cycle and playing a role in symptoms related to PMS.

Additionally, protein intake is vital for thyroid health and directly impacts thermogenesis, the process by which your body generates heat (aka energy) by increasing your metabolic rate. Low basal body temperature is often linked to hypothyroidism, which includes symptoms like weight gain, fertility challenges, and recurrent miscarriages.

Bottom line: Protein is a very well-researched non-negotiable when it comes to optimal hormone health, especially for women in their reproductive years who may have higher protein requirements due to a lower ability to absorb and utilize amino acids for protein synthesis.

While every person's needs will vary slightly based on activity levels, weight, age, sex, and hormone health status, the dietary recommendations indicate that the average person requires 0.8 to 1 gram of protein per pound per day. This averages to 60 to 100 grams of protein per day for women in their reproductive years. If you eat three meals per day, this means that you need about 30 grams of protein per meal. Please note, this is a minimal target to prevent a protein deficiency and not designed to estimate optimal protein intake, which many scientists argue we should increase to no less than 1.2g/kg daily; this can average from 80 to 150 grams of protein per day. **Note:** "Grams of protein" refers to the number of grams of the macronutrient protein, not the weight of the protein source itself. For example, an average chicken breast weighs 174 grams (or about 6 ounces) and has 40 to 50 grams of protein per serving. Thus, you'd be consuming 40 to 50 grams of protein when eating a 174-gram chicken breast.

You'll need to tailor these recommendations for yourself, considering your activity levels, any hormonal imbalances you're struggling with, blood sugar issues, desire to lose weight, and current state of health. At the time of writing this book, I feel a very positive and noticeable difference when consuming an average of 100 grams of protein per day.

FAT

Dietary fat is a crucial element of hormone balance, as it's a building block of all steroid hormones (including estrogen, testosterone, and progesterone) and is used to produce and maintain proper hormone function. It's also necessary for your body to effectively digest and absorb fat-soluble vitamins like A, D, E, and K, which play an important role in hormone regulation and fertility.

Fat has been largely misunderstood and quite controversial (especially if you grew up in the '90s—hello, fat-free everything!), but we now know it plays a vital role in women's fertility, menstrual cycle, pregnancy, and hormone health. In a study of over 3,000 women that assessed diet and PMS,[13] those with the highest intake of fat had a significant reduction in symptoms including fewer food cravings and less bloating, while a study of over 18,000 women found that diets with a higher fat intake, specifically saturated fat, were linked to significantly better ovulatory function, which orchestrates our entire menstrual cycle.[14] Conversely, when dietary fat is limited too much, ovulation can be delayed or cease altogether, disrupting the entire menstrual cycle and impacting everything from fertility to PMS.

What matters (as with everything) is the quality and type of fat, as certain sources are rich in micronutrients and fatty acids key for ovarian hormone production, while others (particularly processed and man-made fats) can cause high levels of inflammation and be detrimental to hormone health.

A Note on Animal Protein vs. Plant Protein

Something that comes up quite a bit in my practice is the dietary dogma surrounding animal protein and plant protein. While I adore plants (and make sure I'm eating them with every meal, as you'll notice in the recipes), I personally prioritize and encourage my female clients to consume animal protein, such as grass-fed red meat and poultry, wild-caught seafood, organ meats, eggs, and gelatin found in bone broth, as these are complete proteins that contain all nine essential amino acids necessary to carry out a variety of functions, from protein synthesis to tissue repair and nutrient absorption.

Some of the amino acids that are found in animal proteins, such as taurine, cysteine, glycine, lysine, and choline, are specifically needed to carry out liver detoxification. Deficiency in these amino acids can increase your liver workload and toxic burden, often resulting in hormonal imbalances such as estrogen dominance. Low lysine intake has also been linked to lower immune function, poor GI function, and increased anxiety, while taurine deficiency can result in menstrual cycle irregularities, miscarriage, and developmental abnormalities during pregnancy. Plant sources are virtually devoid of these amino acids; however, animal sources contain an optimal balance in their most bioavailable form, meaning they're more easily used and assimilated by your body—with your hormones reaping the benefits.

Animal sources are typically much denser in protein than plant sources, so you can eat a smaller amount and achieve a greater overall protein intake. For example, to consume 30 grams of protein you'd need to eat only 4 ounces (or about ½ cup shredded) chicken breast vs. 2 cups of black beans. (And honestly, how many of us are really eating 2 cups of black beans at one sitting?)

We know protein intake is important, but *quality* also matters, with women with higher intakes of animal protein the least likely to report symptoms relating to PMS.[15] While ultimately this choice comes down to your personal preference, cultural background, religion, and lifestyle, if you're struggling with symptoms of hormonal imbalance and lack animal protein in your diet, I'd encourage you to pay attention and keep an open mind moving forward.

While the amount of fat that's right for you will ultimately depend on your caloric needs, Lily Nichols, an RDN and co-author of *Real Food for Fertility,* recommends including a source of fat at each meal and snack, as well as aiming for a daily minimum fat intake of no less than 40 to 45 percent of your calories.[16]

Here's an overview of the types of fats to include in a hormone-healthy diet:

- **SATURATED FATS:** This type of dietary fat is abundant in fatty acids crucial for hormone health regulation, including stearic acid, with high dietary intake linked to a 25 percent reduction in PMS in women.[17] It can be found mostly in animal sources (the fat of beef, pork, lamb, and dairy) as well as some plants (coconut oil, palm oil, and cocoa butter). Saturated fats also contain butyric and caprylic acids, which have been shown to enhance ovarian progesterone synthesis and estradiol and progesterone production, as well as to improve embryo implantation and lower the risk of early pregnancy loss. These fatty acids are found mainly in dairy fats such as butter, cream, and cheese, which may explain the link between consumption of high-fat dairy products and increased fertility in women.

- **MONOUNSATURATED FATS:** This type of fat has also been linked to improved embryo development, fertility, and menstrual cycle health,[18] and is found in abundance in avocado and olive oils, as well as nuts, seeds, pork lard, and poultry fat. It's rich in hormone-healthy fatty acids such as oleic acid, which has been shown to improve insulin sensitivity,[19] reduce hunger and cravings, and boost your overall immune system. The ever-popular Mediterranean diet emphasizes monounsaturated fat intake, which is one reason it's linked to fertility and overall health.[20]

- **POLYUNSATURATED FATS:** Polyunsaturated fats (PUFAs) can be found in both plant and animal sources and contain omega-3 and omega-6 fatty acids. While the anti-inflammatory omega-3 fatty acids abundant in wild-caught fatty fish (salmon, trout, sardines, etc.) and some plant sources (chia, flaxseed, walnuts) are known for their hormone-health benefits—ranging from a decrease in symptoms related to PMS to improvement in insulin sensitivity, blood sugar balance, and egg quality—omega-6 fatty acids have quite the opposite effect. These fatty acids are found in refined vegetable oils such as corn, soy, cottonseed, and safflower and have been linked to decreased fertility rates in women,[21] as they reduce levels of beneficial omega-3 fatty acids in the body and impair both ovarian function and hormone production.

FIBER FROM UNPROCESSED CARBOHYDRATES

Carbohydrates are the final major macronutrient and are found in almost all plant foods, including grains, vegetables, fruits, and legumes. The body can break these long chains of sugar quickly into individual chain links of sugar to be absorbed for almost immediate energy. Carbohydrates are found in abundance in both healthy and processed foods, though my recipes feature mostly whole, complex carbohydrates. These tend to have a lower glycemic index (meaning less of an impact on your blood sugar levels) and a significantly higher micronutrient profile, and offer a plethora of hormone-health benefits due to their dietary fiber.

Dietary fiber is the portion of a plant-derived carbohydrate that cannot be completely broken down by digestive enzymes. It's diverse in composition (soluble, insoluble, prebiotic, etc.), but its main role is to promote a healthy digestive system through a variety of functions and benefits. In this cookbook we focus on whole foods rich in the following types of dietary fiber:

- **SOLUBLE FIBER:** This type of fiber blends with water in your gut, forming a gel-like substance that collects toxins, hormones (such as estrogen), and waste products to safely eliminate them from your body. Soluble fiber has been shown to improve both blood glucose control (linked directly to ovarian function and menstrual cycle health) and lower blood cholesterol. It also feeds your gut microbiome, resulting in an increase in metabolites that work to lower inflammation and may help improve IBS symptoms. Soluble fiber is abundant in oats, peas, beans and legumes, leafy greens, apples, citrus fruits, carrots, barley, and psyllium.

- **INSOLUBLE FIBER:** Insoluble fiber does not blend with water and passes through your digestive system mostly intact. It functions as a broom, sweeping up your GI tract and bulking your stool, speeding up the passage of food and waste through your gut. This type of fiber is typically well tolerated but can potentially irritate the gut for those with IBS or other sensitivities. Foods rich in soluble fiber include whole wheat, nuts and seeds, beans and legumes, cruciferous vegetables like cauliflower and broccoli, root vegetables, and green beans.

- **PREBIOTIC FIBER/RESISTANT STARCH:** Prebiotic fiber, also known as resistant starch, feeds the "good" bacteria in your GI tract to produce health-promoting compounds, such as the short-chain fatty acid butyrate, which enhances intestinal barrier function and mucosal immunity (that is, it protects against inflammation and leaky gut). It can be found in unripe bananas and mangos, chicory root, onions, garlic, legumes, cashews, and raw oats, along with rice, sweet potatoes, or potatoes that have been cooked and then cooled (also known as retrograde resistant starch).

As you can see, consuming adequate dietary fiber impacts our hormones positively in a myriad of ways. It's especially critical when it comes to keeping our estrogen levels in check, which it does by binding to excess estrogen in the large intestine and then safely expelling it via bowel movements. In fact, a good way to tell if we have healthy estrogen levels is how often we're pooping, which should be a minimum of one to three times a day. If not, excess estrogen has nowhere to go and is reabsorbed into your bloodstream, often leading to estrogen dominance, which you've now learned is associated with a variety of uncomfortable symptoms such as PMS, heavy or painful periods, acne, weight gain, fatigue, breast tenderness, depression, and more.

Consuming dietary fiber also increases the production of leptin, our satiety hormone, and reduces ghrelin, our hunger hormone, which helps regulate our appetite and keep cravings at bay (something extremely helpful for those looking to manage their weight). It's an essential part of keeping your gut microbiome healthy, optimizing thyroid hormone conversion and your metabolism as well as nutrient absorption from food and supplements to synthesize hormone production.

The Institute of Medicine recommends 14 grams of dietary fiber per 1,000 calories consumed, which is equivalent to about 28 grams of fiber per day for women consuming a minimum of 2,000 calories daily.

You'll note the majority of the recipes in this book include some protein, fat, and fiber to make them as nutrient-rich and blood sugar–friendly as possible.

Micronutrients

Micronutrients are vitamins and minerals the body needs in small amounts but that are essential for hormone health. They can be consumed via macronutrients (protein, fat, and fiber-rich carbohydrates) and play a variety of roles and functions with our hormones, especially regarding hormone production and regulation, ovulation and fertility, oxidative stress, and endometrial health.

Micronutrient deficiency is a huge contributor to hormonal imbalances in women, with the World Health Organization estimating 67 percent of women in their reproductive years are deficient in one or more essential vitamins and minerals.[22] This is attributed to a diet higher in processed foods (i.e., low in micronutrients) or to undereating/undernourishment, as micronutrients are provided through eating enough real, whole foods. Additionally, women in their reproductive years have higher needs for vitamins and minerals than men or prepubescent girls and postmenopausal women due to the amount of energy it takes to orchestrate ovulation and a healthy menstrual cycle, not to mention pregnancy, childbirth, and lactation.

There are also factors that can inhibit micronutrient absorption, such as certain medications, hormonal birth control, genetic factors, and poor gut health and nutrient absorption. It's up to us to ensure we are eating an abundance of micronutrient-rich foods to balance hormones, keep symptoms at bay, and feel our best. Following is a rundown of the essential micronutrients and their optimal food sources, which you'll of course find in regular rotation throughout the recipes in this cookbook.

VITAMIN A

Vitamin A is required for progesterone production in women and testosterone production in men. Insufficient intake is a known risk factor for early miscarriage and multiple birth defects. Animal foods such as *liver, meat, seafood, eggs, and full-fat dairy* contain true, preformed vitamin A (retinol). And while plant sources like carrots and sweet potatoes are also considered a source of vitamin A, they offer only carotenoids that are less potent and bioavailable for your body to convert.

B VITAMINS

B_1 (thiamine), B_2 (riboflavin), B_3 (niacin), B_5 (pantothenic acid), B_6 (pyridoxine), B_7 (biotin), B_9 (folate or folic acid), and B_{12} (cyanocobalamin) are considered detoxification cofactors. They influence and support our hormones in a myriad of ways, from optimal progesterone production and estrogen-to-progesterone ratio to assisting in a process called methylation, which is vital for female fertility and healthy ovulatory cycles. Foods rich in B vitamins include *liver and other organ meats, meat, fish, shellfish, eggs, lentils and other legumes, bananas, potatoes, and mushrooms.*

VITAMIN C

Vitamin C is essential for optimal progesterone production and fertility in women. It also helps to regulate the adrenal glands and the production of the stress hormone cortisol, as well as to heal your body from stress-related damage. It's abundant in plant sources such as *citrus, bell peppers, tomatoes, papaya, leafy greens, broccoli, Brussels sprouts, strawberries, and melons.*

VITAMIN D

Vitamin D is a fat-soluble hormone that works to regulate estrogen and progesterone as well as insulin and blood sugar, positively impacting ovarian function and the health of our menstrual cycles. Low vitamin D levels are often associated with fertility and pregnancy challenges, as well as an increase in menopausal symptoms. Vitamin D can be found in *fatty fish such as sardines and anchovies, cod liver oil, egg yolks, liver, beef, and mushrooms.*

VITAMIN E

Vitamin E is a powerful antioxidant that is considered anti-estrogenic, meaning it can help reduce negative effects of excess estrogen, a common hormonal imbalance in women. It's also been shown to alleviate period pain and PMS-related symptoms. Foods rich in vitamin E include *sunflower seeds, almonds, peanuts, avocado, and spinach.*

VITAMIN K2

Best known for its role in bone health, K_2 also plays a role in hormone synthesis, improving insulin sensitivity, lowering inflammation, and reducing oxidative stress—all of which are needed to support egg quality and ovulation. It's found in *liver and other organ meats, hard cheeses, egg yolks, and fermented foods like sauerkraut and natto (a fermented soybean).*

MAGNESIUM

A mineral essential to several hormonal and reproductive processes from regulating our circadian rhythm and stress hormone production to stimulating ovulation and thyroid hormone conversion (inactive T4 to its active T3 form), magnesium has been shown to help reduce PMS and menopausal symptoms as well as promote optimal fertility, sleep, and muscle relaxation. Foods rich in magnesium include *leafy greens, nuts and seeds, whole grains like quinoa and brown rice, avocado, and dark chocolate.*

IRON

This mineral is essential for optimal menstrual health, with a higher deficiency risk for women in their reproductive years due to blood loss, which can affect blood flow to the ovaries and impair ovulation. While iron can be found in both plant and animal sources, the type and impact greatly vary, with non-heme iron (from plant sources) found to be absorbed extremely poorly (a rate of 2 to 13 percent), while heme iron (from animal sources) has an absorption efficiency ranging from 25 to 40 percent.[23] The most bioavailable sources include *liver and other organ meats, red meat, poultry, and seafood.*

ZINC

Zinc helps to regulate LH, FSH, and steroid production, making it essential for optimal ovulation, fertility, reproductive cycles, and endometrial function. It also protects the body against oxidative stress–related damage. Zinc deficiencies are associated with multiple fertility and pregnancy challenges, including impaired egg quality, a higher rate of miscarriage, preterm delivery, and birth defects. Foods rich in zinc include *meat, fish, and shellfish.*

SELENIUM

Selenium supports thyroid health, immune function, DNA synthesis, detoxification, and fertility. A deficiency reduces levels of the liver's major detoxification enzyme, glutathione, leading to an increase in oxidative stress, a known contributor to poor egg quality. Foods rich in selenium include *organ meats, seafood, eggs, Brazil nuts, and sesame seeds.*

IODINE

An essential part of thyroid hormone production, iodine regulates metabolism, weight, fertility, and menstrual cycle health. Deficiencies in menstruating women across the globe have skyrocketed in recent years, which has been linked to the rise in plant-based diets. Iodine can be found in *seaweed, along with seafood, eggs, and dairy products.*

DHA

Docosahexaenoic acid (DHA) is a specific type of omega-3 fat that is involved in progesterone and estrogen production, helping to regulate ovulation and menstrual cycles, and plays a crucial role in egg quality, pregnancy, and fetal development. It also helps to lower inflammation and has been shown to be especially beneficial in reducing PMS symptoms, including pain and cramping. *Seafood (especially fatty fish such as salmon and sardines)* is highest in DHA, *along with egg yolks and grass-fed beef.*

CHOLINE

This B vitamin–like compound supports optimal liver function, detoxification and methylation, and estrogen and folate metabolism. Choline has been shown to help increase ovarian function, regulate menstrual cycles, and help mitigate PMS and menopausal symptoms such as hot flashes and night sweats. *Egg yolks and liver* are the most abundant sources of choline, *with trace amounts in plants such as cruciferous vegetables, shiitake mushrooms, peanuts, and almonds.*

AMINO ACIDS

As you learned earlier, amino acids are the building blocks of protein. There are twenty in total, and nine are considered essential, meaning you *must* obtain them from your diet. If you eat a diet rich in *grass-fed, pasture-raised animal protein,* you can rest assured you'll be meeting these needs. However, it is extremely difficult for women following a plant-based diet to obtain adequate amounts of these amino acids, as non-animal sources lack essential amino acids and contain anti-nutrients like phytates, lectins, and tannins, which inhibit amino acid absorption.
If eating meat is not an option for you, I encourage you to emphasize *eggs, seafood (such as oysters and fatty fish), and full-fat dairy products (such as yogurt and cheese),* as well as take a *multivitamin or prenatal vitamin and algae-based DHA supplement* as a way to optimize your protein and nutrient intake.

ELECTROLYTES AND SALT

Electrolytes comprise essential minerals, including sodium (salt), potassium, chloride, calcium, and magnesium, which provide a myriad of functions from supporting energy levels, adrenal health, and fluid balance to maintaining the correct plasma volume in your bloodstream to providing the adequate stomach acid necessary for the absorption of vitamins and minerals and facilitating protein digestion. A low salt intake (less than 1,500 mg per day) is associated with 37 percent lower progesterone levels and a 2.7 times greater risk of anovulation compared to women who consume sufficient salt.[24] It's also been linked to a higher risk for PMS, most likely because a low-salt diet triggers the adrenal glands to release a hormone called aldosterone, leading to fluid and sodium retention.[25] Additionally, low intake of certain electrolytes like calcium and magnesium has been shown to contribute to cycle issues including cramping, breast tenderness, fluid retention (bloating), headaches, and migraines and mood changes.[26]

As you can see, if we want to ensure we're obtaining plenty of nutrients to support optimal hormone balance, we need to take an inclusive approach to food. This all goes back to the idea that if we adopt an add-in mentality and emphasize keeping an open and abundant mindset on food, our hormones and bodies will reap the benefits.

FOODS THAT DON'T SUPPORT HEALTHY HORMONES

While I emphasize an add-in vs. take-away mentality with food—which creates so much more joy and less stress around eating—I would be remiss if I didn't touch on foods that have been found to negatively impact women's menstrual cycles and hormone health.

I encourage you to approach this section with a crowd-out mentality, meaning you should continue to focus on the foods listed in the previous section (and all of the recipes in this book) as they will naturally crowd out the foods listed below. My intention is not to create fear around food, but I *do* want you to have access to all the information so that you can make informed choices that align with your lifestyle and goals.

The following list includes foods (with many more accurately described as "food-like" man-made substances) that do *not* support healthy hormones, so you may want to tread with caution, consume them less often, or avoid them altogether, depending on the circumstance.

VEGETABLE AND SEED OILS

These oils are extracted from seed crops such as *canola (rapeseed), corn, soy, safflower, and cottonseed*. Not only are they refined and processed using an abundance of chemical solvents, they're high in a type of unsaturated fat called omega-6,

> "
>
> IF WE WANT TO ENSURE WE'RE OBTAINING PLENTY OF NUTRIENTS TO SUPPORT OPTIMAL HORMONE BALANCE, WE NEED TO TAKE AN INCLUSIVE APPROACH TO FOOD.

which is extremely vulnerable to oxidation and destabilization when heated (used in cooking), turning into oxidized fats and a major source of toxins (lipid oxidation products, or LOPs).

High intake of oxidized omega-6 fatty acids has been linked to fertility challenges, inflammatory conditions like endometriosis and dysmenorrhea, and depletion of vitamin E, an important antioxidant for fertility, metabolism, and overall hormone health.[27] Most restaurants use these oils in their cooking as they're cheaper, so you're already one step ahead of the game if you cook most meals at home. (If you don't already, you can start with this book!) You'll want to be wary of *fried foods like French fries or doughnuts,* and check ingredient labels when purchasing snack foods like *chips and crackers, baked goods, dressings, sauces, and nondairy alternatives.*

TRY THESE INSTEAD: Extra virgin olive oil, avocado oil, unrefined coconut oil, sesame oil.

MAN-MADE TRANS FATS AND PARTIALLY HYDROGENATED OILS

This type of trans fat is made through a process called hydrogenation, where liquid vegetable oils (like those listed on page 50) are converted into a solid, like shortening or margarine. These fats are highly inflammatory and have been linked to everything from diabetes, cancer, and heart disease to endometriosis and fertility problems. Research has shown that in women of reproductive age, every 2 percent increase in trans-fat consumption is linked to a 73 percent greater risk of anovulation (infertility due to lack of ovulation).[28] Because these fats have virtually no benefits, only posing health risks, I encourage you to steer clear of them altogether. They can often be found in *processed and fried foods* (as they extend shelf life) such as *fast food, doughnuts, store-bought cookies, cakes and pastries, and frosting.*

TRY THESE INSTEAD: Tallow, lard, grass-fed butter, ghee.

REFINED CARBOHYDRATES

While you previously learned about the benefit of whole, unrefined sources of carbohydrates that are rich in fiber, refined carbohydrates have been stripped of fiber and micronutrients and processed into flours or isolated starches. The result is a product of pure starch that is void of virtually all nutrients, causes major spikes in blood sugar, and has been increasingly identified as the main culprit in blood sugar and metabolic issues. These can contribute to menstrual health issues ranging from severe PMS to ovulatory dysfunction and PCOS. Refined carbohydrates include anything made from white or enriched flour such as *bread, bagels, crackers, chips, pizza, pasta, noodles, pretzels, breakfast cereals, and "instant" rice or other quick-cooking starches.*

TRY THESE INSTEAD: Bread made from nuts (almond, coconut, etc.), pasta made from beans or legumes, brown rice, quinoa, whole oats, millet, flax meal, yams, potatoes.

GLUTEN AND GRAINS

Gluten is a protein found in certain grains such as *wheat, rye, and barley* that has been linked to a host of gut-related disorders (intestinal permeability) as well as autoimmune diseases like celiac and Hashimoto's. Many people are not able to digest or properly break down these large proteins, so that they pass through the gut lining and into the bloodstream, where the immune system attacks them, causing an inflammatory response. Additionally, some people cannot tolerate grains well (even gluten-free ones), due to the lack of a gene called AMI-1, which creates the digestive enzyme amylase helping to break down and digest grains. Gluten sensitivity should be addressed on a case-by-case basis, where you take into consideration your own needs. However, if you experience symptoms such as stomach cramps, nausea, indigestion, sneezing or runny nose, hives or skin rashes, headaches, or fatigue after consuming gluten, grains, or both, I encourage you to remove them from your diet for a period of time to see if symptoms improve. You will note that this cookbook is entirely gluten-free. This is because my mom has celiac disease, and both my eldest daughter and I are extremely sensitive to gluten, so I personally do not cook with it.

TRY THESE INSTEAD: Flour derived from nuts (almond, coconut), potatoes, cassava, yams, squash, flax meal, and ground seeds.

ADDED SUGARS

Piggybacking on refined carbohydrates, refined sugar is a subcategory that also provides little to no nutritional value and has detrimental effects on our hormone health. Diets high in sugar have been repeatedly linked with menstrual health issues (such as PMS), ovulatory disorders (including PCOS), insulin resistance, and thyroid and adrenal function issues.[29] Added sugars also disrupt mineral metabolism in the body, specifically iron, copper, and zinc, which you're now aware play a vital role in hormone health. Refined sugar has a variety of confusing names and types and is hidden in processed foods as well as those often deemed healthy like *dried fruit and fruit juices.* Make sure to read the ingredient labels on any packaged food you purchase such as *candy, sweetened beverages, soda, nondairy milk, sauces, jams, cookies, and crackers,* and note both the total grams of sugar (4 grams = 1 teaspoon) along with the ingredient list itself, looking for terms such as *sugar, evaporated cane juice, any sort of syrup, maltodextrin, or anything ending in "ose"* (e.g., sucrose and fructose).

TRY THESE INSTEAD (IN SMALL QUANTITIES): Maple syrup, dates, raw honey, coconut sugar.

NOTE: While I avoid added or refined sugars as much as I can, you'll notice in the recipes that I do not avoid them altogether! I have quite the sweet tooth, but I opt for unrefined sources that contain trace amounts of minerals and nutrients, such as maple syrup, coconut sugar, and dates. I also use them in smaller quantities and pair them with protein and fat to curb a potential blood sugar spike. To completely cut out sugar altogether is just not realistic for me, or most people, so I try to take a mindful and minimal approach, as well as follow the pillars outlined in eating for blood sugar balance (see page 37) to minimize any hormone disruption.

ARTIFICIAL SWEETENERS

These sugar alternatives rely on chemicals that trick your taste buds into registering a very sweet flavor (100 times sweeter than real sugar) and encourage both sugar cravings and sugar dependence. This can lead to a dysregulation of sweet taste buds and overeating. Additionally, recent research has shown that artificial sweeteners interact with microbes in your gut, leading to an elevation in blood sugar and decrease of good bacteria, which is directly linked to hormone balance.[30] They've also been shown to impact thyroid function (remember, 20 to 30 percent of thyroid conversion happens in the gut).[31] Artificial sweeteners include *aspartame, sucralose, saccharin, acesulfame potassium, and neotame.*

TRY THESE INSTEAD (IN SMALL QUANTITIES): Stevia, sugar alcohols, monk fruit.

ALCOHOL

While I enjoy the occasional cocktail or glass of wine, alcohol intake is a known hormone disruptor and a key culprit in hormonal imbalances and symptoms. We know this thanks to scientific studies that associate even one alcoholic drink per day with an over 5 percent rise in estrogen (and four or more drinks per day with a 60 percent increase!),[32] along with a decline in progesterone, testosterone, and luteinizing hormones. These changes are enough to throw off your menstrual cycle, resulting in impaired ovarian function and diminished ovarian reserve, along with higher rates of infertility. Alcohol has also been shown to suppress thyroid and liver function and increase cortisol and insulin secretion, leading to issues with detoxification, blood sugar regulation, and adrenal function. It's a known anti-nutrient, meaning it depletes vitamins and minerals necessary for hormone production. As with every guideline in this book, I encourage you to pay attention to how it affects you. If you are dealing with menstrual cycle irregularities, sleep issues, or hormonal imbalances and regularly consume alcohol, cutting back or minimizing intake may be a simple yet profoundly impactful shift you can make.

TRY THIS INSTEAD: Swap out a cocktail for one of the mocktail recipes in this book! They are delicious, fun, and festive alternatives.

CAFFEINE

I absolutely love enjoying a cup of coffee as part of my morning ritual (after a blood sugar–balancing breakfast!). However, it's important to acknowledge that caffeine stimulates cortisol production, so if you're already dealing with stress or symptoms of high cortisol or adrenal fatigue, reducing your intake or eliminating it could help you reduce symptoms. An increase in cortisol production is often linked to a decrease in progesterone levels (due to their sharing the same precursor hormone, pregnenolone), which can result in symptoms ranging from a shortened luteal phase (and thus difficulty conceiving) to exacerbated PMS symptoms. Consuming caffeine also results in a spike in your glucose and insulin response, leading to blood sugar dysregulation. This is why I always encourage you to have any source of caffeine (including tea, energy drinks, sodas, etc.) with or after a meal rich in protein, fat, and fiber, and never on an empty stomach (which has a disastrous effect on blood sugar levels). Lastly, as with alcohol, high caffeine intake places an additional burden on your liver and depletes micronutrients essential for balanced hormones. Ultimately, this is another one that boils down to personal preference, but reducing or limiting intake can go a long way in supporting your hormones.

TRY THESE INSTEAD: Single-shot espresso (instead of a double shot) or decaf, matcha, herbal teas, chicory coffee, mushroom coffees or teas, bone broth hot chocolate (page 110), or a golden milk latte (page 274).

CONVENTIONAL ANIMAL PROTEIN AND DAIRY

While animal protein and full-fat dairy consumption are key for optimized hormones, quality is extremely important. Sourcing pasture-raised and grass-fed meat, wild-caught seafood, and minimally processed, full-fat dairy ensures you're absorbing ample quantities of essential micronutrients and amino acids that play a huge role in liver function and hormone production. Conventional meat, poultry, and dairy products often test positive for antibiotics, pesticides, and synthetic growth hormones, while farmed fish are typically contaminated with PCBs, dioxins, and other chemicals, all of which have been shown to negatively impact hormones. While this often comes down to budget and accessibility, it's something to pay attention to and prioritize if you can. I also include recipes that call for less expensive cuts of meat in this cookbook (chuck roast, pork shoulder, etc.) to help you get more bang for your buck.

TRY THESE INSTEAD: Pasture-raised poultry, grass-fed red meat, wild-caught seafood, and organic grass-fed butter and dairy.

CONVENTIONAL SOY AND CORN

Among all food crops in the United States, soy and corn are the most heavily sprayed with pesticides such as glyphosate (also known as Roundup), a weed killer and known toxin and endocrine disruptor. The US Department of Agriculture estimates that 94 percent of these crops are also genetically modified to make them withstand high levels of glyphosate.[33] Soy has also been linked to high levels of heavy metals, including aluminum and cadmium, negatively impacting fertility and menstrual cycle health. It also contains phytoestrogens called isoflavones, and long-term ingestion has been shown to delay ovulation and lower progesterone. I rarely use soy and corn in my own cooking, but when I do (as with the high-protein pudding, page 160), and the GOAT corn salad, page 187), I opt for organic and minimally processed whole-food sources to negate any potential negative effects (i.e., corn on the cob vs. corn chips, etc.).

TRY THESE INSTEAD: Organic fermented soy (miso, tempeh), organic or heirloom corn, and soy and corn plant alternatives (in milks, chips, wraps, etc.) such as cassava root, almond, hemp, taro, and macadamia.

At the end of the day, opting for real, whole, and nutrient-dense foods and limiting man-made, processed, or chemically engineered foods is one of your best bets for supporting optimal hormone health. Cooking more meals at home (I hope via this cookbook) also gives you more control over ingredients and quality, making it a very impactful habit when it comes to supporting your hormones.

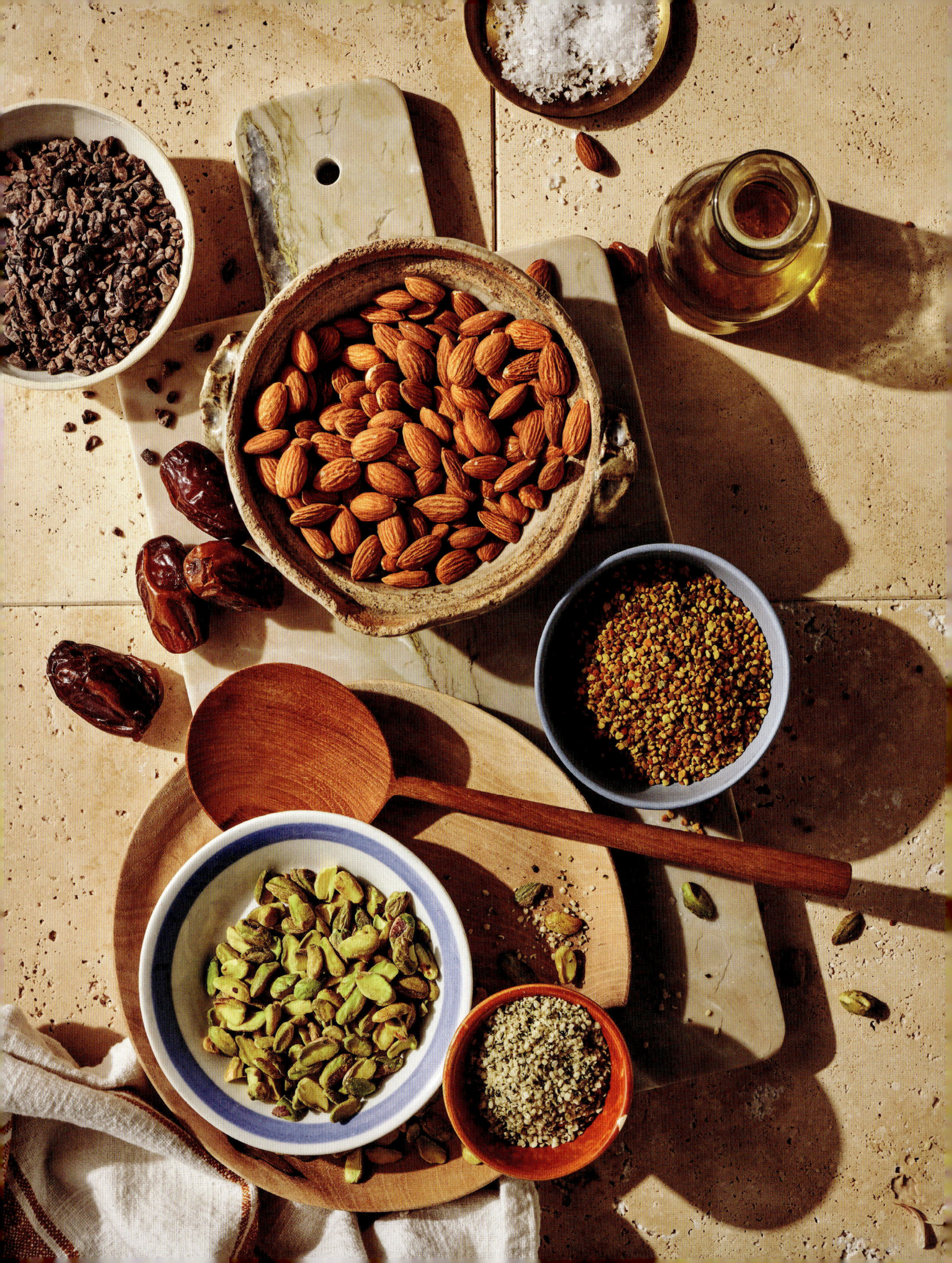

PART TWO

100 Recipes to Support, Balance, and Nourish Your Hormones

SO YOU CAN FEEL YOUR ABSOLUTE BEST

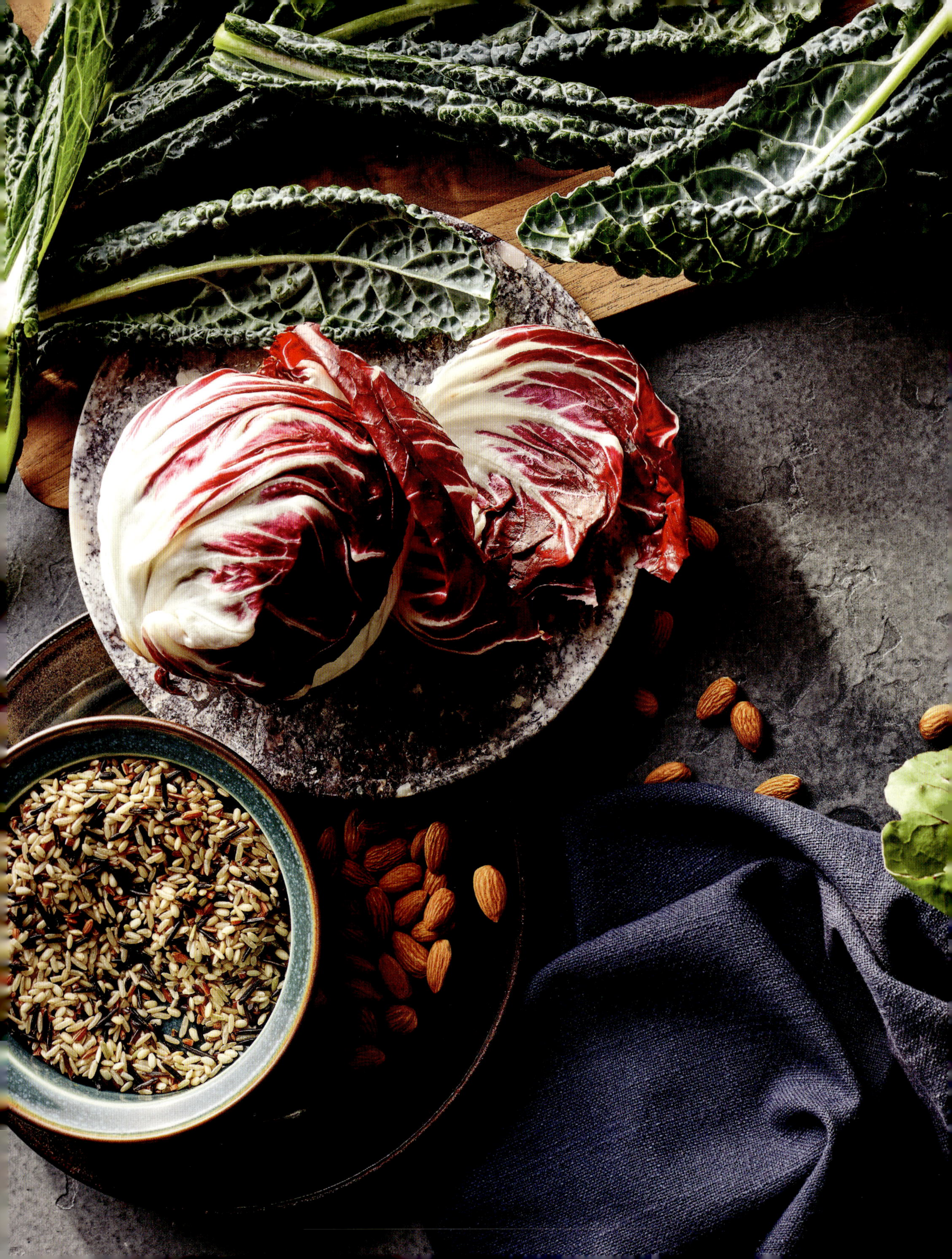

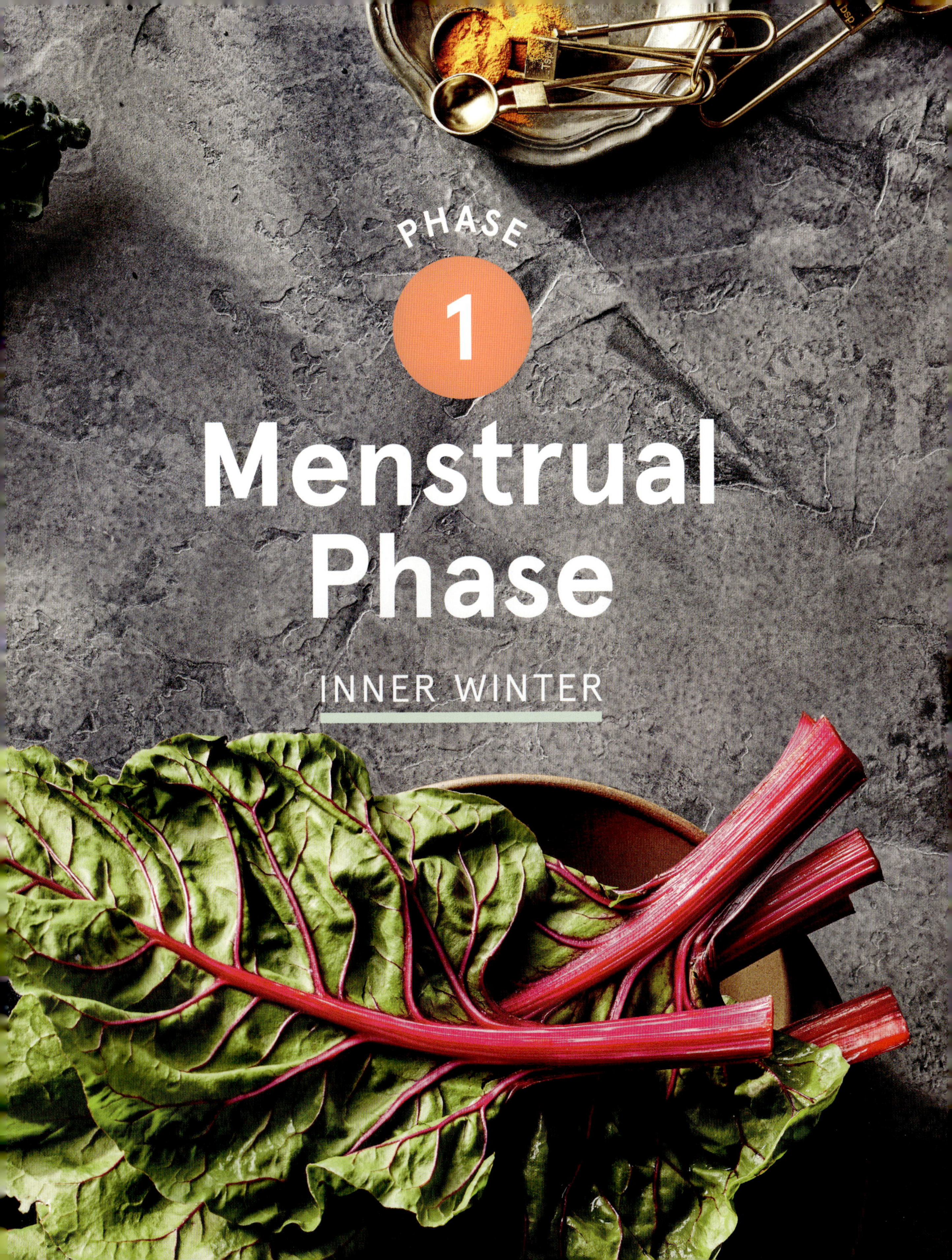

PHASE 1

Menstrual Phase

INNER WINTER

RECIPES

WHAT'S HAPPENING

The first day of your period marks the beginning of your menstrual phase, typically lasting anywhere from 3 to 7 days. It is the result of a normal inflammatory process that prompts the disintegration of the functional layer of the endometrium (no longer needed for egg implantation) and the regeneration of a new layer in preparation for implanting an embryo in the upcoming cycle.

It's an energy-intensive phase involving tissue injury and restoration, and as such it makes sense for you to feel more tired, withdrawn, vulnerable, and tender (especially in your abdomen). That does not mean it should feel painful or debilitating in any way (physically or emotionally). If you do experience any of these symptoms it is often linked to one or more hormonal imbalances. Please remember, painful periods are all too common, but they are not normal, and they should *not* be accepted as a normal part of your life.

In addition to the tissue degeneration taking place, all of your sex hormones (including estrogen, progesterone, and testosterone) are at their lowest levels, impacting your mood, confidence, sleep, energy, and libido. These shifts align with the winter season, embodying an essential time to hunker down and hibernate, rest, and replenish. When we tune in and listen to these cues, we preserve energy, replenish lost nutrients, and ultimately set ourselves up for a symptom-free cycle.

PILLARS OF EATING FOR YOUR MENSTRUAL PHASE

One of the very best ways to support your hormones during this time is with food! Nutrient repletion is critical now, as you're losing minerals due to blood loss (and you now know these nutrients are the very building blocks of hormones). The following foods and eating habits are deeply restorative and reflect our natural cravings and physiological needs during this phase.

Optimal Foods to Support Your Menstrual Phase

IRON-RICH FOODS (WITH AN EMPHASIS ON ANIMAL PROTEINS)

Because your body is undergoing an intense process of shedding the uterine lining, it's especially important to emphasize foods that are rich in iron, which is deeply restorative to the blood and kidneys, particularly heme iron from animal proteins, the most bioavailable form. **Optimal sources include:**

- Liver and other organ meats
- Grass-fed red meat (beef, bison, buffalo, lamb)
- Wild-caught fatty fish (sardines, salmon, tuna, mackerel, anchovies)
- Shellfish (oysters, clams, mussels, shrimp)
- Poultry
- Organic tofu (make sure it is organic and non-GMO and use sparingly)
- Legumes

PRO TIP: You can also cook food in a cast-iron pan, which may increase the iron of non-heme sources by up to 16 percent.[1]

VITAMIN C–RICH FOODS

Vitamin C helps your body dissolve and absorb iron, particularly from non-heme (plant-based) sources. It's also involved in suppressing inflammation and helps to offset oxidative stress. **Optimal sources include:**

- Cruciferous vegetables
- Bell peppers
- Leafy greens
- Parsley
- Papaya/guava
- Dark-colored berries
- Citrus

MINERAL-RICH FOODS

Minerals such as magnesium, zinc, calcium, and iron are essential to hormone production and function, and they can work to combat common menstrual phase symptoms such as cramping, headache, dizziness, fatigue, and inflammation. Because we excrete these minerals with our uterine lining, it's especially important to consume an abundance during this phase. **Optimal sources include:**

- Liver and other organ meats
- Red meat
- Bone broth
- Shellfish
- Sardines
- Dark leafy greens
- Sea vegetables (nori, dulse, kombu, kelp, seaweed)
- Nuts and seeds (particularly pumpkin, flaxseed, chestnuts, peanuts)
- Legumes (kidney and adzuki beans)
- Cruciferous vegetables
- Dark chocolate
- Sea salt

FOODS HIGH IN B VITAMINS

B vitamins—particularly B_6 (pyridoxine) and B_9 (folic acid)—support optimal progesterone production, which is crucial to reducing period pain and PMS prior to your period, as well as balancing blood sugar levels and thwarting energy dips and cravings. **Optimal sources include:**

- Liver and other organ meats
- Poultry
- Tuna
- Wild-caught salmon
- Kidney beans
- Buckwheat
- Wild rice
- Mushrooms
- Ricotta and cottage cheese

FOODS HIGH IN OMEGA-3 FATTY ACIDS

As you previously learned, these fatty acids are considered highly anti-inflammatory and can help lower prostaglandins associated with cramping and period pain. **Optimal sources include:**

- Wild-caught salmon
- White fish (cod, halibut, flounder)
- Oily fish (sardines, anchovies)
- Pasture-raised eggs
- Spirulina
- Walnuts
- Hemp seeds
- Chia seeds
- Flaxseed

ANTI-INFLAMMATORY HERBS AND SPICES

Herbs and spices have been used in traditional Chinese medicine for over 2,000 years, and are now clinically proven to help reduce cramping, nausea, bloating, fatigue, and headaches, as well as to boost immunity and digestion and promote cycle regularity. **Optimal herbs and spices to incorporate in your menstrual phase include:**

- Nettle
- Red raspberry leaf
- Ginger
- Turmeric
- Chamomile

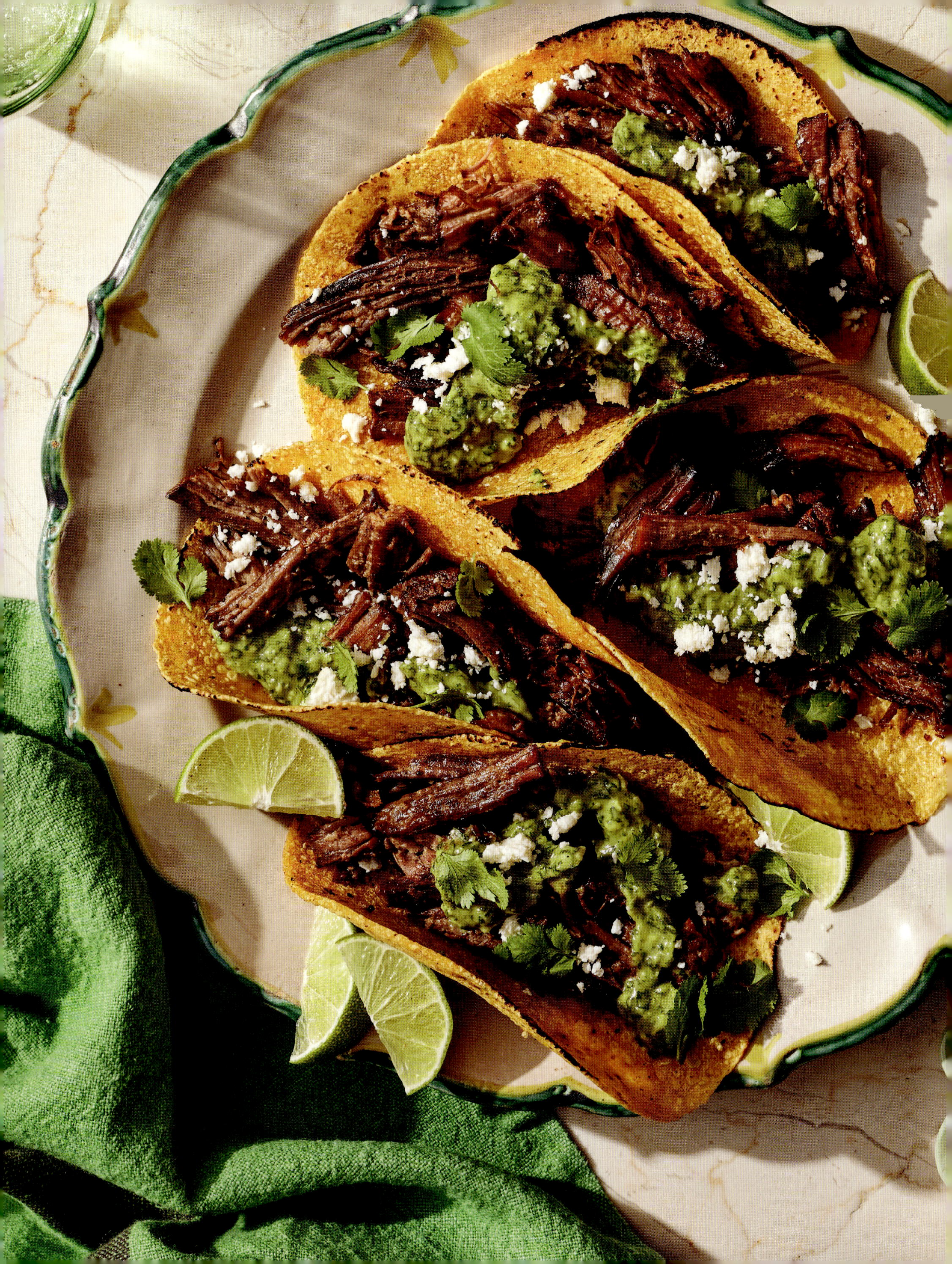

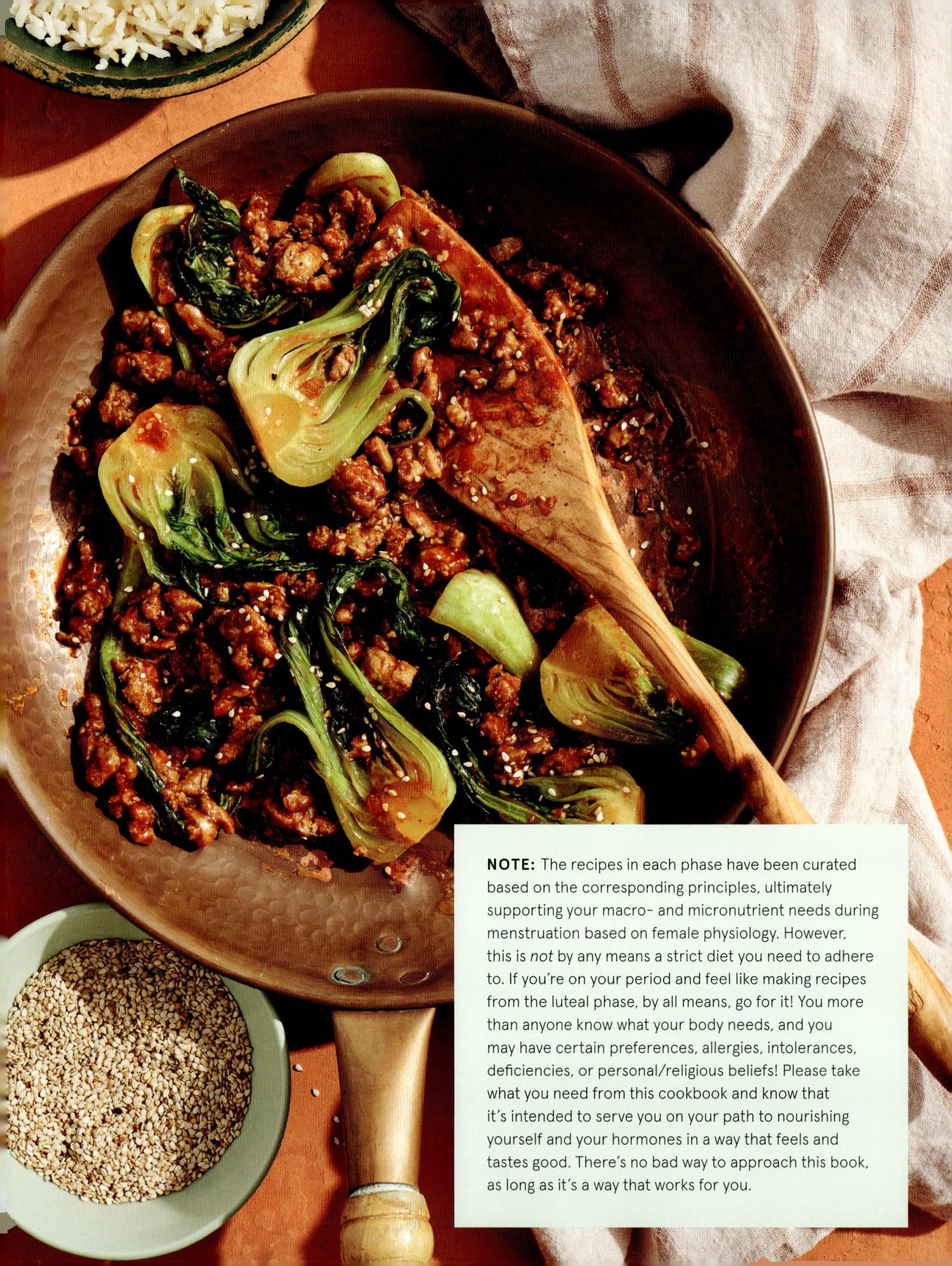

NOTE: The recipes in each phase have been curated based on the corresponding principles, ultimately supporting your macro- and micronutrient needs during menstruation based on female physiology. However, this is *not* by any means a strict diet you need to adhere to. If you're on your period and feel like making recipes from the luteal phase, by all means, go for it! You more than anyone know what your body needs, and you may have certain preferences, allergies, intolerances, deficiencies, or personal/religious beliefs! Please take what you need from this cookbook and know that it's intended to serve you on your path to nourishing yourself and your hormones in a way that feels and tastes good. There's no bad way to approach this book, as long as it's a way that works for you.

COOKING AND EATING TIPS TO SUPPORT YOUR MENSTRUAL PHASE

PRIORITIZE PROTEIN FROM ANIMAL SOURCES

I've said it before and I'll say it again: High-quality protein sourced from animals is one of the most bioavailable sources of the micronutrients and amino acids needed for functions vital to your hormones. Along with being building blocks that structurally make up hormones, amino acids assist in everything from protein synthesis and tissue repair to nutrient absorption and liver detoxification. They're also the most bioavailable sources of iron, which we need to replenish due to blood loss (even more so if dealing with heavy bleeding, which is often linked to anemia, or iron deficiency).

OPT FOR WARM, SLOW, AND WELL-COOKED FOODS

According to traditional Chinese medicine, your period is the coldest part of your cycle (think winter!) due to a slight drop in basal body temperature. Additionally, an increase in progesterone during your luteal phase (the phase right before your period) can restrict blood flow, leading to coldness in your extremities. Warm, well-cooked foods (think soups, stews, casseroles, slow cooker meals, etc.) will help to increase blood flow and circulation (which helps with cramping), often contain more nutrients (especially meat slow cooked on the bone), and are also considered easier to digest and extract nutrients from.

OPTIMIZE HYDRATION WITH SALT AND ELECTROLYTES

You know how important it is to drink water regularly, but to maintain proper fluid levels you'll want to also prioritize electrolytes and salt. These are essential minerals—sodium, potassium, chloride, calcium, and magnesium—that provide a myriad of functions we discussed on page 50. Low salt intake has been associated with a higher risk for PMS, most likely because it triggers the adrenal glands to release a hormone called aldosterone, which leads to fluid and sodium retention. If you experience fluid retention leading up to and during the first few days of your menstrual phase, it's likely you need to consume more salt, not less.

Recipe Icons

To help you with your planning and preparation of meals, for every recipe you'll find a group of icons representing different aspects of the recipe to help you quickly identify the ones that work within your dietary preferences and needs. They are:

GF = **GLUTEN-FREE**

DF = **DAIRY-FREE**

V = **VEGAN**

V = **VEGETARIAN**

P = **PALEO**
(encompassing grain-free, dairy-free, and refined-sugar-free ingredients; also noted in recipes with paleo-friendly options)

S = **STAPLE**
(something that I make often, usually due to the simplicity, flexibility, or timing of the recipe)

BF = **BUDGET-FRIENDLY**

Note: These icons appear if there are optional or alternative ingredients that are compliant with the label; i.e., a recipe may be labeled dairy-free if it includes Greek yogurt *and* a dairy-free alternative like coconut yogurt.

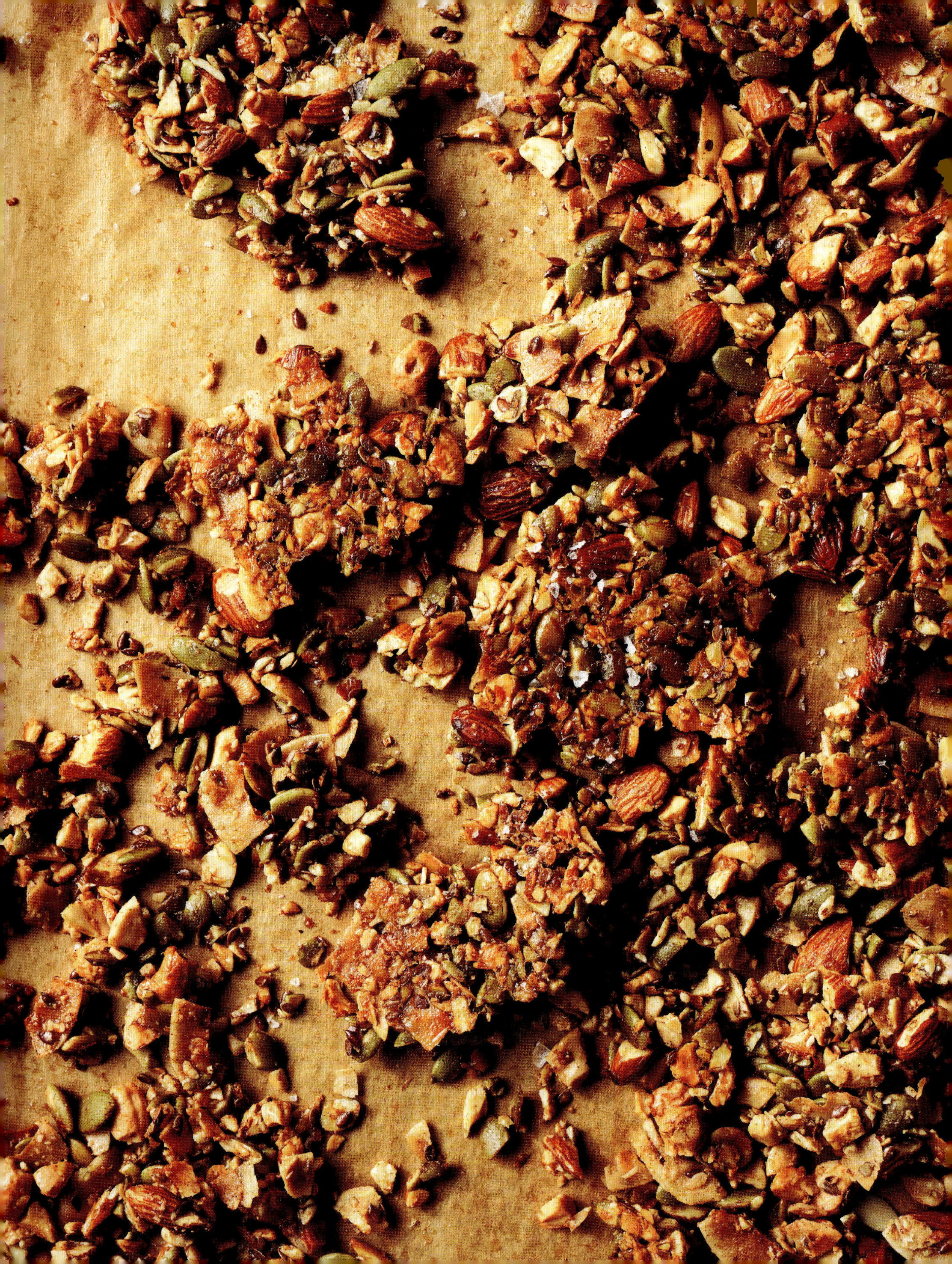

Seed-Cycle Maple Cinnamon Granola

PREP: 5 MINUTES COOK: 25 MINUTES SERVES 6–8

GF DF V P S BF

If there's one thing I make without fail *every. single. week,* it's this seed-cycle granola. It's crunchy, aromatic, and delicious—and the perfect topping for yogurt bowls, chia pudding, and even dessert. It's also functional, incorporating the growing trend of seed cycling, a way to support the female endocrine system through its hormone fluctuations by consuming different seeds during different phases of your cycle.

Theoretically, eating pumpkin seeds and flaxseeds rich in phytoestrogens during the first half of the menstrual cycle (the menstrual, follicular, and ovulatory phases) can help to balance estrogen levels, increasing or decreasing them as needed. This helps to regulate other hormones such as FSH, which is needed for ovulation to occur.

During the second half of your cycle (the luteal phase), a switch to incorporating sunflower and sesame seeds, which are rich in gamma-linolenic acids that work to support progesterone levels, will help to reduce inflammation and PMS.

While the evidence on seed cycling is largely anecdotal, there is plenty of science-backed research to support the benefits of consuming seeds regularly, so even if you decide to forgo seed cycling itself, you'll still sneak in plenty of nutrients with this granola recipe.

1 cup raw organic cashews

1 cup raw organic almonds, Brazil nuts, or pecans

1 cup raw organic pumpkin seeds (use sunflower seeds after ovulation/during luteal phase)

2 tablespoons flaxseeds (use sesame seeds after ovulation/during luteal phase)

1 cup unsweetened coconut flakes

1 heaping teaspoon cinnamon

½ teaspoon sea salt

2 heaping tablespoons unrefined organic coconut oil, melted

⅓ cup pure maple syrup

1 teaspoon pure vanilla extract

Flaky sea salt, for topping

1. Preheat the oven to 325°F and line a large baking pan with parchment paper.

2. Add all the nuts and seeds to a food processor and pulse several times to chop them into a crumbly texture (make sure not to overmix, as you want some larger chunks for clusters). Transfer to a medium mixing bowl and stir in the coconut flakes, cinnamon, and ½ teaspoon sea salt.

3. In a separate small bowl, whisk together the coconut oil, maple syrup, and vanilla until smooth. Pour this mixture over the dry ingredients and stir well until fully combined.

4. Spread the mixture in a single layer on the lined baking sheet (you want it to clump together to achieve those clusters). Bake for 12 to 15 minutes. Gently turn the granola over (keep it very gentle to ensure the clusters stay intact). Bake for another 12 to 15 minutes, until golden brown.

5. Let the granola cool at room temperature; it will crisp up as it cools. Sprinkle with flaky sea salt. Store in an airtight container at room temperature for up to 1 week.

MENSTRUAL PHASE BENEFITS

Rich in minerals • Anti-inflammatory

Upgraded Spinach-Feta Breakfast Wrap

PREP: 10 MINUTES COOK: 10 MINUTES MAKES 4 WRAPS (PESTO SERVES 6–8)

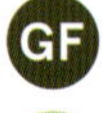
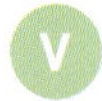

Back in my 20s, egg whites were all the rage, and every time I embarked on a Frappuccino run, I ordered a spinach and feta wrap and felt like: *health goals*. For this cookbook I decided it was time the wrap got a hormone-healthy upgrade, specifically by including the egg yolks, which contain anti-inflammatory omega-3 fatty acids that help to lower prostaglandins associated with cramping and period pain. I like to make a batch of wraps (four or six at a time) and freeze them, individually wrapped in foil, for quick reheat-and-go options. While the pesto adds loads of flavor, if you're looking to save time you can swap it out for 2 tablespoons chopped sun-dried tomatoes, adding them to the spinach to cook.

Sun-Dried Tomato Pesto

- **8 ounces organic sun-dried tomatoes, oil drained**
- **⅓ cup raw organic cashews**
- **½ cup fresh basil leaves**
- **2 tablespoons nutritional yeast**
- **1 teaspoon balsamic vinegar**
- **4 cloves garlic, minced**
- **½ teaspoon sea salt**
- **½ cup extra virgin olive oil**

Wrap

- **4 large gluten-free (such as brown rice or cassava flour) tortillas**
- **2 tablespoons grass-fed ghee or avocado oil**
- **4 cups organic spinach, roughly chopped**
- **8 large pasture-raised eggs plus 4 egg whites**
- **2 teaspoons garlic powder**
- **1 teaspoon sea salt**
- **½ cup crumbled feta cheese**
- **Avocado oil spray**

1. *For the sun-dried tomato pesto:* Combine all of the ingredients except the olive oil in a food processor. Cover with a lid and run the food processor while slowly drizzling the olive oil through the hole in the lid. Stop to scrape the sides with a spatula if needed, then let run until the pesto is creamy and smooth. Set aside.

2. Preheat the oven to 400°F.

3. *For the wraps:* Line a small baking sheet with parchment paper and lay the tortillas flat on the pan. Spread the sun-dried tomato pesto evenly over each tortilla and set aside.

4. Melt the ghee in a medium skillet over medium heat. Stir in the spinach and sauté until slightly wilted, 1 to 2 minutes.

5. Whisk together the eggs and egg whites in a medium bowl until well combined, then stir in the garlic powder and sea salt. Pour the mixture into the pan with the spinach and scramble for 4 to 5 minutes, until the eggs are gently cooked through.

6. Use a large spatula to transfer one-fourth of the egg mixture to the center of one tortilla and spread evenly. Sprinkle one-fourth of the feta cheese evenly over the eggs, then fold the right and left sides of the tortilla inward, 1 to 2 inches over the filling. Fold the bottom of the tortilla over the filling, then roll up, tucking as you roll. Continue rolling until the wrap is seam side down. Repeat to make four wraps. Spray the tortillas lightly with avocado oil. Bake the wraps for 5 to 10 minutes, flipping halfway through, until crispy and golden. Cut in half and enjoy.

NOTE: Any leftover sun-dried tomato pesto can be stored for up to 1 week in the fridge to use on toast, sandwiches, pasta, bowls, or scrambles.

MENSTRUAL PHASE BENEFITS

High in protein and amino acids • High in vitamin C • Anti-inflammatory

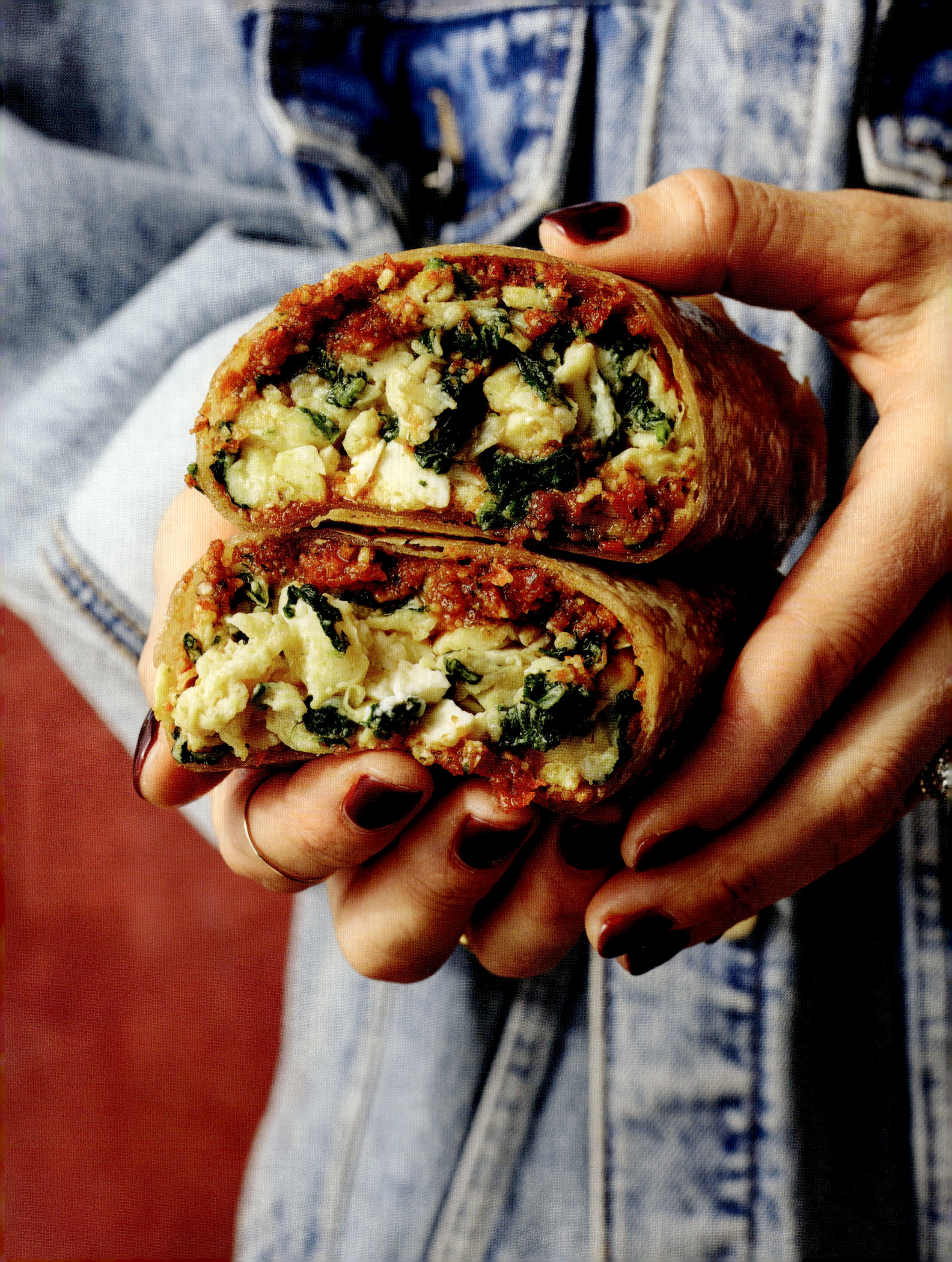

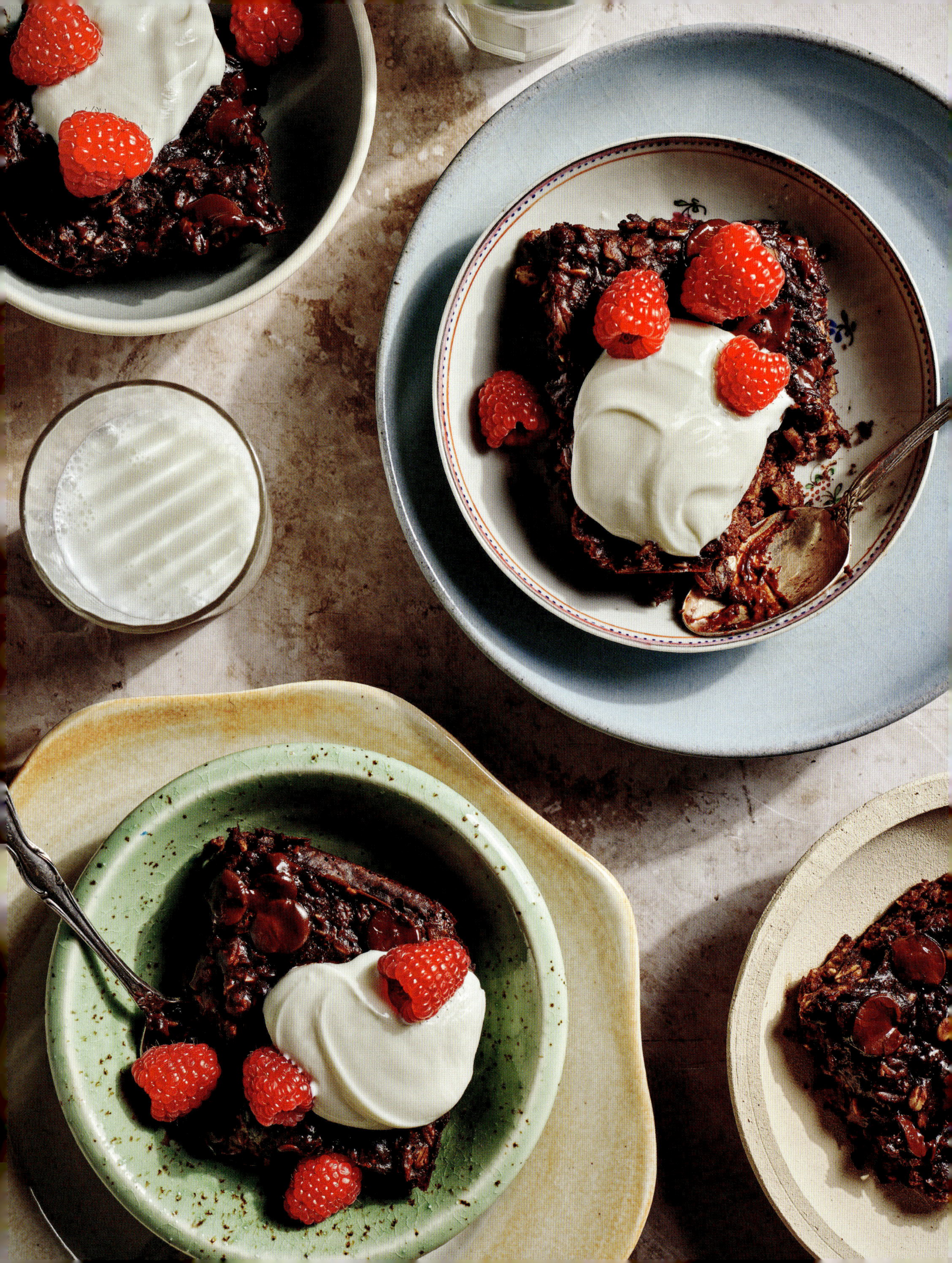

Brownie Batter Baked Oats

PREP: 10 MINUTES COOK: 35 MINUTES SERVES 6–8

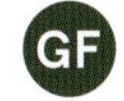

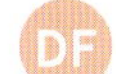

S

BF

I adore this recipe when I'm on my period as it's warm and cozy, sneaks in plenty of protein to keep my blood sugar stable, and makes almost a week's worth of breakfasts, meaning more rest and downtime during this energy-intensive phase! Studies suggest that eating between 40 and 120 grams of dark chocolate daily during your period may help reduce pain due to its high magnesium content, which is easy—and delicious—to do with this breakfast.

- **2 tablespoons flaxseeds plus 5 tablespoons warm water (or 2 eggs, whisked)**
- **2½ cups nondairy milk (I like unsweetened almond milk)**
- **½ cup pure maple syrup**
- **⅓ cup creamy nut butter**
- **1 teaspoon pure vanilla extract**
- **2 cups gluten-free oats**
- **1 cup cauliflower rice (or additional oats)**
- **½ cup dark chocolate chips, plus more for topping**
- **½ cup cacao powder**
- **1 teaspoon baking powder**
- **½ teaspoon sea salt**
- **1 teaspoon decaf instant espresso (can use regular if needed), optional**
- **2 to 4 servings collagen peptides (for a protein boost), optional**
- **Fresh berries, full-fat organic Greek yogurt, and maple syrup, for topping, optional**

1. Preheat the oven to 350°F and coat a 9 by 13-inch baking pan with avocado oil spray.

2. Whisk the flaxseeds and warm water together in a small bowl and let set for a few minutes until it gels, creating a binder. Combine the flaxseed mixture (or 2 whisked eggs), milk, maple syrup, nut butter, and vanilla in a large mixing bowl and mix well. Stir in the oats, cauliflower rice, chocolate chips, cacao powder, baking powder, salt, instant espresso (if using), and collagen peptides (if using). Pour into the prepared baking pan and top with more chocolate chips if desired.

3. Bake for 30 to 35 minutes, until the liquid has been absorbed. Let cool for a few minutes before serving.

4. Option to top with berries, yogurt, and/or a drizzle of maple syrup if you like.

NOTE: For a 30-gram protein power breakfast, don't skip the collagen peptides, use protein oats, and serve with full-fat, organic Greek yogurt.

MENSTRUAL PHASE BENEFITS

Rich in magnesium • High in B vitamins • Slow cooked for maximum nutrient absorption and digestion

Creamy Buckwheat Porridge + Blackberry Chia Compote

PREP: 2 MINUTES COOK: 10 MINUTES SERVES 2

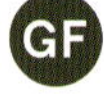

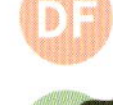

While I was growing up, Cream of Wheat was a breakfast staple in our household, and I loved the way my mom prepared it—piping hot, thick and creamy, and swirled with melted butter and sweet brown sugar. I wanted to re-create this nostalgic dish but include plenty of nutrients to elevate both the health and flavor factors. This buckwheat version contains much more protein and fiber than the original, along with plenty of B vitamins to keep energy stable and antioxidants to fight inflammation and reduce pain or cramping.

Blackberry Chia Compote

- **1 cup organic blackberries, rinsed**
- **2 tablespoons water**
- **1 to 2 tablespoons pure maple syrup**
- **2 tablespoons chia seeds**

Creamy Buckwheat Porridge

- **1 (13.5-ounce) can full-fat unsweetened coconut milk (or 1½ cups other nondairy milk of choice)**
- **¼ teaspoon sea salt**
- **½ cup dry buckwheat cereal**
- **2 tablespoons pure maple syrup, plus more for topping**
- **1 teaspoon pure vanilla extract**
- **1 teaspoon cinnamon**
- **1 to 2 servings protein powder or collagen peptides (optional)**
- **Grass-fed ghee or vegan butter, for topping**
- **Creamy nut butter, coconut flakes, or chopped nuts and seeds, for topping (optional but delicious)**

1. *For the compote:* Combine the blackberries, water, and maple syrup in a small pot and bring to a boil, using a large spoon to mash the berries. Reduce to a simmer and cook, continuously stirring and mashing the berries, for 10 minutes, until the mixture has a thick, jam-like consistency. Remove from the heat and stir in the chia seeds. Let sit until ready to use.

2. *For the porridge:* While the compote is cooking, combine the coconut milk and salt in another small pot and bring to a boil. Stir in the buckwheat cereal, maple syrup, vanilla extract, and cinnamon and reduce to a simmer. Cook, stirring frequently, for 5 to 10 minutes, until the cereal is thick and creamy. Remove from the heat. If using, stir in the protein powder or collagen peptides.

3. Divide the cereal between two large bowls and top with the compote and ghee or vegan butter. If you like, add nut butter, more maple syrup, and any other toppings of choice.

NOTE: The porridge comes together quickly and is best served immediately, but the chia compote makes a large portion that will keep in the fridge for a week. It's great with yogurt bowls, oatmeal, and chia pudding.

MENSTRUAL PHASE BENEFITS

Anti-inflammatory • High in B vitamins • Slow cooked for maximum nutrient absorption and digestion

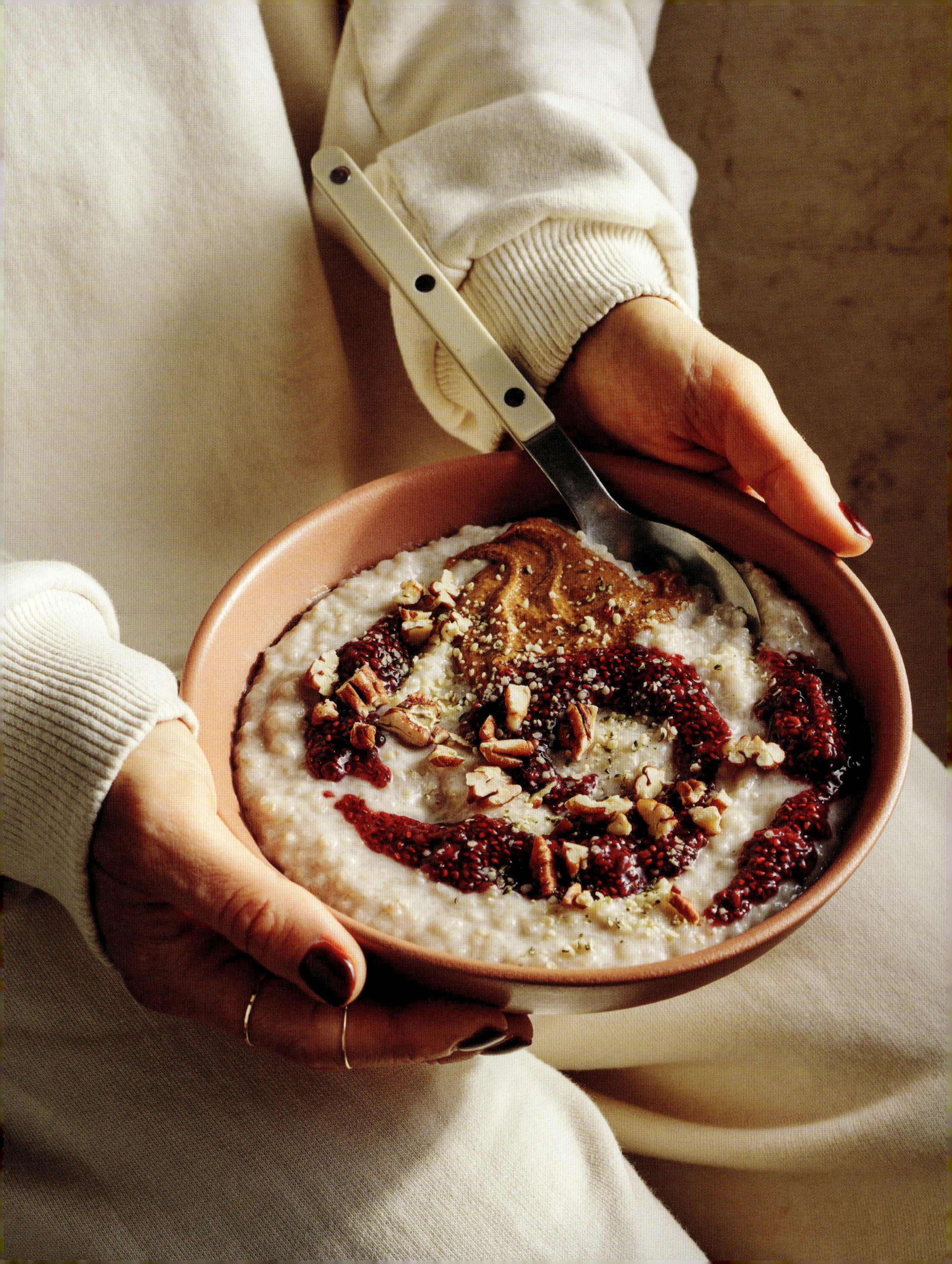

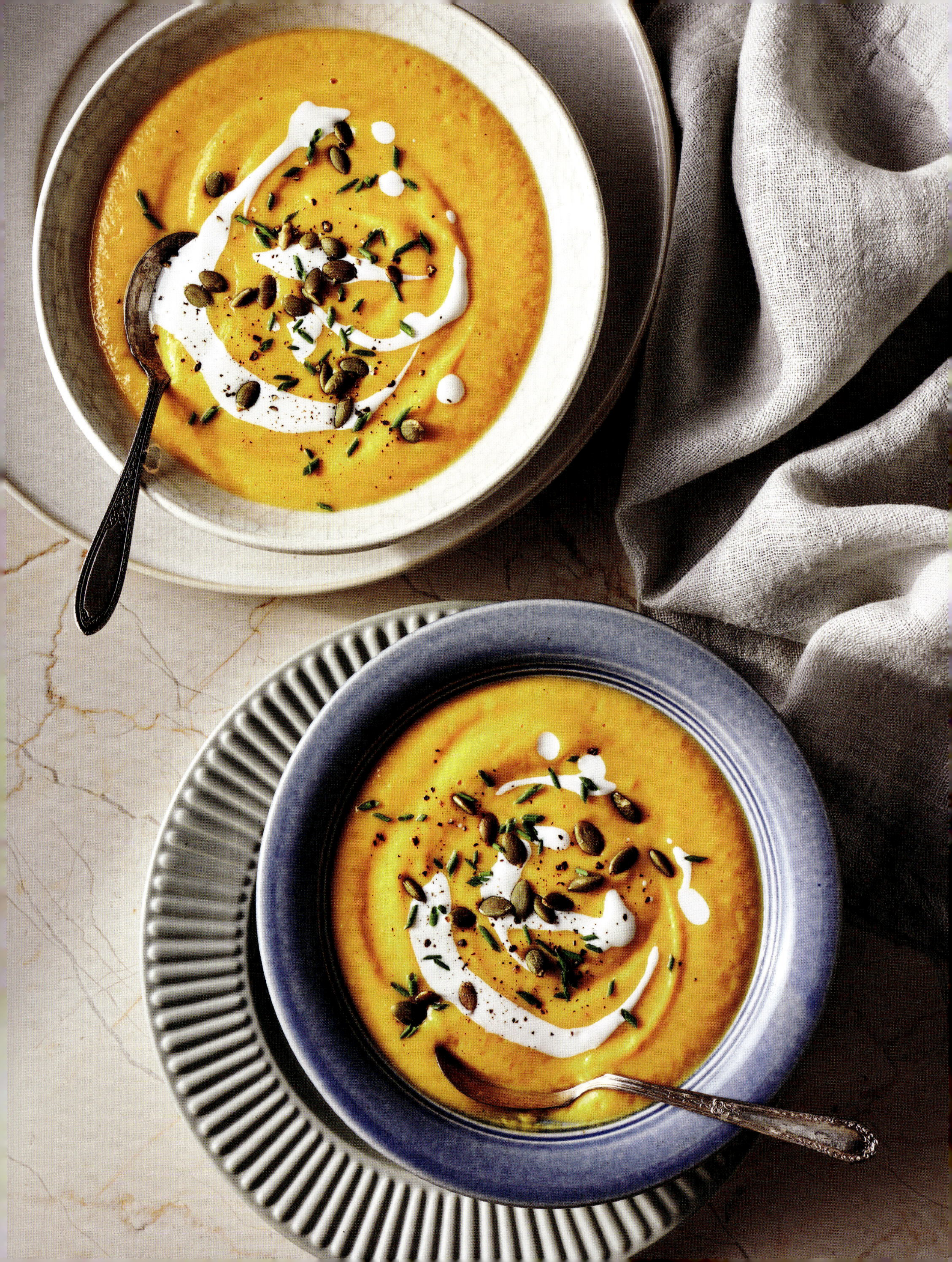

Creamy Roasted-Squash Blender Soup

PREP: 10 MINUTES COOK: 45 MINUTES SERVES 4

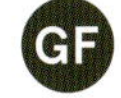

BF

This soup is the GOAT of easy soups, especially when you don't feel like peeling or chopping a ton of vegetables. Instead, all you have to do is roast squash halves on a sheet pan with most of the other ingredients, which creates layers of depth and flavor, then add it all to a blender and—voilà!—you get the creamiest, coziest bowl of soup. I like to use bone broth and add unflavored collagen peptides for a boost of protein and amino acids.

- **2 medium kabocha squash (also known as Japanese pumpkins), 1 large butternut squash, or 4 small acorn squash**
- **4 tablespoons avocado oil, divided**
- **1½ teaspoons sea salt, divided**
- **1 sweet onion, cut into large chunks**
- **4 to 6 whole garlic cloves, peeled**
- **1 (8-ounce) block feta cheese, crumbled**
- **¼ cup minced fresh thyme or 2 teaspoons dried thyme**
- **Black pepper to taste**
- **4 cups bone broth (try using the Super Simple Homemade Bone Broth on page 109)**
- **2 tablespoons raw honey or pure maple syrup**
- **2 to 4 servings collagen peptides (optional)**
- **Coconut cream or yogurt, minced fresh chives, and toasted pepitas, for topping (optional)**

1. Preheat the oven to 400°F and line a large baking sheet with parchment paper.

2. Halve the squash lengthwise and scoop out and discard the seeds. Drizzle the flesh (inside) of the squash with 2 tablespoons of the avocado oil and sprinkle with ¼ teaspoon of the salt. Place the squash cut side down on the lined pan, then place the onion pieces, garlic cloves, and feta around the squash. Drizzle everything with the remaining 2 tablespoons avocado oil and sprinkle with the thyme, remaining 1¼ teaspoons salt, and pepper to taste. Roast for about 45 minutes, or until the onion and feta are golden brown and the squash is cooked through. Let cool slightly.

3. Pour the bone broth into a high-speed blender and add the roasted onion, garlic cloves, and feta. Scoop out all of the cooked flesh of the squash and add to the blender. Drizzle in the honey and collagen peptides (if using), then blend, starting slow and increasing in speed until the soup is creamy and well mixed. (If you don't have a high-speed blender, you can use an immersion blender by transferring the ingredients to a large pot or bowl and blending.) If you like, top with yogurt, fresh chives, and toasted pepitas.

NOTE: If you're unable to digest dairy well, omit the feta, then swap out 1 cup of the bone broth for coconut cream to attain that extra velvety texture.

MENSTRUAL PHASE BENEFITS

High in vitamin C • Anti-inflammatory • Abundant in collagen, gelatin, and amino acids

Cream of Mushroom, Chicken, and Wild Rice Soup

PREP: 10 MINUTES   COOK: 1 HOUR, OR 6–8 HOURS IN A SLOW COOKER   SERVES 6

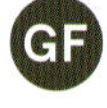

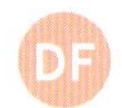

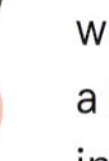

Nostalgic and comforting, this soup will give you all the fuzzy feels, not to mention plenty of vitamins (B and D) that work to replenish red blood cells and boost immunity, and antioxidants that fight off oxidative stress. I love making a big pot on day 1 of my period, then reheating leftovers throughout the week for quick and nourishing meals. I've included both stovetop and slow cooker options depending on your preference!

- **2 tablespoons grass-fed ghee or avocado oil**
- **1½ pounds organic boneless, skinless chicken thighs, rinsed and patted dry (you can substitute chicken breasts)**
- **2 teaspoons sea salt, divided**
- **Black pepper to taste**
- **1 small yellow onion, diced**
- **2 large stalks celery, diced**
- **2 large carrots, peeled and diced**
- **2 cups white mushrooms, sliced**
- **4 cloves garlic, minced**
- **1 cup organic wild rice, rinsed**
- **3 bay leaves**
- **9 sprigs fresh thyme or 1½ teaspoons dried thyme**
- **6 cups chicken bone broth (try using Super Simple Homemade Bone Broth on page 109)**
- **1 (13.5-ounce) can full-fat unsweetened coconut milk**
- **1 tablespoon arrowroot starch**
- **Grated Parmesan for topping (optional)**

TO MAKE ON THE STOVETOP

1. Melt the ghee or avocado oil in a large pot or Dutch oven over medium-high heat. Use tongs to add the chicken to the pot and sprinkle with 1 teaspoon of the salt and black pepper to taste. Sear both sides of the chicken until browned, 3 to 4 minutes per side. Remove the chicken from the pan with tongs and set aside on a plate.

2. Reduce the heat to medium and add the onion, celery, carrots, and mushrooms to the pan and sauté for 3 to 4 minutes, until softened. Stir in the garlic and remaining 1 teaspoon salt and sauté for another minute, until fragrant. Stir in the chicken, wild rice, bay leaves, thyme, and bone broth and bring to a boil. Reduce the heat to low and simmer for 45 minutes, until the rice is completely cooked and tender.

3. Transfer the chicken with tongs to a medium bowl and shred with two forks. Fish out the bay leaves and thyme sprigs and discard. Stir the chicken back into the pot.

4. Mix the coconut milk with the arrowroot starch to create a slurry (this will thicken the soup and give it that extra creamy texture). Stir the slurry into the soup and simmer for 5 to 10 more minutes, until thickened and creamy. Remove from the heat and let cool for a few minutes before serving. Top with Parmesan if desired.

TO MAKE IN THE SLOW COOKER

5. Omit the ghee or avocado oil. Add the chicken, onion, celery, carrots, salt, pepper, garlic, wild rice, bay leaves, thyme, and bone broth to the slow cooker. Cover and cook on low for 6 to 8 hours, adding the mushrooms during the last 30 minutes of cooking.

6. Transfer the chicken with tongs to a medium bowl and shred with two forks. Fish out the bay leaves and thyme sprigs and discard. Return the meat to the soup.

7. Mix the coconut milk with the arrowroot starch to create a slurry (this will thicken the soup and give it that extra creamy texture). Stir the slurry into the soup and cook for 5 to 10 minutes, until thickened and creamy. Top with Parmesan if desired.

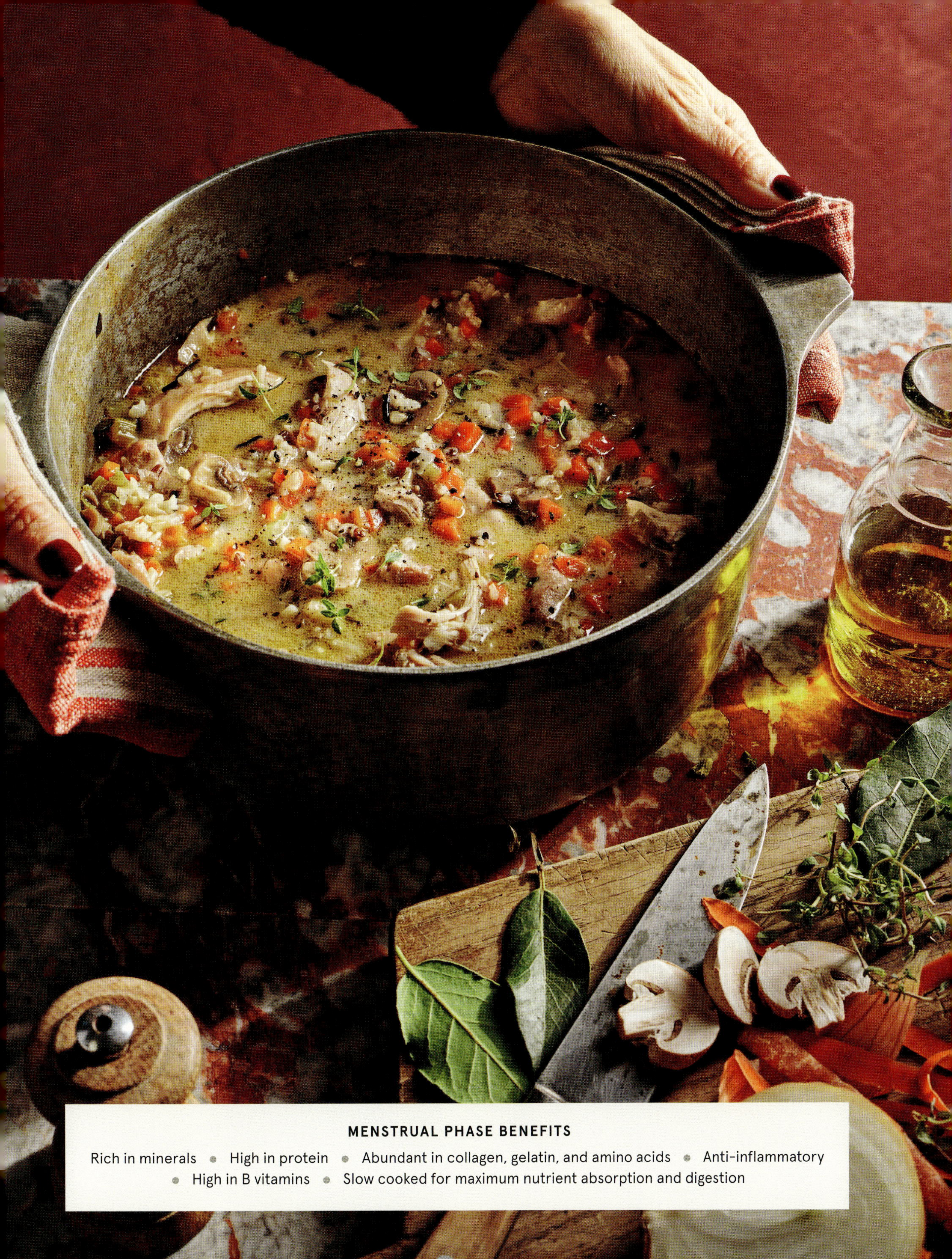

MENSTRUAL PHASE BENEFITS

Rich in minerals • High in protein • Abundant in collagen, gelatin, and amino acids • Anti-inflammatory • High in B vitamins • Slow cooked for maximum nutrient absorption and digestion

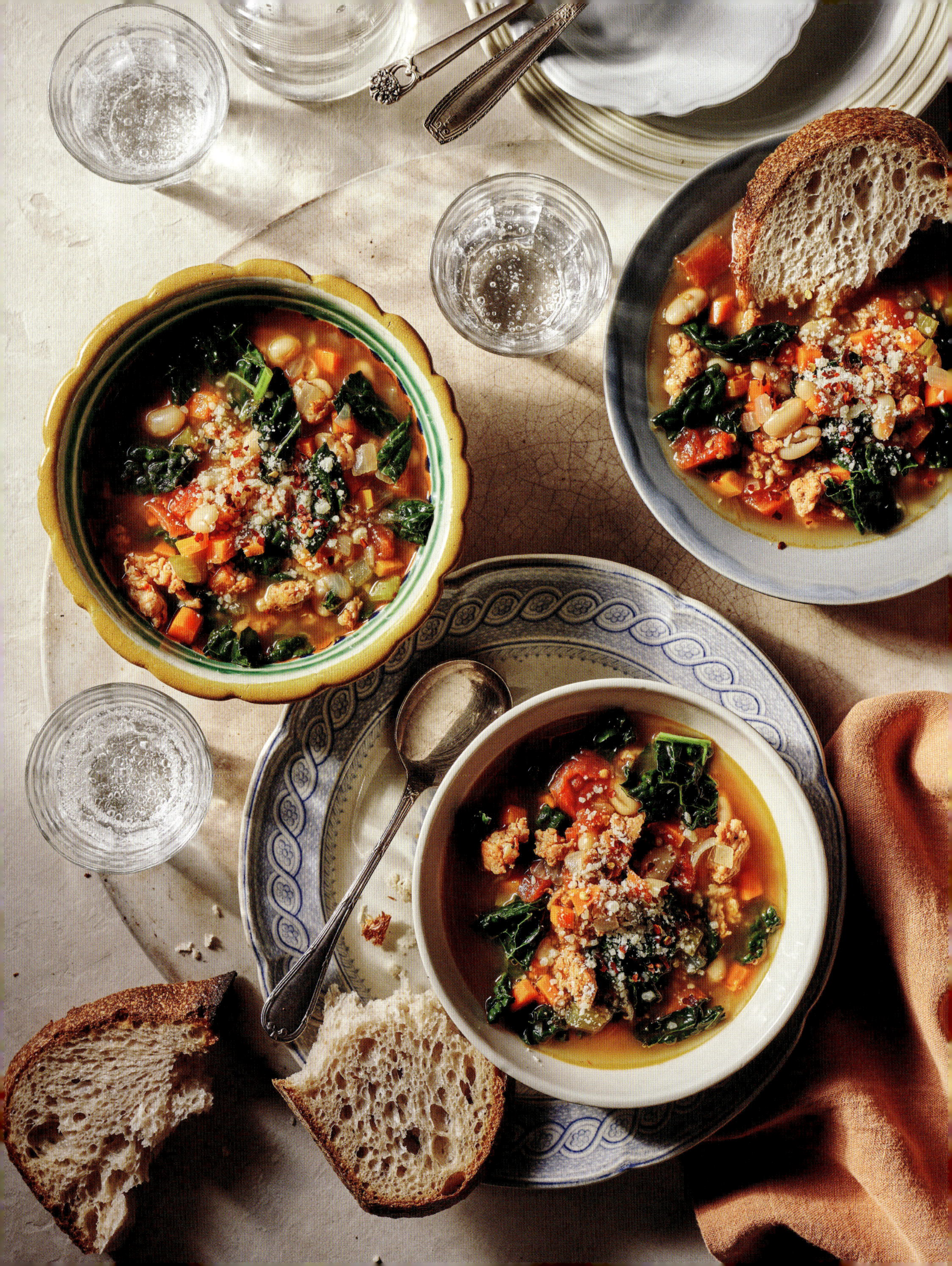

Hearty Tuscan Kale and White Bean Soup

PREP: 15 MINUTES COOK: 30 MINUTES SERVES 4–6

This is the soup I make whenever I'm feeling a little bit under the weather, kind of like a chicken noodle soup, but *more* flavorful and loaded with immunity-boosting ingredients like garlic, bone broth, carrots, parsley, and kale. I love it as a preemptive measure during the menstrual phase, when our immune system downshifts and we're more susceptible to catching a cold.

GF

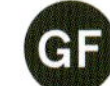

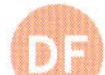

- 2 tablespoons avocado oil or grass-fed ghee
- 1 pound organic Italian chicken sausage, casings removed
- 1 yellow onion, diced
- 2 or 3 large carrots, peeled and diced (1 cup)
- 2 celery stalks, diced
- 4 cloves garlic, minced
- 1½ teaspoons sea salt, plus more to taste
- Black pepper to taste
- ¼ cup white wine (optional; the alcohol burns off with cooking)
- 1 (15-ounce) can diced tomatoes
- 6 cups bone broth (try using the Super Simple Homemade Bone Broth on page 109)
- 1 (15-ounce) can cannellini beans, rinsed and drained
- 1 bunch lacinato kale, stems removed, leaves rinsed and chopped
- ½ cup chopped fresh flat-leaf parsley
- Shaved Parmesan or pecorino and red chile flakes, for serving (optional)

1. Heat the avocado oil or ghee in a large pot over medium heat. Add the sausage and cook, breaking it into small pieces with a spatula, until browned, 3 to 5 minutes. Add the onion, carrots, and celery and sauté for 5 minutes, until the veggies are soft. Stir in the garlic, salt, and pepper and sauté for another minute. If using the wine, stir it in to deglaze the pot. Add the tomatoes and bone broth, cover the pot, and bring to a boil. Reduce the heat and simmer for 20 minutes, until the veggies are cooked through.

2. Stir in the beans and kale and simmer for another 5 minutes, until the kale is wilted. Add the parsley, then remove the soup from the heat. Season with additional salt and pepper to taste and serve with Parmesan or pecorino and red chile flakes if you like.

MENSTRUAL PHASE BENEFITS

Rich in iron and minerals • High in protein • Abundant in collagen, gelatin, and amino acids • High in vitamin C • High in B vitamins

Spicy Kimchi Fried Rice

PREP: 15 MINUTES, PLUS OVERNIGHT COOK: 15 MINUTES SERVES 4

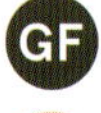
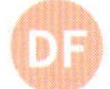
BF

This recipe is such a great way to dip your toes into kimchi, which is fermented cabbage that has loads of flavor and probiotics to help your gut metabolize excess estrogen. Topping the kimchi fried rice with nori helps to replenish and remineralize your body with key nutrients like iodine, zinc, and iron. This is another tasty leftovers-for-breakfast option, especially when topped with a yolky fried egg.

1½ cups jasmine rice, rinsed in cold water three times and drained

2 cups bone broth

1 cup kimchi, chopped, juices drained and reserved

1 to 2 tablespoons gluten-free gochujang paste (depending on spice tolerance)

2 tablespoons coconut aminos or other gluten-free soy sauce

1 tablespoon fish sauce

1 teaspoon sesame oil

4 strips uncured bacon, diced

3 tablespoons avocado oil, divided

4 green onions, diced

1 cup frozen organic peas

1 cup shelled cooked edamame

Sea salt and pepper to taste

4 to 8 pasture-raised eggs

1 sheet of nori, folded into quarters and thinly sliced

Sesame seeds, sriracha, and diced green onions, for topping (optional)

1. *At least 1 day prior, make the rice (this is important for texture; see Notes):* Cook the rice according to package instructions, using the bone broth for the liquid. Let cool for 30 minutes, then store in an airtight container in the fridge until ready to use, or up to 3 days.

2. Whisk together the juice from the kimchi with the gochujang, coconut aminos, fish sauce, and sesame oil in a small bowl and set aside.

3. Heat a large wok or skillet over medium-high heat. Add the diced bacon and stir-fry until brown and crispy, 4 to 5 minutes. Use a slotted spoon to transfer the bacon to a paper towel–lined plate to absorb excess grease and set aside.

4. Add 1 tablespoon of the avocado oil to the pan with the bacon grease. Stir in the drained kimchi and green onions and cook until the kimchi begins to caramelize, 4 to 5 minutes. Transfer the mixture to the plate with the bacon and set aside.

5. Add 1 tablespoon of the avocado oil to the skillet and stir in the rice, using a spatula to break up any clumps. Cook until warmed through and beginning to toast, 3 to 4 minutes. Stir in the cooked bacon, kimchi, and green onions. Drizzle the kimchi juice mixture over the top and mix well to combine. Add the green peas and cooked edamame and season with salt and pepper to taste. When the fried rice is well mixed and seasoned, cook undisturbed over medium-high heat for 1 to 2 minutes, which will create a delicious crispy crust. Remove from the heat and set aside.

6. In another skillet, heat the remaining 1 tablespoon avocado oil over medium-high heat. Add as many eggs as you prefer and cook sunny side up until the whites are opaque and the yolk is still runny.

7. Scoop the kimchi rice into large bowls and top with a fried egg or two. Garnish with the sliced nori along with sesame seeds, sriracha, and green onions if you like.

NOTES: I recommend using jasmine rice, which isn't too sticky and holds its shape well. You want to cook the rice at least one day in advance so it will stale a bit to develop some crunch, otherwise it will get mushy when cooked. Or, if you know you'll be ordering some takeout prior, purchase an extra carton of rice to save cooking time.

MENSTRUAL PHASE BENEFITS

Rich in iron and minerals • Abundant in amino acids • High in B vitamins

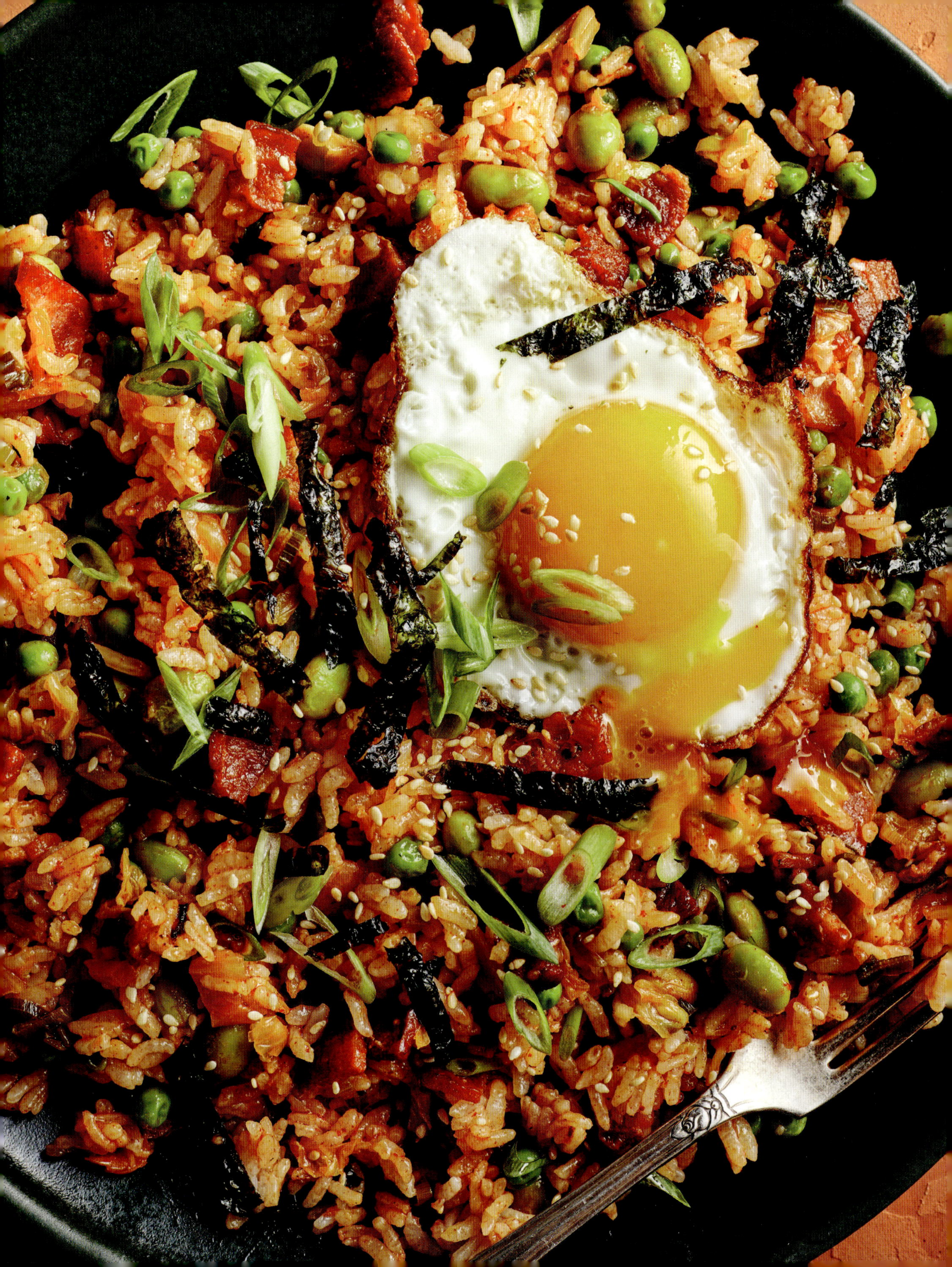

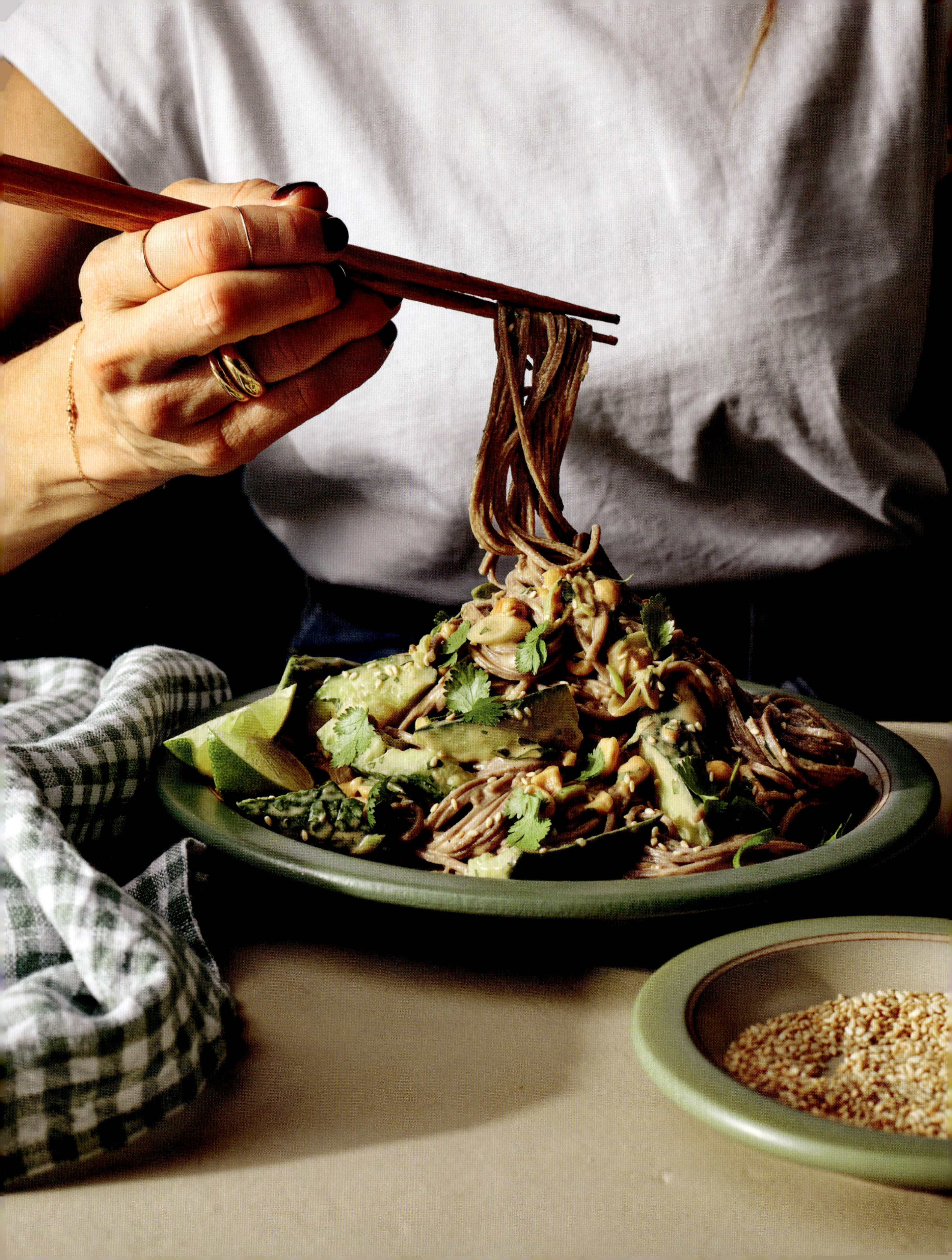

Saucy Peanut Noodles + Smashed Cucumbers

PREP: 10 MINUTES COOK: 10 MINUTES SERVES 4

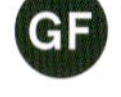
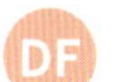

This recipe was literally one of the only meals (i.e., not crackers or cereal) I could stomach during my first trimester with my third baby girl, Frankie. I would eat it cold, and felt comfort in knowing it contained a vegetable, as well as some protein and fiber from the buckwheat noodles and peanut sauce. While I wasn't having a cycle at the time of recipe conception, I now enjoy this one during menstruation, as the buckwheat noodles are loaded with vitamins, minerals, and antioxidants that can prevent the formation of blood clots and reduce inflammation, while the hydrating cucumbers mitigate bloat.

Creamy Peanut Sauce

- **¾ cup unsweetened creamy organic peanut butter**
- **⅓ cup coconut aminos**
- **¼ cup full-fat canned coconut milk (or water)**
- **¼ cup rice vinegar**
- **3 tablespoons pure maple syrup**
- **2 teaspoons minced fresh ginger**
- **2 cloves garlic, minced**
- **1 teaspoon sriracha, plus more depending on spice preference**

Noodles

- **1 (8-ounce) package organic 100 percent buckwheat soba noodles (the package should list only one ingredient!)**
- **2 organic English cucumbers, rinsed and patted dry**
- **¼ cup chopped cilantro leaves**
- **3 green onions, white and green parts, thinly sliced on a bias**
- **¼ cup crushed peanuts**
- **Sesame seeds, lime wedges, and chili oil, for serving (optional)**

1. Bring a large pot of water to a boil.

2. *For the peanut sauce:* While you wait for the water to boil, combine all the peanut sauce ingredients in a high-speed blender and pulse until creamy and smooth. Set aside.

3. *For the noodles:* Add the noodles to the boiling water and give them a quick stir, making sure all the noodles are submerged. Let the water return to a boil, then reduce the heat to a simmer and cook according to package instructions, typically 5 to 8 minutes, until the noodles are fully cooked. While the noodles are cooking, fill a large bowl with cold water and set aside. You'll use this once the noodles have finished cooking.

4. To smash the cucumbers, lay a large knife flat against one cucumber and smash it with firm pressure using your other hand (like you would a garlic clove). The cucumber should crack open into four sections. Repeat along the full length of the cucumber. Once it's completely cracked into four long pieces, cut at a 45-degree angle into bite-size pieces. Repeat with the second cucumber and set aside.

5. Drain the noodles, then dump into the bowl of cold water. Use your hands to rub the noodles, washing off excess starch. (This prevents the noodles from turning into a gummy blob. If you want to serve warm, see Note.)

6. Drain the noodles again, and toss in a large bowl with the peanut sauce. Stir in the smashed cucumbers, cilantro, green onions, and peanuts. If desired, top with sesame seeds and serve immediately with lime wedges and chili oil.

NOTE: During my period I almost always like to heat the noodles back up in a bowl of hot water to serve warm. However, if I make these at a different phase, such as follicular or ovulatory, I prefer to leave them chilled.

MENSTRUAL PHASE BENEFITS

Anti-inflammatory • Rich in minerals

White Beans + Tinned Fish on Toast

PREP: 10 MINUTES   COOK: NONE   SERVES 4

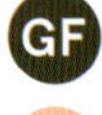

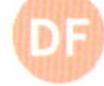

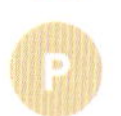

BF

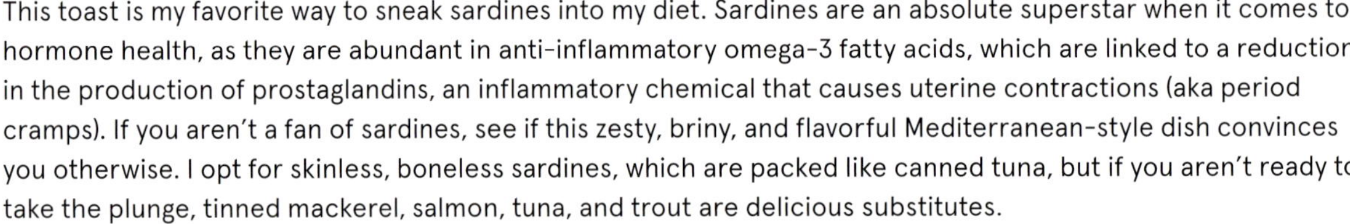

This toast is my favorite way to sneak sardines into my diet. Sardines are an absolute superstar when it comes to hormone health, as they are abundant in anti-inflammatory omega-3 fatty acids, which are linked to a reduction in the production of prostaglandins, an inflammatory chemical that causes uterine contractions (aka period cramps). If you aren't a fan of sardines, see if this zesty, briny, and flavorful Mediterranean-style dish convinces you otherwise. I opt for skinless, boneless sardines, which are packed like canned tuna, but if you aren't ready to take the plunge, tinned mackerel, salmon, tuna, and trout are delicious substitutes.

- 2 tablespoons extra virgin olive oil
- 2 tablespoons fresh lemon juice
- 1 teaspoon Dijon mustard
- 1 teaspoon sea salt
- Black pepper to taste
- 2 (4-ounce) cans wild-caught boneless, skinless sardines (packed in extra virgin olive oil), drained and smashed into bite-size chunks with a fork
- 1 (15-ounce) can organic cannellini beans, rinsed and drained
- ½ cup halved pitted Castelvetrano olives (or use kalamata)
- ⅓ cup oil-packed sun-dried tomatoes, chopped
- ⅓ cup finely minced flat-leaf parsley
- ¼ cup minced red onion
- Toasted gluten-free sourdough, extra virgin olive oil, microgreens, and flaky sea salt, for serving

1. To make the dressing, whisk together the olive oil, lemon juice, mustard, salt, and pepper in a small bowl.

2. Combine the sardines and beans in a medium mixing bowl. Add the olives, sun-dried tomatoes, parsley, and red onion. Drizzle the dressing over the top and stir everything together. Let sit while you prepare the toast.

3. Scoop a generous portion of the sardine mixture on top of each piece of toast and top with olive oil, microgreens, and flaky sea salt.

NOTE: This is a great meal prep option for lunch throughout the week as the sardine mixture will hold for 2 to 3 days in the fridge. I love it with toast, but it's also tasty in lettuce wraps or as a spread for gluten-free crackers.

MENSTRUAL PHASE BENEFITS

Anti-inflammatory • High in B vitamins • Rich in minerals • High in protein

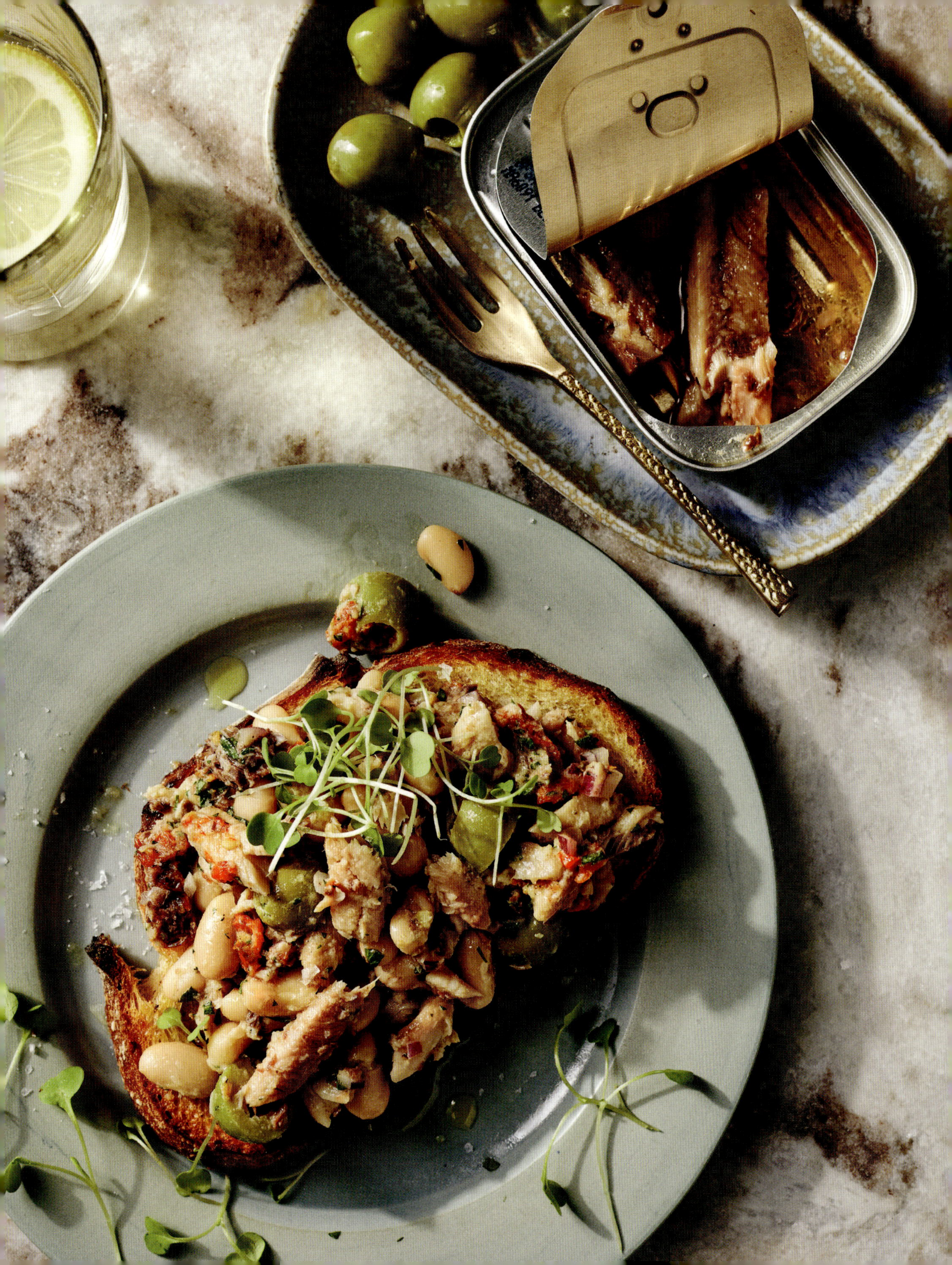

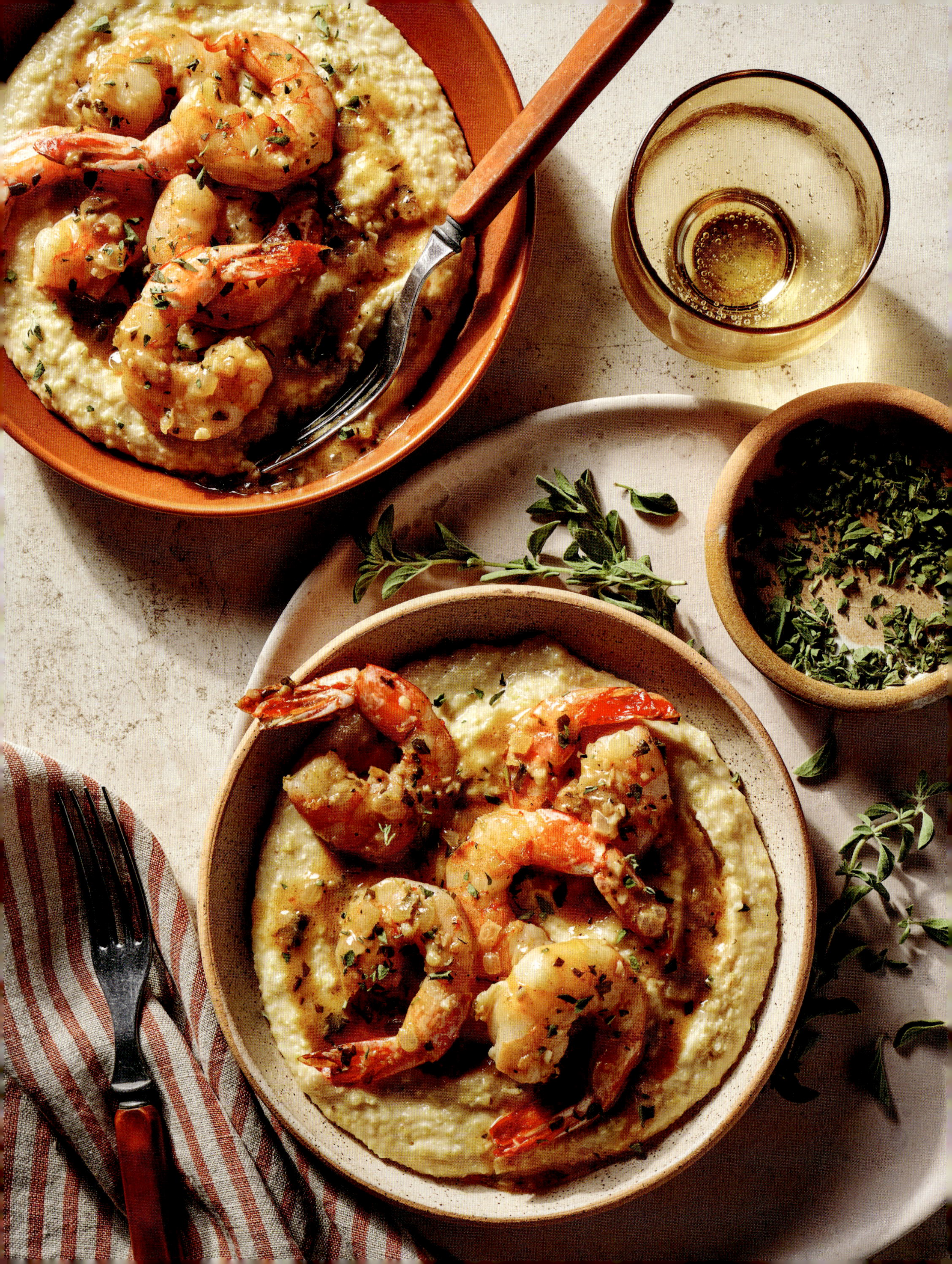

Cajun-Spiced Shrimp + Creamy Polenta

PREP: 5 MINUTES COOK: 25 MINUTES SERVES 4

GF
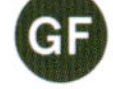

This meal tastes restaurant-worthy but comes together surprisingly quickly—making it a great weeknight dinner option. It's also rich in protein, B vitamins, minerals, omega-3 fatty acids, and vitamin D, which work to reduce inflammation and cramping, replenish lost nutrients, and promote optimal blood flow and circulation. Serving the shrimp over creamy polenta feels cozy, and adds some complex carbohydrates to stabilize your serotonin level and mood. **PRO TIP:** Cook the shrimp in a cast-iron skillet to naturally increase the iron content.

Creamy Polenta

- **2 cups bone broth**
- **2 cups unsweetened nondairy milk such as almond or cashew (or use more bone broth)**
- **1 cup polenta**

Cajun-Spiced Shrimp

- **2 tablespoons avocado oil**
- **1½ pounds wild-caught Argentinian or Patagonian Pink shrimp, peeled, deveined, and patted dry**
- **¼ cup grass-fed ghee, butter, or vegan butter**
- **½ yellow onion, diced**
- **4 cloves garlic, minced**
- **2 tablespoons chopped fresh oregano, plus more for topping**
- **1 heaping tablespoon Cajun seasoning**
- **½ teaspoon sea salt**
- **Black pepper to taste**
- **1 cup bone broth**
- **½ cup full-fat canned coconut milk**
- **Juice of ½ lemon**

To Serve

- **2 to 4 tablespoons grass-fed ghee, butter, or vegan butter**
- **1 teaspoon sea salt**
- **½ cup grated Parmesan, plus more for topping (optional)**

1. *For the polenta:* Combine the broth and milk in a medium pot and bring to a boil. Gently whisk in the polenta, cover the pot, and turn the heat to low. Simmer, stirring every few minutes, for 15 to 20 minutes, until the mixture pulls away from the sides of the pot and has a creamy, tender texture.

2. *For the shrimp:* Heat the avocado oil in a large cast-iron or steel skillet over medium-high heat. Add the shrimp in an even layer and cook, turning once, until just turning golden, about 1 minute per side. The shrimp should not be completely cooked through, as they will finish cooking in the sauce. Remove from the pan and set aside.

3. Add the ghee or butter to the same skillet and reduce the heat to medium. When the ghee has melted, add the onion and garlic and cook, stirring occasionally, until the onion is cooked through, 3 to 4 minutes. Add the oregano, Cajun seasoning, salt, and pepper and stir until fragrant, about 1 minute. Pour in the bone broth, coconut milk, and lemon juice and stir, bringing the mixture to a boil. Reduce to a simmer and let the mixture cook until reduced by about half, another 3 to 4 minutes.

4. Return the seared shrimp to the pan, stir well, and cook for another 2 to 3 minutes, until the shrimp are completely cooked through (registering an internal temperature of 145°F). Remove from the heat and set aside.

5. *To serve:* When the polenta is finished cooking, immediately remove from the heat and stir in the ghee or butter, salt, and Parmesan.

6. Scoop generous portions of polenta into wide, shallow bowls, then top with generous portions of the shrimp and creamy sauce. Option to garnish with more fresh herbs like oregano and Parmesan.

MENSTRUAL PHASE BENEFITS

Rich in iron and minerals • High in protein • Anti-inflammatory • High in B vitamins

Maple-Rosemary Roast Chicken + Buttery Mashed Potatoes

PREP: 10 MINUTES COOK: 1 HOUR 20 MINUTES SERVES 4–6

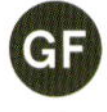

DF
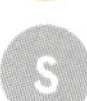

BF

While roasting a whole chicken might sound a bit intimidating, it's actually pretty straightforward and yields so much flavor—not to mention plenty of collagen-rich amino acids, thanks to slowly cooking the meat on the bone. This recipe has been a staple in my household for years, and I almost always make it right before my period.

- **⅓ cup pure maple syrup**
- **¼ cup ghee or vegan butter**
- **6 sprigs fresh rosemary, needles from half of the sprigs minced (about 3 tablespoons)**
- **4 cloves garlic, minced**
- **1 whole (3- to 5-pound) organic pasture-raised chicken, neck and giblets removed (if included), rinsed and patted dry**
- **Sea salt and black pepper to taste**

Buttery Mashed Potatoes

- **2 pounds (4 to 6) Yukon gold potatoes, peeled and cut into chunks**
- **Sea salt**
- **½ cup nondairy milk (I prefer almond milk, but coconut, cashew, or oat will work)**
- **¼ cup ghee or vegan butter, plus more for serving**
- **Black pepper to taste**

1. Preheat the oven to 400°F.

2. Combine the maple syrup, ghee or vegan butter, minced rosemary, and garlic in a small saucepan. Bring to a boil, then remove immediately from the heat.

3. Generously season the chicken with salt and pepper, then tuck the remaining rosemary sprigs into the cavity (feel free to add more garlic or other herbs like thyme here as well).

4. Place the chicken, breast side up, in a large Dutch oven or 9 by 13-inch baking dish. Evenly pour the maple syrup mixture all over the chicken. Slide the pan into the oven and roast for 20 minutes. Reduce the oven temperature to 350°F and continue to roast the chicken, basting every 10 to 15 minutes with the maple mixture, for about 1 hour, or until the thickest part of the breast registers 160°F.

5. *For the potatoes:* While the chicken is roasting, peel the potatoes and chop into large chunks. Place in a large pot and add water to cover. Salt the water, cover, and bring to a boil. Cook for 15 to 20 minutes, until the potatoes are tender. Drain well, then use a fork to mash with the nondairy milk, ghee or vegan butter, 1 teaspoon salt, and pepper. Cover and keep warm until the chicken is ready.

6. Transfer the chicken to a large cutting board and let it rest until slightly cooled, about 10 minutes. Carve with a knife or use your hands to pull apart. Serve the chicken with the mashed potatoes (topped with more ghee) and any other sides of choice.

NOTE: Make sure to save all of the bones, storing them in an airtight glass container in the fridge for up to 5 days, so you can use them to make the Super Simple Homemade Bone Broth (page 109) and Bone Broth Hot Chocolate (page 110).

MENSTRUAL PHASE BENEFITS

Rich in iron and minerals • High in protein • Abundant in collagen, gelatin, and amino acids • High in B vitamins • Slow cooked for maximum nutrient absorption and digestion

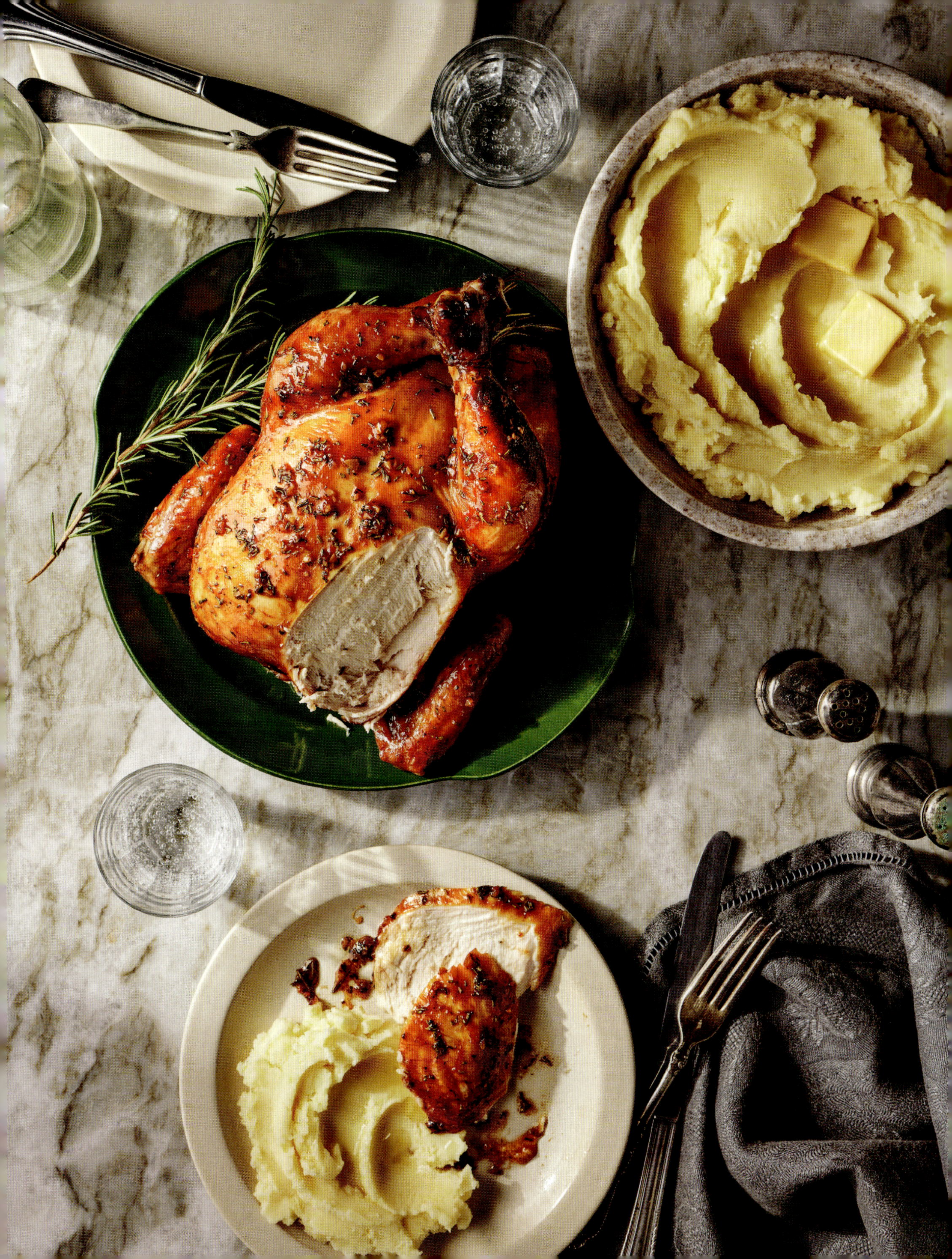

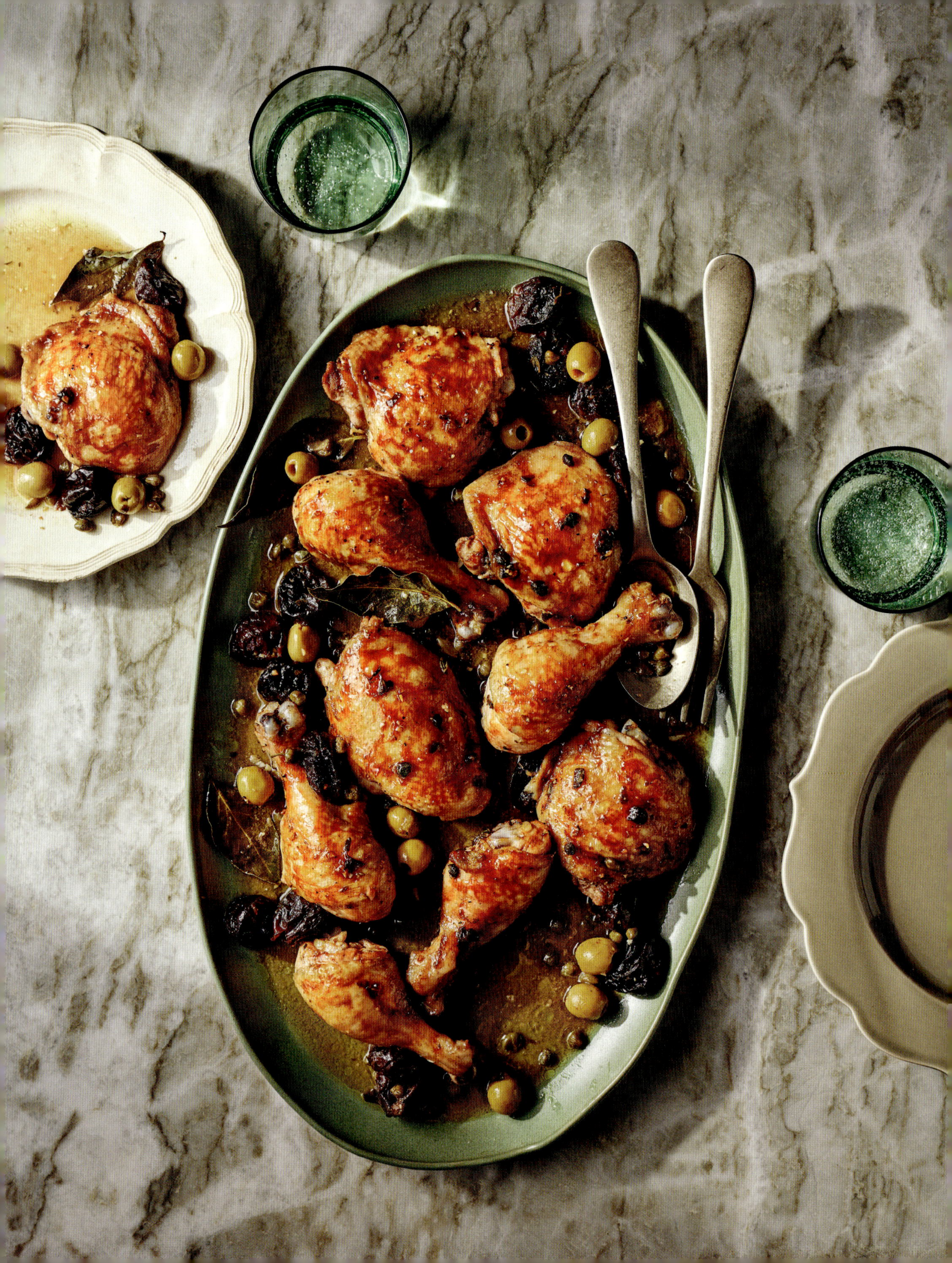

Mom's Mediterranean Chicken Marbella

PREP: 10 MINUTES, PLUS OVERNIGHT MARINATING   COOK: 1 HOUR   SERVES 6–8

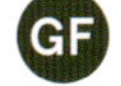

DF

When I was growing up, my mom would make this dish often, and it became the ultimate comfort food for me as an adult—I'd request it for dinners when I was home from college, for birthday celebrations, and after I had my babies. The slowly cooked chicken provides tons of flavor as well as protein-rich amino acids and collagen and gelatin, which aid in hormone synthesis and tissue repair. But my favorite parts of this dish are the juicy olives and prunes, which plump up with the fragrant sauce (and boost digestion). Serve over rice to soak up more of the sauce!

- ½ cup extra virgin olive oil
- ½ cup red wine vinegar
- 1 cup pitted prunes
- ½ cup pitted Spanish olives
- ½ cup capers with their juices
- ¼ cup dried oregano
- 4 cloves garlic, minced
- 1 teaspoon sea salt
- ½ teaspoon black pepper
- 6 bay leaves
- 6 pasture-raised organic bone-in chicken thighs
- 6 pasture-raised organic bone-in drumsticks
- 1 cup coconut sugar
- 1 cup white wine (most of the alcohol will burn off with cooking but it's important for flavor!)
- ¼ cup chopped fresh parsley, for garnish
- Wild rice, for serving (optional)

1. In a large bowl, stir together the olive oil, vinegar, prunes, olives, capers, oregano, garlic, salt, pepper, and bay leaves until well combined. Add the chicken and use your hands to mix evenly. Cover tightly and marinate overnight (or a minimum of 8 hours) in the fridge.

2. Preheat the oven to 350°F. Arrange the chicken in a shallow 13 by 18-inch baking pan and spoon the marinade over evenly. Sprinkle the chicken with the coconut sugar and drizzle with the white wine. Bake for 50 to 60 minutes, basting frequently, until the chicken is golden brown and registers an internal temperature of 165°F. Fish out and discard the bay leaves. Garnish with parsley and serve with wild rice if desired.

NOTE: If serving over wild rice, make sure to cook it according to package instructions while the chicken is baking.

MENSTRUAL PHASE BENEFITS

Rich in iron and minerals • High in protein • Abundant in gelatin, collagen, and amino acids • Slow cooked for maximum nutrient absorption and digestion

BBQ Pulled Pork–Stuffed Sweet Potatoes + Coleslaw

PREP: 15 MINUTES COOK: 4 HOURS, OR 8–10 HOURS IN A SLOW COOKER SERVES 6

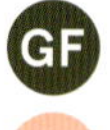
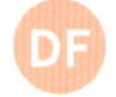
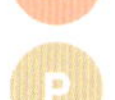
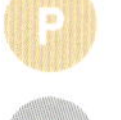
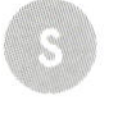

Some things just taste better stuffed into sweet potatoes, and pulled pork is one of them! This recipe is a repeat offender in our household as it's incredibly filling and flavorful, thanks to the juicy, slightly sweet, and tangy shredded pork and buttery melt-in-your-mouth sweet potatoes, with coleslaw adding some acidity and brightness to round out the dish. It also packs in tons of protein and fiber, helping to replenish lost nutrients and optimize digestion, *and* it makes great leftovers! See the Note if you want to use your pressure cooker or slow cooker to cook the pork.

Pulled Pork

- **2 tablespoons coconut sugar**
- **1 tablespoon smoked paprika**
- **1 tablespoon sea salt**
- **1 teaspoon cumin**
- **1 teaspoon garlic powder**
- **1 teaspoon onion powder**
- **4 pounds pork shoulder, cut into 4 to 6 large pieces**
- **2 tablespoons avocado oil**
- **1½ cups bone broth**

Sweet Potatoes

- **6 small to medium orange-fleshed sweet potatoes (such as garnet yams), whole, rinsed and patted dry**

Coleslaw

- **½ cup avocado oil mayonnaise**
- **2 tablespoons pure maple syrup**
- **2 tablespoons apple cider vinegar**
- **1 teaspoon Dijon mustard**
- **1 teaspoon sea salt**
- **1 (16-ounce) package organic coleslaw mix**

To Serve

- **2 cups barbecue sauce (look for a brand with minimal ingredients and that is refined-sugar-free)**
- **2 to 4 tablespoons grass-fed ghee (optional)**

1. Preheat the oven to 300°F.

2. *For the pulled pork:* In a small bowl, combine the coconut sugar, paprika, salt, cumin, garlic powder, and onion powder. Rub the mixture evenly into the pork pieces. Heat the avocado oil in a Dutch oven over medium-high heat. In batches, add the pork and sear, turning, until browned, 1 to 2 minutes per side.

3. Return all of the pork to the Dutch oven and add the bone broth. Cover, transfer to the oven, and cook for 3 hours. Uncover and cook for 1 to 2 additional hours, until the pork is completely tender but crisped up around the edges.

4. *For the sweet potatoes:* Meanwhile, at the 2-hour mark, start the sweet potatoes. Line a large baking sheet with parchment paper and place the whole sweet potatoes on the sheet. Bake for 1 hour, then flip and bake for another 30 minutes to 1 hour, until the sweet potatoes are completely soft and fragrant. Slit each one in half lengthwise and let cool.

5. *For the coleslaw:* When the pork and sweet potatoes are almost finished cooking, mix the mayonnaise, maple syrup, vinegar, mustard, and salt together in a large bowl. Add the coleslaw mix and stir well to combine.

6. *To serve:* Transfer the pork to a medium bowl and use two forks to shred. It should fall apart easily. Stir in the barbecue sauce and season with more salt and pepper if needed.

7. Brush a bit of ghee onto the cut side of each sweet potato half for extra buttery flavor if desired, then heap on a generous amount of pulled pork. Top with the coleslaw, or serve it on the side.

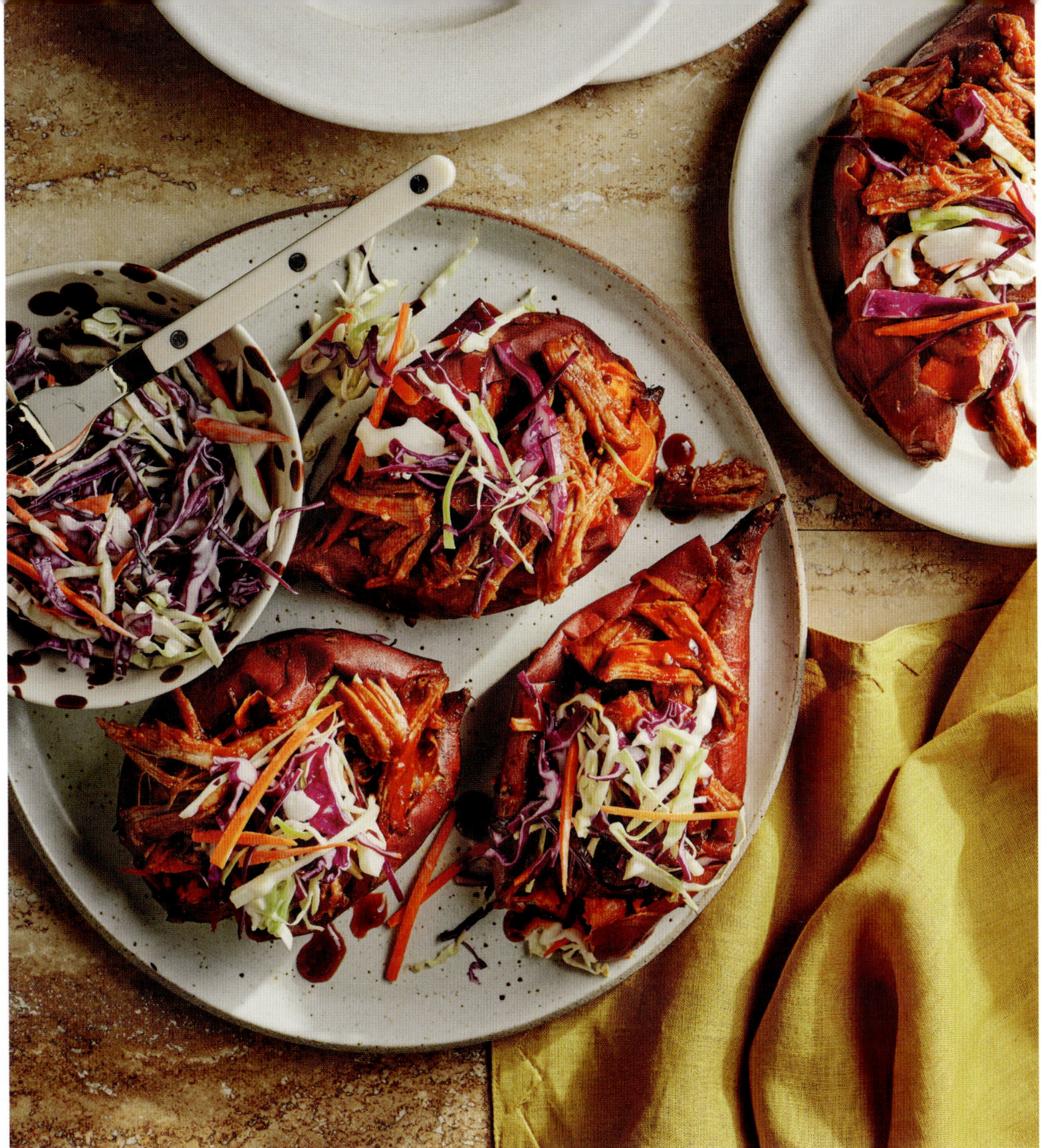

NOTE: To cook the pork in a slow cooker or pressure cooker, first sear the seasoned pork in a large stovetop skillet or utilize the sauté method in the pressure cooker. For the slow cooker, combine the pork and bone broth in the cooker and set it for 4 to 6 hours on high, or 8 to 10 hours on low (the longer, the more tender). For the pressure cooker, combine the pork and bone broth in the cooker and set to high pressure for 1 hour, then allow the pressure to manually release for 10 to 15 minutes. Follow the remaining instructions accordingly, and make sure to give yourself 2 hours to cook the sweet potatoes.

MENSTRUAL PHASE BENEFITS

High in protein and amino acids • Anti-inflammatory • High in vitamin C • Slow cooked for maximum nutrient absorption and digestion

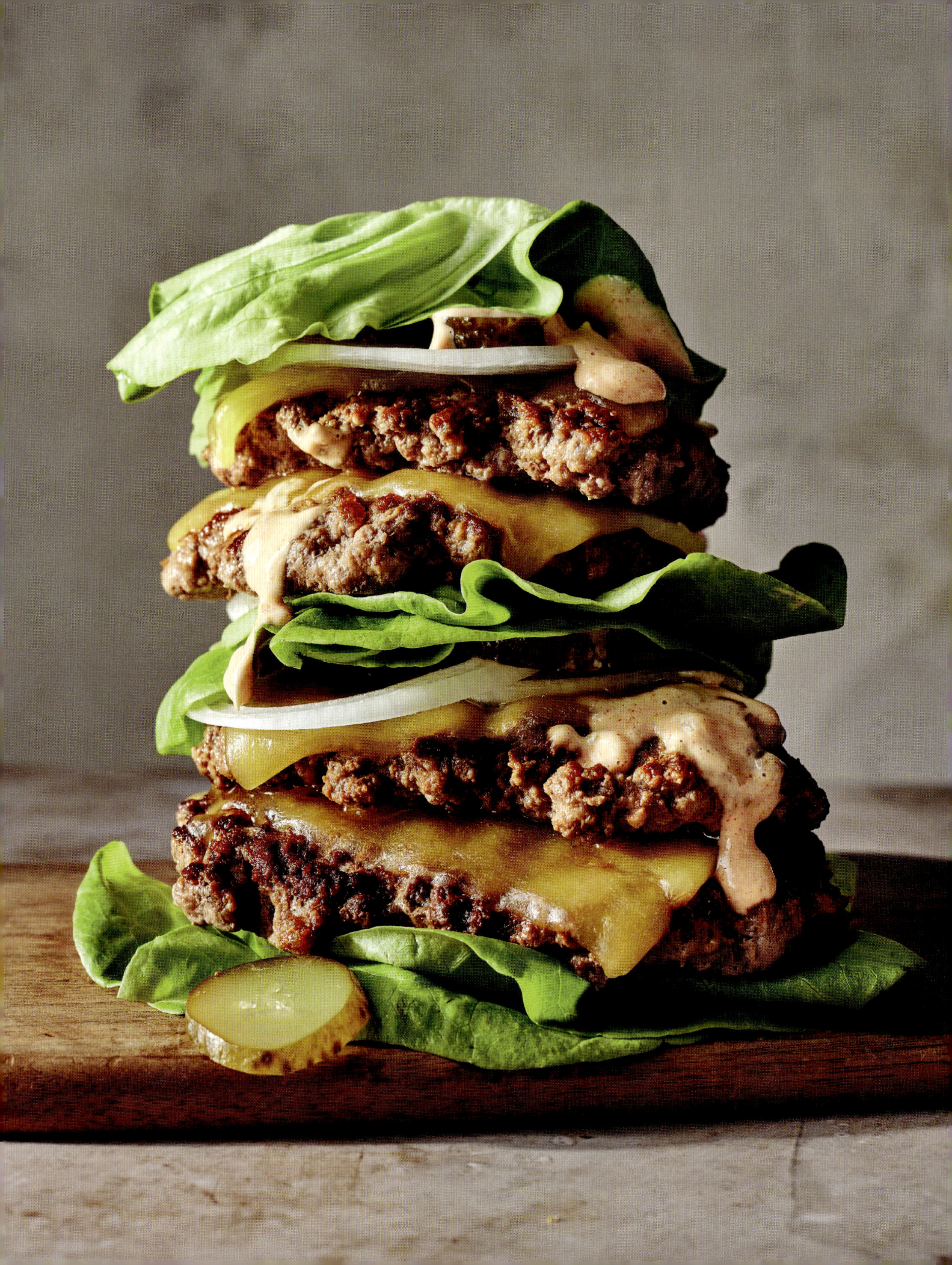

Lettuce-Wrapped Smash Burgers + Secret Sauce

PREP: 10 MINUTES COOK: 15 MINUTES SERVES 4

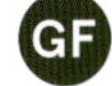

S

There is almost nothing I crave more than a good burger, especially during my period when my body naturally gravitates toward iron-rich red meat. Smashing beef patties on a super hot pan or grill increases the Maillard reaction, forcing the juices of the meat upward, creating more flavor, less dryness, and a delicious crunchy crust. Double stack 'em (hello, protein!), layer with dill pickles, cheese, and lettuce, and—whatever you do—don't skip the secret sauce! You can also swap out the lettuce wraps for toasted, gluten-free buns, or make a deconstructed burger bowl with more lettuce and the Root Veggie Fries on page 252.

Secret Sauce

- **½ cup avocado oil mayonnaise**
- **2 tablespoons organic refined-sugar-free ketchup (or barbecue sauce)**
- **2 tablespoons sweet pickle relish (or dill pickle relish)**
- **2 teaspoons yellow mustard**
- **2 teaspoons gluten-free Worcestershire sauce**
- **1 teaspoon white or apple cider vinegar**
- **½ teaspoon paprika**
- **½ teaspoon garlic powder**
- **½ teaspoon onion powder**
- **½ teaspoon sea salt**
- **1 to 2 tablespoons finely minced onion (optional)**

Burgers

- **1½ pounds ground grass-fed beef, formed into 8 balls of equal size**
- **Garlic powder**
- **Sea salt and black pepper**
- **Yellow mustard (optional)**
- **4 ounces raw organic cheddar, thinly sliced or shredded**
- **8 large bibb or green-leaf lettuce leaves, rinsed and patted dry**
- **4 large dill pickles, thinly sliced (or pickle chips)**
- **¼ cup thinly sliced white onion**

1. *For the secret sauce:* Whisk together all the ingredients in a small bowl and set aside.

2. *For the burgers:* Heat a large skillet or griddle over high heat for 1 to 2 minutes (you want the pan piping hot). Place two of the beef balls in the pan and smash each as thinly as you can using a stiff metal spatula. Season the patties generously with garlic powder, salt, and pepper and drizzle with mustard (if you like), then let them cook until the top surface begins to appear cooked, about 1 minute. Scrape up the patties with the spatula, flip, and cook for another 30 seconds. Add a portion of cheddar to the top of one of the patties and let melt another 30 seconds or so. Transfer both patties to one of the lettuce leaves, stacking one on top of the other. Repeat to cook the remaining beef balls, making eight patties, two for each burger.

3. Top each burger stack with sliced pickles and onions and drizzle generously with secret sauce. Add the top lettuce "bun" and enjoy immediately.

MENSTRUAL PHASE BENEFITS

Rich in iron and minerals • High in protein • Abundant in amino acids • High in B vitamins

Slow-Cooked Chuck-Roast Tacos + Avocado Chimichurri

PREP: 10 MINUTES　　COOK: 4½ HOURS　　SERVES 4–6

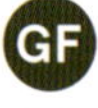
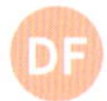

This is one of those standout meals that taste like you've spent countless hours preparing them, when in reality slow cooking a chuck roast is an easy, mostly hands-off method that tenderizes the beef's connective tissues and fat. The result is an abundance of flavor and easily digestible nutrients such as collagen, gelatin, and amino acids. I love that it makes a large amount of beef, which often equates to tasty leftovers (a must in breakfast tacos!) and less active cooking time when I'm on my period. Don't skip the herbaceous chimichurri, which cuts through the richness of the meat with bright and zesty notes. See the Note if you want to use your pressure cooker or slow cooker.

Chuck Roast

1 teaspoon chili powder

1 teaspoon garlic powder

1 teaspoon onion powder

1 teaspoon smoked paprika

1 teaspoon coriander

1 teaspoon sea salt, plus more to taste

3 pounds grass-fed boneless beef chuck roast

½ cup freshly squeezed orange juice

½ cup beef bone broth

1 large yellow onion, cut into quarters

Black pepper

Avocado Chimichurri

1 large bunch (about 2 cups) fresh cilantro

1 large bunch (about 2 cups) fresh flat-leaf parsley

1 small or ½ large avocado, pitted, peeled, and chopped

½ jalapeño, seeded

4 cloves garlic, minced

Juice of 3 limes (about 6 tablespoons)

2 tablespoons pure maple syrup

1 teaspoon sea salt

¼ cup avocado oil or extra virgin olive oil

2 to 4 tablespoons water, to thin

For Serving

Organic corn, cassava, or almond flour tortillas

Diced avocado, minced cilantro, cotija cheese, or full-fat organic sour cream (optional)

1. *For the chuck roast:* Preheat the oven to 325°F. In a small bowl, combine the chili powder, garlic powder, onion powder, paprika, coriander, and salt. Rub the mixture evenly over all sides of the roast.

2. Combine the orange juice, bone broth, and quartered onion in a Dutch oven, nestle the seasoned roast inside, and cover. Roast for 4 hours. The meat should easily shred into large chunks using forks. If it's not falling apart, return to the oven and roast for 30 minutes longer.

3. Increase the oven temperature to 425°F and line a large baking sheet with parchment paper. Shred the meat and spread evenly onto the sheet. Pour some of the cooking liquid (⅓ to ½ cup) over the meat and generously sprinkle with salt and pepper. Return to the oven and roast for 10 to 15 minutes, until the meat is crispy and caramelized.

4. *For the chimichurri:* While the meat is finishing in the oven, combine all the chimichurri ingredients in a food processor and mix until creamy, adding water if needed. Set aside until ready to serve.

5. *To assemble the tacos:* If you have a gas stove, you can heat each tortilla over an open flame for about 1 minute per side. Alternatively, lightly coat a pan with oil, place over medium heat, and fry the tortillas one by one.

6. Generously scoop the chuck roast into the tortillas and drizzle with the chimichurri. Finish with additional toppings of choice.

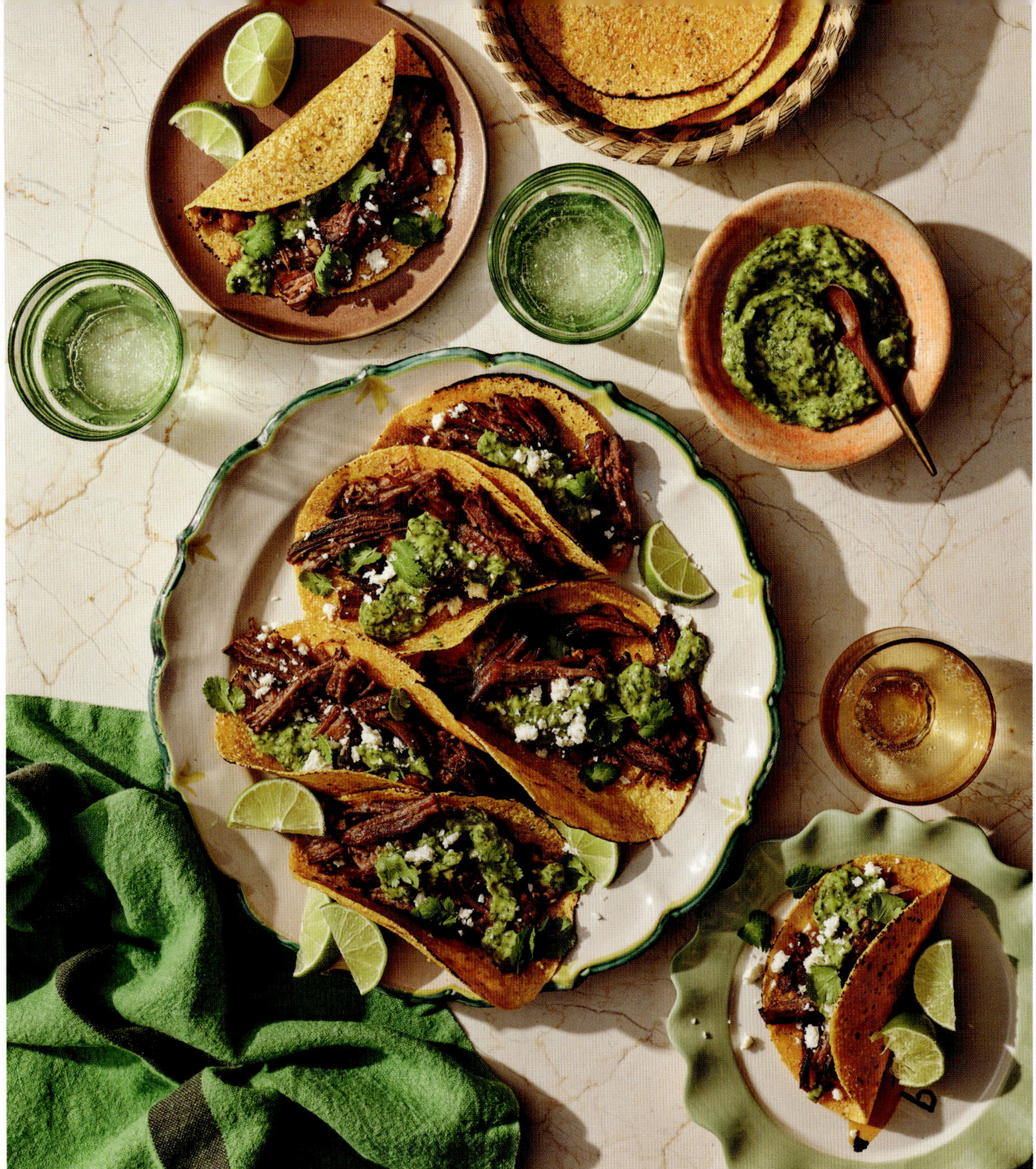

NOTE: To make chuck roast in a pressure cooker or slow cooker, cut the roast in half and season with the spice mixture. Place the halves in the pressure cooker or slow cooker, along with the orange juice, beef bone broth, and onion. Set the pressure cooker timer for 1 hour and 10 minutes, or the slow cooker timer for 6 hours on high or 8 hours on low. When done, shred the meat with two forks. Follow the instructions in step 3 to caramelize and crisp the meat in a 425°F oven.

MENSTRUAL PHASE BENEFITS

Rich in iron and minerals • High in protein • Abundant in collagen, gelatin, and amino acids • High in B vitamins • Slow cooked for maximum nutrient absorption and digestion

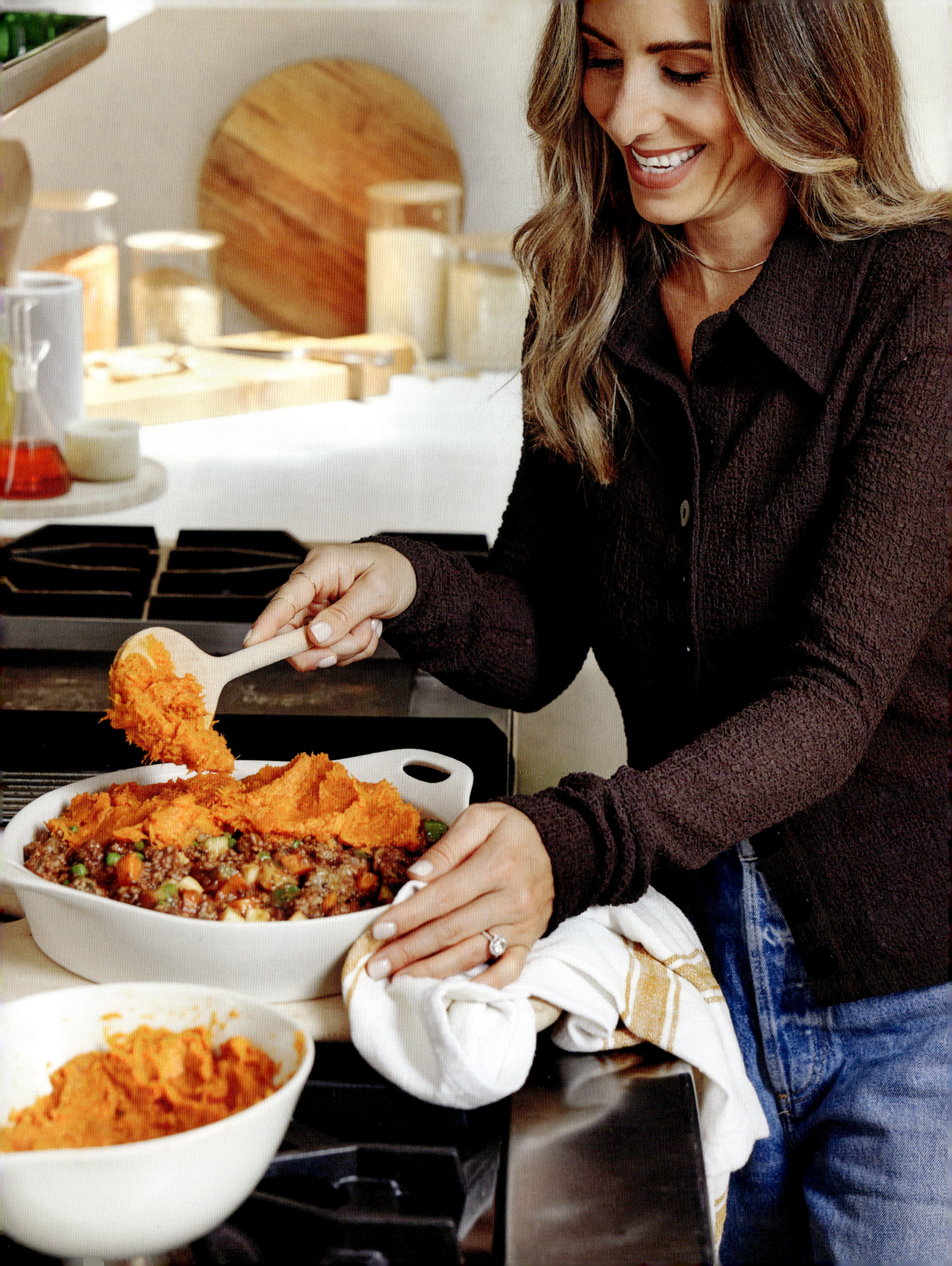

Hidden-Liver Sweet-Potato Shepherd's Pie

PREP: 15 MINUTES   COOK: 1½–2½ HOURS   SERVES 6–8

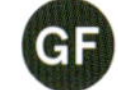

After having my third baby and a postpartum hemorrhage scare, I was looking for easy ways to replenish lost nutrients and wanted a recipe with a high concentration of bioavailable vitamins and minerals. While liver might sound off-putting, a little goes a long way, and using a pound of ground beef mixed with 3 ounces of liver neutralizes the liver taste while still allowing me to reap all of the benefits. Just trust me when I say this dish is so delicious, no one will ever guess its secret ingredient! **PRO TIP:** Save yourself an extra step by looking for a brand such as Ancestral Blends that premixes the beef and liver.

Sweet Potato Topping

- **4 large sweet potatoes**
- **¼ cup grass-fed ghee, melted**
- **1 teaspoon smoked paprika**
- **1 teaspoon chili powder**
- **1 teaspoon sea salt**
- **Black pepper to taste**

Filling

- **2 tablespoons grass-fed ghee or avocado oil**
- **1 medium yellow onion, diced**
- **1 pound mix of grass-fed ground beef and beef liver (see headnote)**
- **3 large carrots, peeled and diced**
- **1 zucchini, diced**
- **½ cup frozen green peas**
- **4 cloves garlic, minced**
- **2 sprigs fresh rosemary, needles minced**
- **2 sprigs fresh thyme, leaves minced**
- **2 teaspoons Italian seasoning**
- **1½ teaspoons chili powder**
- **1 teaspoon sea salt**
- **Black pepper to taste**
- **2 tablespoons tomato paste**
- **⅔ cup no-sugar-added tomato sauce**

1. *To start the sweet potatoes:* Preheat the oven to 400°F. Place the whole sweet potatoes on a baking sheet and roast for 1 to 2 hours (depending on the size), until soft and cooked through. Slice open with a knife and set aside to cool while you make the filling.

2. *For the filling:* Reduce the oven temperature to 375°F. Heat the ghee or avocado oil in a 9-inch oven-safe skillet over medium heat. (You can use a pan that is not oven-safe, but you'll need to transfer the filling to a baking dish before baking.) Add the onion and sauté until translucent, 3 to 5 minutes. Add the ground meat, carrots, zucchini, peas, garlic, rosemary, thyme, Italian seasoning, chili powder, salt, and pepper and cook, stirring frequently, until the meat is browned and veggies are soft, 15 to 20 minutes. Stir in the tomato paste and tomato sauce and remove from the heat.

3. While the filling is cooking, scoop out the flesh of the baked sweet potatoes into a food processor or medium mixing bowl and add the ghee, paprika, chili powder, salt, and pepper. Blend in the processor or use a handheld mixer in the bowl to mix until the topping is creamy and smooth.

4. If using an oven-safe skillet, use a spatula to evenly spread the sweet potato mixture on top of the filling in the skillet. (If your skillet is not oven-safe, transfer the filling to a 9 by 9-inch baking dish and spread the sweet potato mixture evenly on top.) Bake for 12 minutes, until the filling is bubbling and the sweet potato topping has slightly browned around the edges. Let cool for 5 to 10 minutes before serving.

NOTE: I like to bake the sweet potatoes the night before and store them in the fridge to cut down on cooking time on serving day.

MENSTRUAL PHASE BENEFITS

Rich in iron and minerals • High in protein • Abundant in collagen, gelatin, and amino acids • High in vitamin C • High in B vitamins

The Legendary Bison Butternut Squash Chili

PREP: 15 MINUTES   COOK: 30–60 MINUTES   SERVES 8

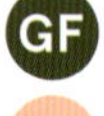

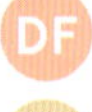
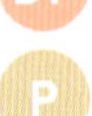
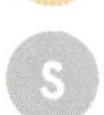
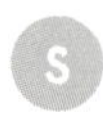

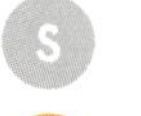
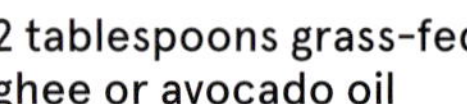

This recipe is never not getting rave reviews (hence its name) and is an especially amazing meal to incorporate into your menstrual phase, as bison is rich in protein and the micronutrients (like iodine, iron, selenium, and zinc) that must be replenished due to blood loss. (It's also a great postpartum meal for new moms for the same reason!) But I'm pretty confident everyone will love a hearty, cozy bowl of this chili, whether menstruating or not.

- 2 tablespoons grass-fed ghee or avocado oil
- 1 medium yellow onion, diced
- 2 pounds grass-fed ground bison
- 2 tablespoons tomato paste
- 6 cloves garlic, minced
- 2 tablespoons chili powder
- 2 teaspoons cumin
- 2 teaspoons sea salt
- ½ teaspoon cinnamon
- ½ teaspoon red chile flakes or cayenne pepper
- Black pepper to taste
- 2 bay leaves
- 1 medium butternut squash, peeled and chopped into 1-inch cubes
- 1 (15-ounce) can fire-roasted tomatoes
- 1 (15-ounce) can diced tomatoes
- 4 cups beef bone broth
- 2 cups spinach, roughly chopped
- Vegan or regular sour cream, shredded cheddar cheese, chopped fresh cilantro, diced green onion, and diced avocado, for topping (optional)

1. Heat the ghee or avocado oil in a large pot over medium heat. Add the onion and cook for 3 to 5 minutes, until translucent. Add the bison and cook, stirring frequently, until browned, about 5 minutes. Add the tomato paste, garlic, chili powder, cumin, salt, cinnamon, chile flakes, pepper, and bay leaves and stir for an additional minute, until fragrant.

2. Stir in the squash, tomatoes, and bone broth, then cover and bring to a boil. Reduce the heat and simmer for a minimum of 30 minutes or up to 1 hour, until the squash is soft and tender.

3. Discard the bay leaves. Stir in the spinach and remove the pot from the heat. The spinach will wilt easily while the chili is still hot. Serve with toppings of choice.

NOTE: To make in a slow cooker, follow the first step in a skillet on the stovetop, then transfer to a slow cooker. Add the remaining ingredients (except the spinach) and cook on high for 3 to 4 hours or low for 6 to 8 hours. Stir in the spinach with 5 to 10 minutes remaining.

MENSTRUAL PHASE BENEFITS

Rich in iron and minerals • High in protein • Abundant in collagen, gelatin, and amino acids • High in vitamin C • High in B vitamins • Slow cooked for maximum nutrient absorption and digestion

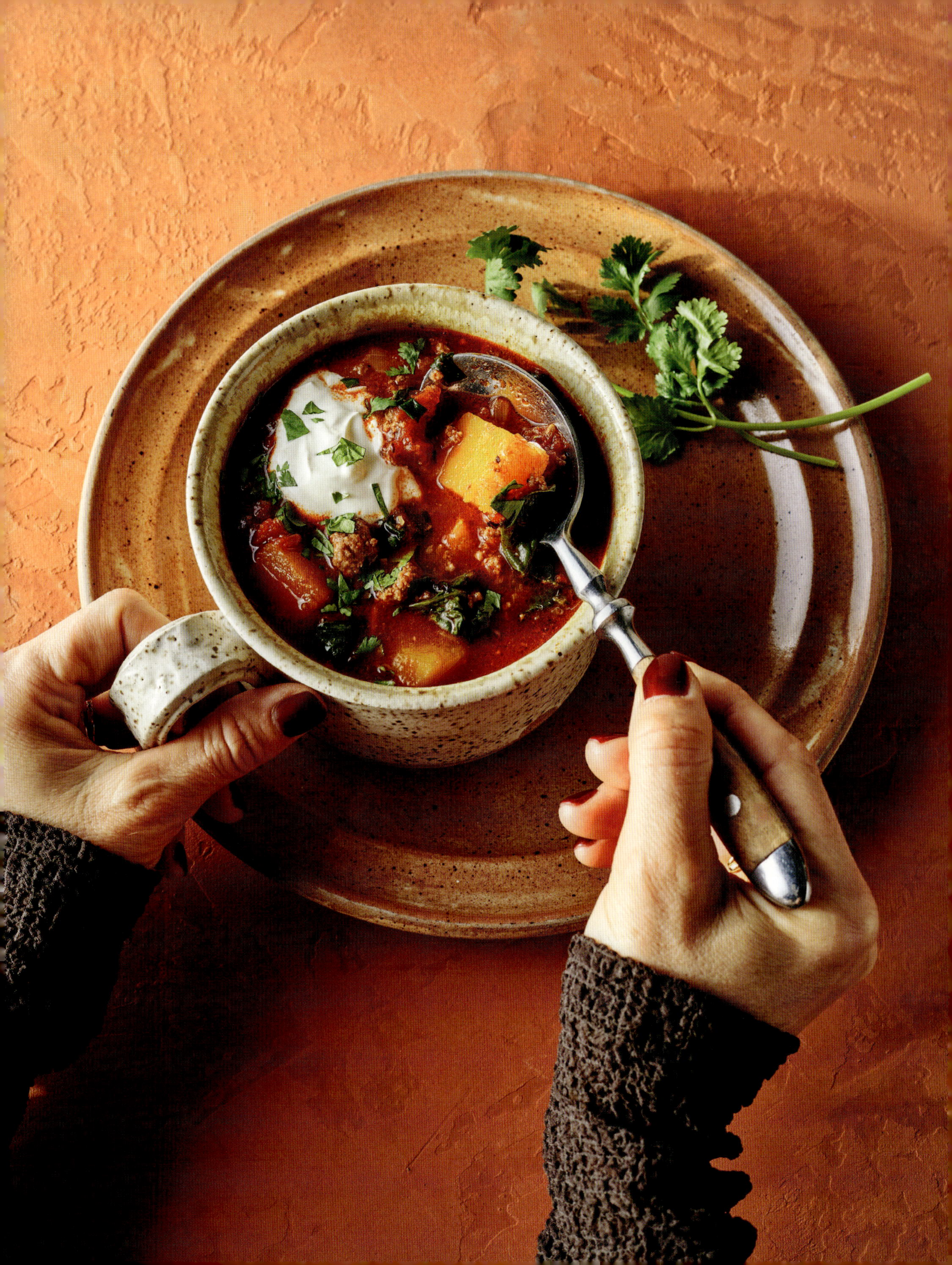

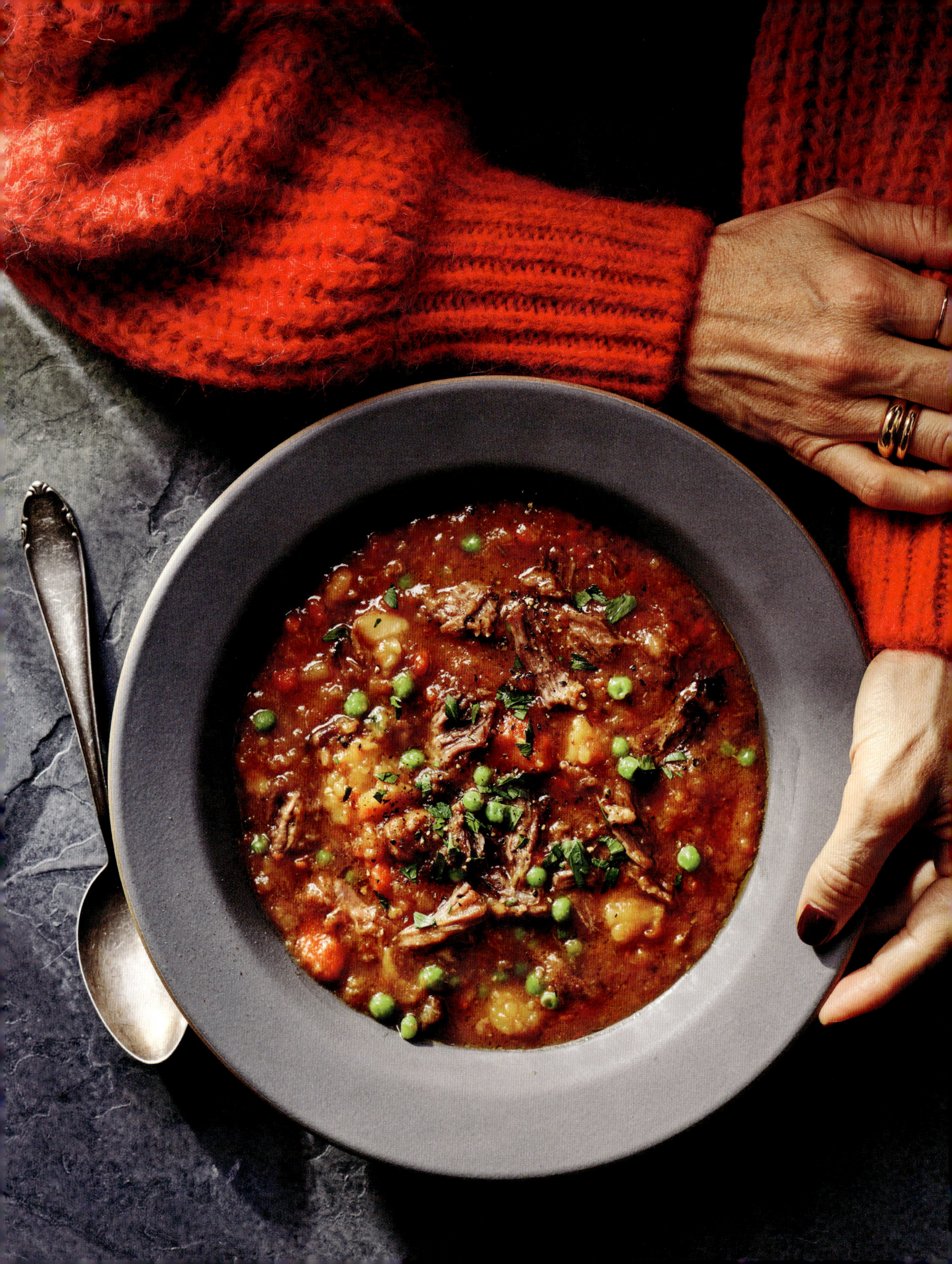

Cozy and Classic Irish Lamb Stew

PREP: 20 MINUTES COOK: 3–4 HOURS SERVES 6–8

GF

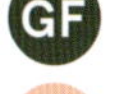

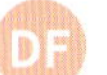

This is a beloved recipe of my mom's, and when I asked her to share it with me for the book, she sent me a picture of the recipe written on the back of a napkin. Apparently, many years ago when my parents traveled to Ireland, they had this stew at a local pub and loved it so much the chef jotted down the recipe for them. So, yeah, this stew is about as OG as it gets! I've tweaked it a bit to increase the nutrient density, but it's still simple, cozy, and "classic"—hence the name.

- 2 tablespoons avocado oil
- 2 pounds lamb stew meat, or 3 pounds (8 to 10) bone-in lamb loin chops
- Sea salt and black pepper to taste
- 1 yellow onion, diced
- 4 medium carrots, peeled and cut into small rounds (2 cups)
- 1 to 2 parsnips, peeled and cut into small rounds (1 cup)
- 6 cloves garlic, minced
- 6 sprigs fresh rosemary, needles minced
- 6 cups beef bone broth
- 1 to 2 Yukon Gold potatoes, peeled and cut into large chunks (2 cups)
- 1 cup frozen organic peas
- Chopped fresh flat-leaf parsley, for topping (optional)

1. Heat the avocado oil in a large pot or Dutch oven over medium-high heat. In batches if necessary, add the stew meat or chops, liberally seasoning them with salt and pepper, and sear until all sides are browned, 2 to 3 minutes per side. As the meat browns, transfer with tongs to a large plate.

2. Reduce the heat to medium and add the onion, carrots, parsnips, garlic, and rosemary to the pot. Stir everything well, then cover the pot and let the vegetables "sweat" (get soft) for 10 to 20 minutes, stirring occasionally, until the veggies are soft and the rosemary is fragrant. Return the browned lamb to the pot and add the bone broth and potatoes. Sprinkle in more salt (about 2 teaspoons) and black pepper and bring the liquid to a boil. Reduce the heat, cover, and simmer for 3 to 4 hours, until the meat is completely tender and falls off the bone.

3. If using lamb chops, use tongs to transfer to a bowl. Using two forks, shred the lamb meat from the bones, then return the shredded meat to the stew; discard the bones.

4. Stir in the peas and let them cook for 2 to 3 minutes. Remove the pot from the heat and let sit for 5 to 10 minutes before serving. Top with parsley if desired.

NOTE: If you can find pre-cut lamb stew meat it will save you an extra step. However, I prefer using lamb chops because the bones add more flavor as well as gut- and liver-supportive amino acids, collagen, and gelatin.

MENSTRUAL PHASE BENEFITS

Rich in iron and minerals • High in protein and amino acids • High in B vitamins • Slow cooked for maximum nutrient absorption and digestion

Protein Peanut Butter–Chocolate Cereal Bars

PREP: 10 MINUTES, PLUS 1 HOUR CHILLING   COOK: NONE   SERVES 16

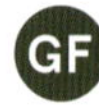

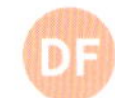

My sweet tooth knows no bounds, but I'm always trying to sneak protein and nutrients into my treats whenever I can, to effectively satisfy my craving *and* keep my blood sugar stable. These no-bake cereal bars manage to do all of that, and they're a go-to when I'm on my period thanks to the low-maintenance approach *and* magnesium-rich dark chocolate ganache.

- **1½ cups creamy nut butter (I prefer peanut butter or almond butter)**
- **⅔ cup pure maple syrup**
- **½ cup vanilla protein powder (or collagen peptides)**
- **1 teaspoon pure vanilla extract**
- **½ teaspoon sea salt**
- **1 (7-ounce) box (about 4½ cups) gluten-free cereal (I love the Lovebird brand; see Note)**
- **12 ounces (2 cups) dark chocolate chips**
- **½ cup coconut cream (or the solid that separates from the liquid in a can of full-fat coconut milk; see the Note on page 110)**
- **Flaky sea salt for topping (optional)**

1. Line an 8 by 8-inch baking pan with parchment paper.

2. In a large mixing bowl, whisk together the nut butter, maple syrup, protein powder, vanilla extract, and sea salt until well combined. Add the cereal and mix with a spatula until well combined. Spoon the mixture into the lined pan and spread until even.

3. Melt the chocolate chips in a microwave-safe bowl in 30-second increments, stirring each time, until mostly melted. (If you don't have a microwave, you can melt the chocolate in a small pan over low heat.) Whisk in the coconut cream until the mixture is thick, shiny, and creamy.

4. Pour the melted chocolate evenly over the cereal base. Chill for 1 hour in the fridge, then cut evenly into 16 squares. Sprinkle with flaky sea salt if desired. Store in an airtight container in the fridge for up to 5 days.

NOTE: Make sure to choose a cereal brand with minimal ingredients so you avoid excess sugar or inflammation. Lovebird cereals are made with ingredients like cassava flour and honey.

MENSTRUAL PHASE BENEFITS

Rich in minerals • High in B vitamins

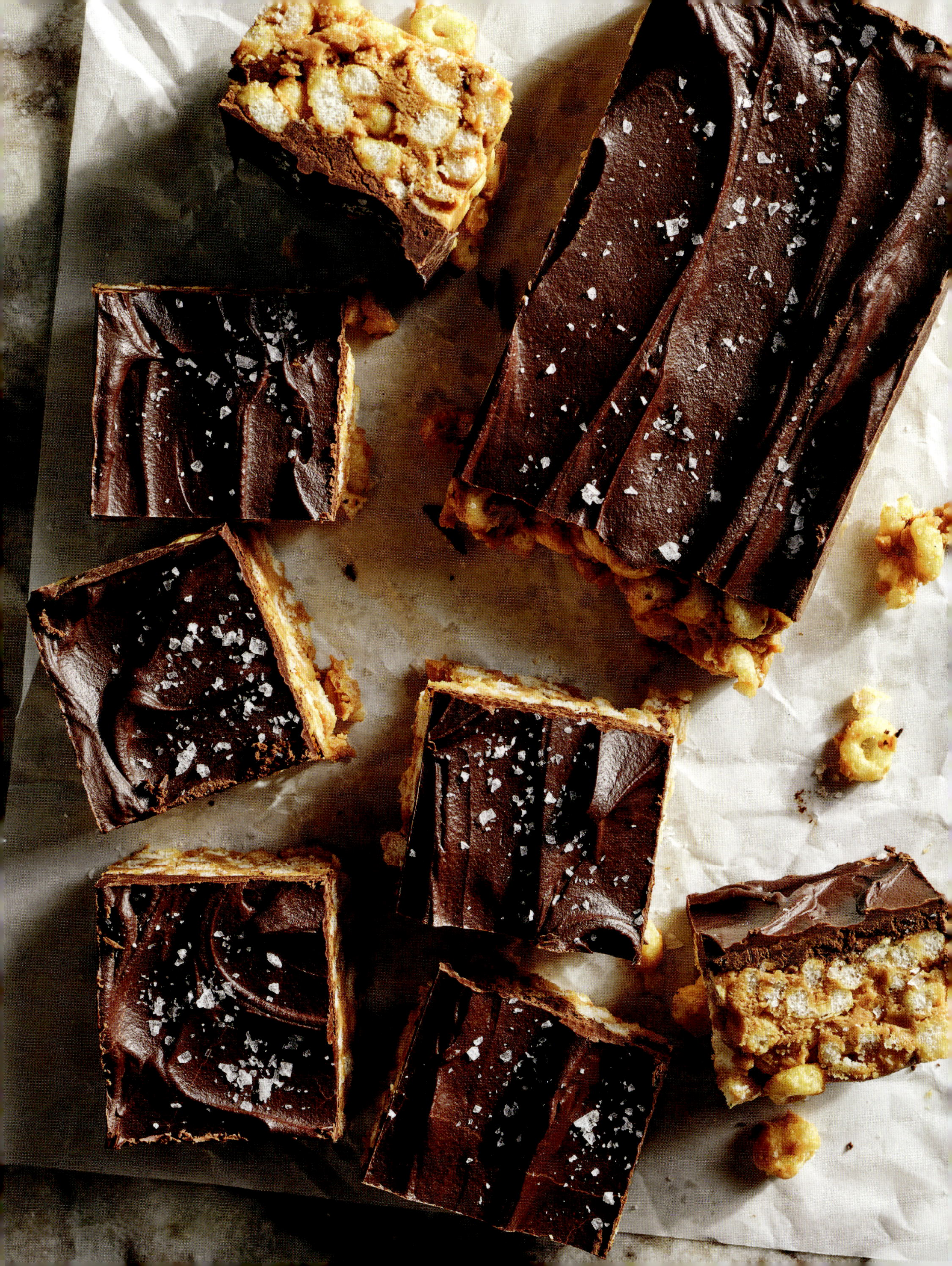

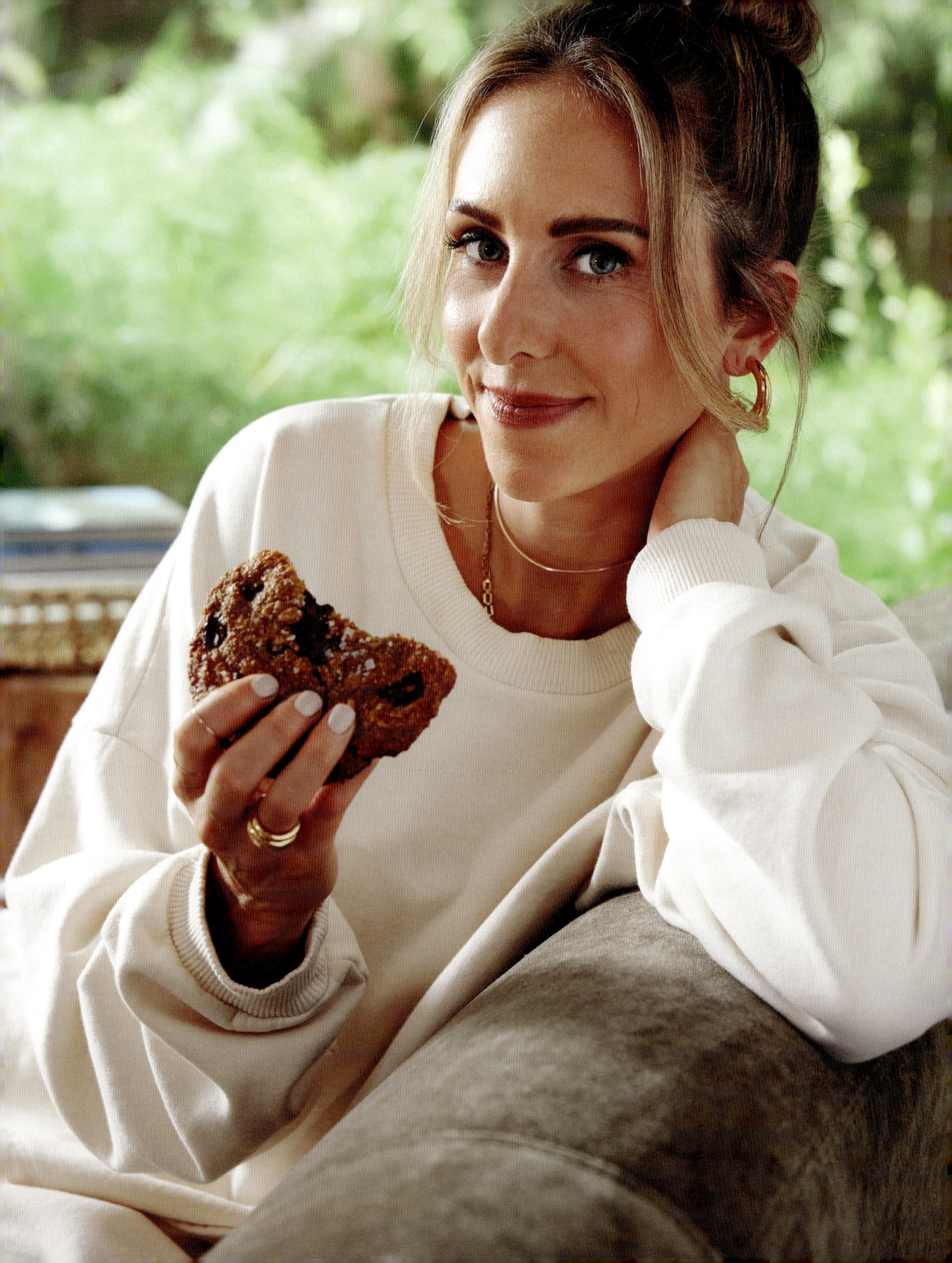

Energy-Boosting Dark Chocolate Chunk Oatmeal Cookies

PREP: 10 MINUTES, PLUS 2 HOURS CHILLING   COOK: 10–14 MINUTES   SERVES 12

GF DF

S

These cookies have become low-key famous in our inner circle due to their perfect texture—crunchy on the outside, soft on the inside, and studded with melty chunks of dark chocolate and chewy oats, then sprinkled with flaky sea salt. But the most amazing part is that they contain a secret, nutrient-dense ingredient called brewer's yeast, which is an excellent source of B vitamins that combat fatigue during a very energy-intensive phase. In this case, you really can have your cookies and eat them too!

Important note: Make sure to prep the dough and chill it in the fridge at least 2 hours (or up to 24 hours) before you need to bake the cookies. This will significantly optimize the texture, helping them get that crunchy outer layer and chewy, soft inside.

- **1 cup organic coconut sugar**
- **⅓ cup unrefined organic coconut oil, at room temperature (or use grass-fed butter, but the cookies will not be dairy-free)**
- **2 large pasture-raised eggs**
- **1 teaspoon pure vanilla extract**
- **1⅔ cups blanched almond flour**
- **¼ cup debittered gluten-free brewer's yeast**
- **½ teaspoon cinnamon**
- **½ teaspoon sea salt**
- **½ teaspoon baking soda**
- **¾ cup gluten-free rolled oats (I love using protein oats for an extra protein boost)**
- **1¼ cups dark chocolate chunks or chips**
- **½ cup chopped walnuts (optional)**
- **Flaky sea salt, for topping**

1. Combine the coconut sugar and softened coconut oil in a large mixing bowl or stand mixer. Beat until well combined. Add the eggs and vanilla extract and continue to mix until well combined. Add the almond flour, brewer's yeast, cinnamon, sea salt, and baking soda and beat. Using a wooden spoon or spatula, fold in the rolled oats, chocolate chunks or chips, and walnuts (if using) until evenly mixed in the dough. Cover the bowl with a lid and let the batter chill in the fridge for a minimum of 2 hours or up to 24 hours.

2. Preheat the oven to 350°F and line a large baking sheet with parchment paper.

3. Use either your hands or a cookie dough scooper (I prefer the scooper as it keeps each cookie uniformly shaped and consistent) to form the dough into 12 balls. Evenly arrange the dough balls in three or four rows on the lined pan, making sure to leave enough space between the balls as the cookies will expand quite a bit. Use your hand to flatten each ball a bit until it resembles more of a cookie shape, then sprinkle the tops with flaky sea salt. Bake for 10 to 14 minutes, until the cookie edges are golden brown and the chocolate is melty. Let the cookies cool for 15 minutes, allowing them to firm up. Store in an airtight container at room temperature for up to 5 days.

NOTE: Make sure to buy a certified non-GMO, gluten-free, debittered brewer's yeast so your cookies have no bitter aftertaste.

MENSTRUAL PHASE BENEFITS

High in B vitamins

Citrus Ginger Immunity Booster

PREP: 2 MINUTES COOK: 5 MINUTES SERVES 1

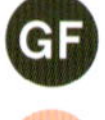

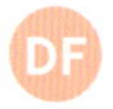

Years ago, when I lived in Seattle, I would frequent a health food restaurant in my neighborhood for their flu buster—a steaming-hot, slightly sweet and tart beverage filled with anti-inflammatory, antimicrobial, antifungal, and antibacterial ingredients that sound gross but tasted altogether delicious (like liquid sunshine). Sadly, the restaurant has shut down, but the memory lives on with my homage recipe, which I often make during menstruation, when I'm more likely to feel run-down or catch a cold due to a downshift in my immune system.

1½ cups freshly squeezed orange juice

Juice of 1 small lemon (about 1 tablespoon)

¼ small white onion, chopped (2 to 3 tablespoons)

2 cloves garlic, minced

1 teaspoon minced fresh ginger

1 to 2 tablespoons raw honey

Dash of cayenne pepper (optional)

1. Combine the orange and lemon juice in a small pot and warm over medium heat while preparing the rest of the ingredients, 1 to 2 minutes. Add the onion, garlic, and ginger and bring to a simmer. Reduce the heat to low and let steam for 5 minutes.

2. Pour the mixture into a high-speed blender and add the honey. Blend until the mixture is creamy, well combined, and frothy. Pour into a mug (it will be hot!) and top with an optional sprinkle of cayenne pepper. Enjoy immediately.

NOTE: Try pairing this immunity booster with a non-heme-iron-rich meal (i.e., with iron from plant sources); the high vitamin C content will naturally help to increase absorption.

MENSTRUAL PHASE BENEFITS

High in vitamin C • Anti-inflammatory

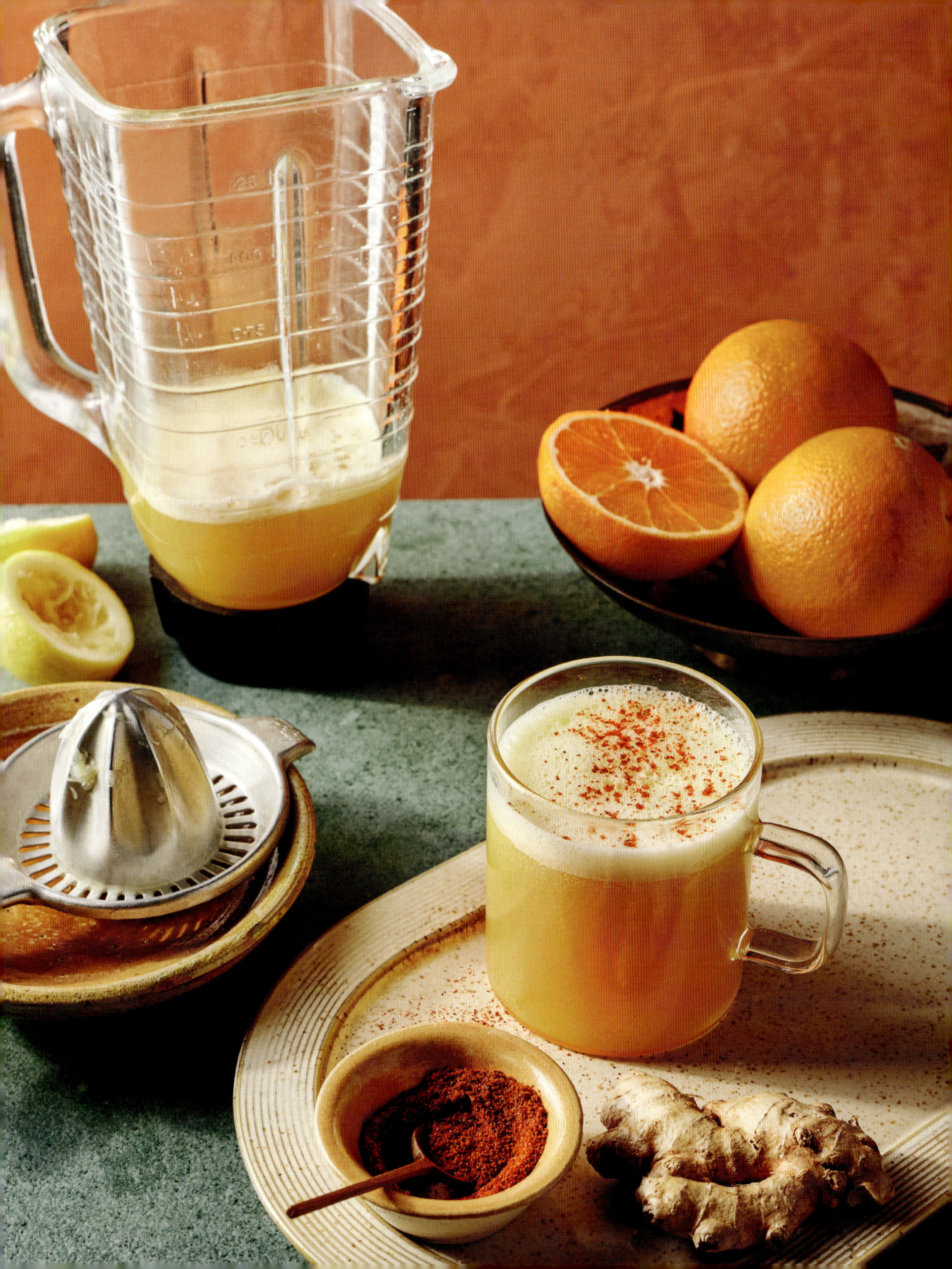

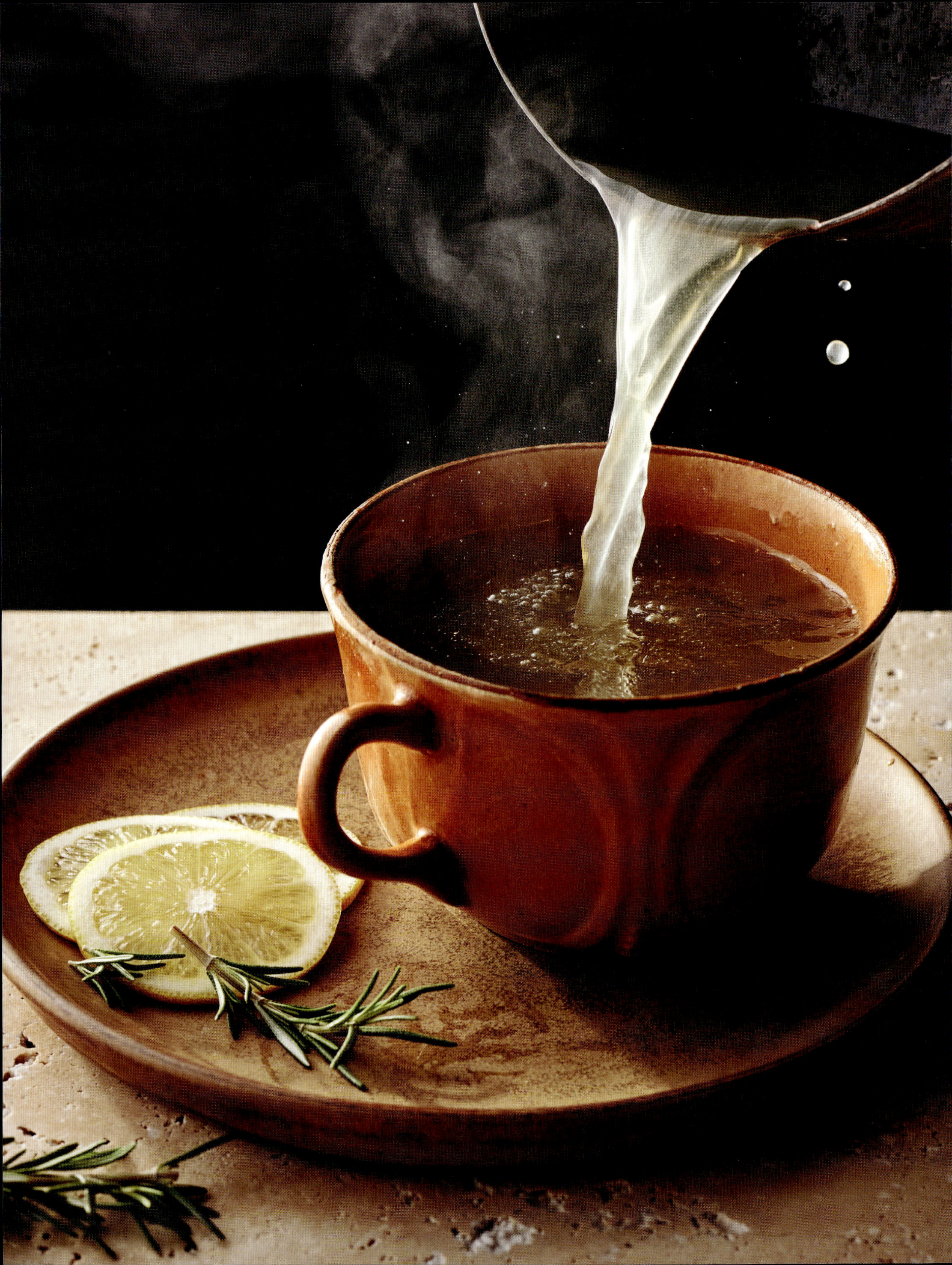

Super Simple Homemade Bone Broth

PREP: 10 MINUTES   COOK: 10–12 HOURS   MAKES 6–8 CUPS

The obsession with bone broth is real, and for good reason! Not only does it add major flavor to soups, grains, slow cooker meals, and even hot chocolate (page 110), but it's loaded with amino acids that reduce oxidative stress, support healthy connective and reproductive tissue, boost GI and immune function, and promote the secretion of female reproductive hormones (orchestrating everything from ovulation to embryo implantation). It's also rich in minerals that tend to get depleted due to blood loss, which is why I include it in so many recipes during this phase! This homemade broth is easy to make and versatile, so you can use it in both sweet and savory dishes. Or just sip it on its own throughout the day for a tasty, protein-rich pick-me-up.

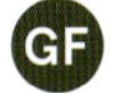

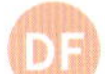

BF

Bones, skin, and carcass of a pasture-raised, organic whole chicken (see Note)

12 cups cold filtered water

2 tablespoons apple cider vinegar

1 lemon, sliced

6 sprigs fresh rosemary

Sea salt and black pepper to taste

1. Place the carcass (including bones and skin) in a large pot, Dutch oven, or slow cooker. Add the filtered water and vinegar. If cooking on the stovetop, bring to a boil over medium heat, then reduce to low and simmer for 10 to 12 hours. If cooking in a slow cooker, cook on low for 10 to 12 hours. (I find 12 hours is ideal to get a more flavorful, collagen-rich broth.)

2. Add the lemon to the pot or slow cooker 1 hour before the chicken is finished cooking.

3. Add the rosemary 30 minutes before the chicken is finished cooking.

4. Season with salt and black pepper, then strain through a fine-mesh sieve or strainer into a large bowl or container; discard the solids. Place the container or bowl upright in a larger bowl filled with ice water to quickly cool the broth to room temperature. Transfer to wide-mouth glass jars with sealable lids. If freezing, make sure to leave at least 1 inch of room at the top of the jar, which will allow the liquid to expand without breaking the glass, and store upright.

5. Store the jars in the fridge for up to 5 days, or in the freezer for 1 to 2 months. You can also store the bone broth in silicone ice cube tray molds in the freezer. Bone broth typically gelatinizes when refrigerated due to the collagen, but once you reheat it will liquify just like a store-bought broth.

NOTE: You can either use your leftover bones from roasting a whole chicken (such as the Maple-Rosemary Roast Chicken on page 86) or purchase raw bones from a specialty or general butcher shop. You can sometimes also find pre-packaged bones at grocery stores.

MENSTRUAL PHASE BENEFITS

Rich in iron and minerals • High in protein • Abundant in collagen, gelatin, and amino acids • Slow cooked for maximum nutrient absorption and digestion

Gut-Healthy Bone Broth Hot Chocolate + Coconut Whipped Cream

PREP: 10 MINUTES COOK: 5 MINUTES SERVES 12

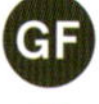

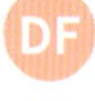

Creamy, dreamy, protein-rich, and delicious—this hot chocolate truly has it all. It's become one of my favorite menstrual phase rituals because not only does it taste indulgent, but the bone broth packs in collagen, gelatin, amino acids, and minerals that help to reduce inflammation and cramping, boost gut health and immune function, and promote a healthy, symptom-free period. I promise you do not taste the bone broth—but you do reap its amazing health benefits. It's perfect any time of day—cold mornings, as an afternoon pick-me-up, or as a post-dinner dessert. Try using your homemade bone broth (page 109) in this recipe, it's *so* good.

Coconut Whipped Cream

1 (13.5-ounce) can full-fat unsweetened coconut cream, chilled in the fridge for 24 hours (or see Note)

¼ cup organic confectioners' sugar (you can sub maple syrup, but it won't quite attain a super fluffy texture)

1 teaspoon pure vanilla extract

¼ teaspoon sea salt

Hot Chocolate Mix

1 cup organic cacao powder

1 cup coconut sugar

1 cup roughly chopped dark chocolate

2 tablespoons arrowroot starch

2 teaspoons cinnamon

1 teaspoon pure vanilla extract

½ teaspoon sea salt

Single Serving Hot Chocolate

¼ cup hot chocolate mix

¾ cup chicken bone broth

¾ cup organic whole milk or nondairy milk (try the Coconut Cashew Milk on page 274)

1 serving collagen peptides or protein powder (optional)

Coconut whipped cream and chocolate shavings, for serving

1. *For the coconut whipped cream:* Combine all the whipped cream ingredients in a large mixing bowl and whip with a handheld mixer (or a stand mixer) until fluffy. Store in an airtight container in the fridge until ready to use, up to 5 days.

2. *For the hot chocolate mix:* Combine all of the ingredients in a food processor and pulse until fine and well mixed; it should resemble a powder. Store in an airtight container in the pantry for 2 to 3 months.

3. *To make one serving:* Combine the hot chocolate mix, bone broth, and milk of choice in a small pot. Whisk over medium heat for 3 to 5 minutes, until the milk is thick and steaming and the mix is completely dissolved. Option to whisk in a scoop of collagen peptides or protein powder.

4. Serve with a generous dollop of coconut whipped cream and top with chocolate shavings.

NOTE: Instead of the coconut cream, you can chill two 13.5-ounce cans of coconut milk in the fridge for 24 hours, until the milk separates into solid on top and liquid at the bottom. Scoop out the solid cream and discard the liquid.

MENSTRUAL PHASE BENEFITS

Rich in minerals • High in protein • Abundant in collagen, gelatin, and amino acids

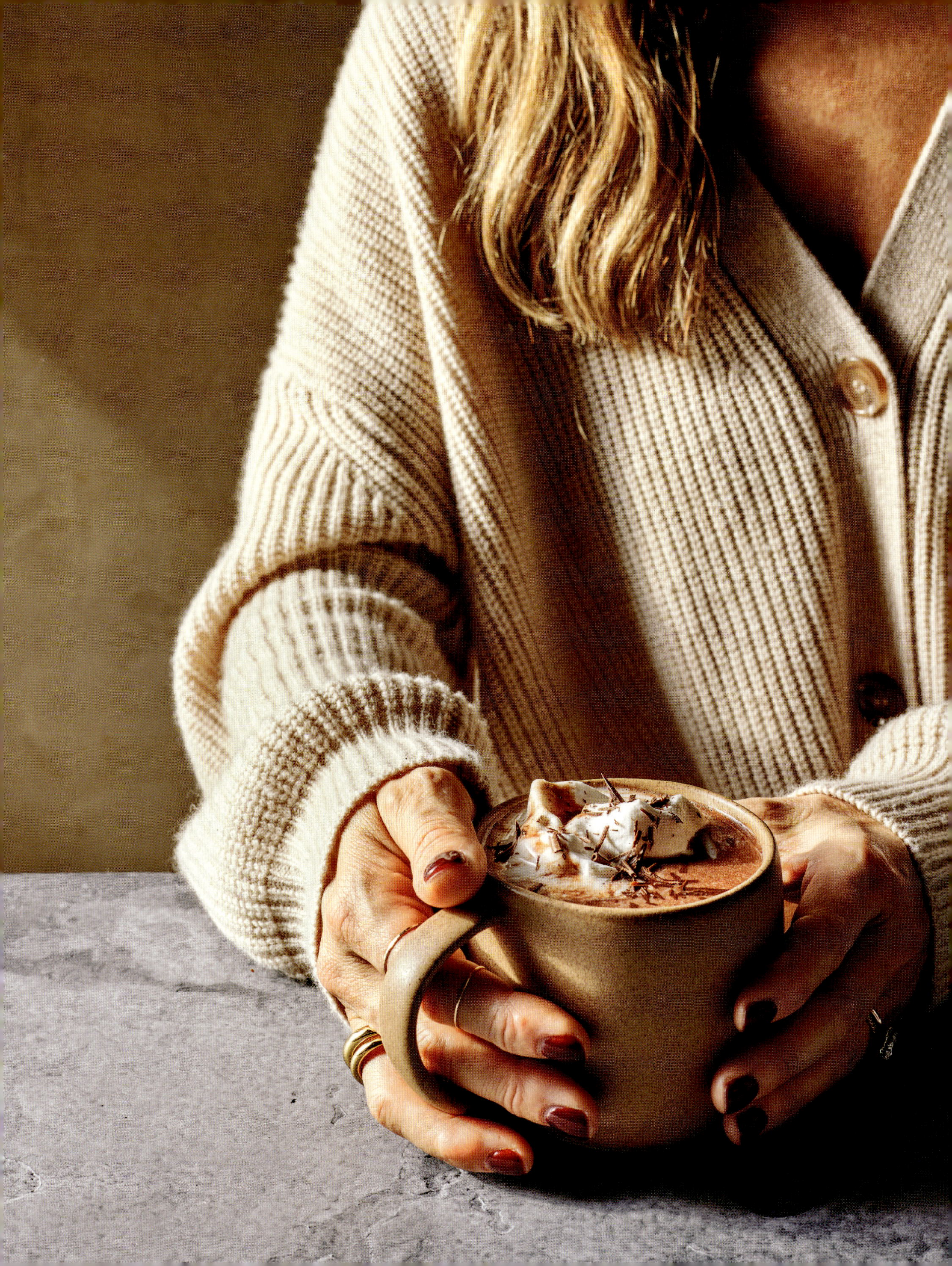

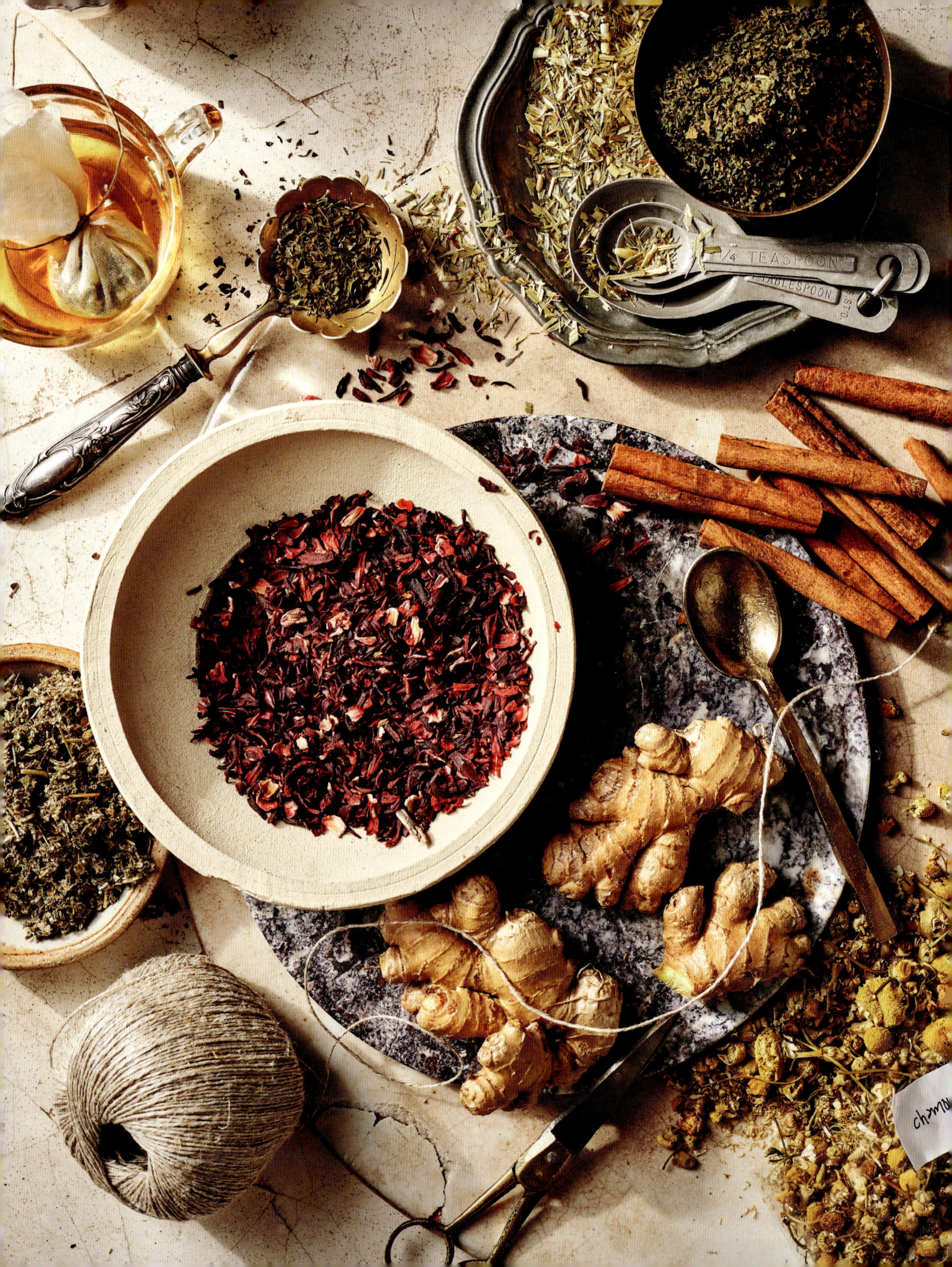
/4 TEASPOON
TABLESPOON

Hormone Healthy Herbal Infusion 4 Ways

PREP: 2 MINUTES COOK: 10 MINUTES MAKES 2 CUPS, OR 1 INDIVIDUAL SERVING

Incorporating herbs into your routine is a tradition that has been upheld for centuries across many cultures (think traditional Chinese medicine, Ayurvedic medicine, etc.) and one I think we could all continue to benefit from! I like to rotate herbs based on the phases of the menstrual cycle, with each herb uniquely suited to reduce common symptoms and promote hormonal harmony. Below you'll find the specific loose-leaf herbal formulas I use for each phase as well as how to brew them for optimal flavor and benefits.

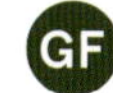
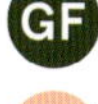
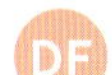
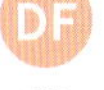
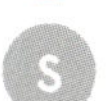

2 cups water

Herbal formula based on your cycle phase

Raw honey, squeeze of lemon, and nondairy milk or cream (optional)

Add the water to a pot or teakettle. Add the herbal blend to an infuser and place inside the pot. Cover with a lid and bring to a boil, then immediately remove from the heat and let steep for 5 to 10 minutes. Pour the liquid into a mug. Option to add raw honey, lemon, milk, or cream.

NOTE: I encourage buying herbs in loose-leaf form and brewing in a teapot with an infuser rather than using tea bags whenever possible. This ensures you're getting higher-quality herbs and a stronger, better flavor while avoiding microplastics that can leak into your tea from the bag itself. I like to purchase bulk herbs grown sustainably and organically, from brands such as Starwest Botanicals and Mountain Rose Herbs.

HERBAL FORMULAS

MENSTRUAL PHASE

- **Chamomile** to help reduce cramping and inflammation, aid in sleep and relaxation
- **Ginger** to reduce cramping and increase blood flow and circulation

Herbal blend: 1½ teaspoons chamomile flowers plus ½ teaspoon grated or minced fresh ginger per serving

FOLLICULAR PHASE

- **Nettle** to replenish minerals lost post-bleed and reduce excess estrogen (especially helpful for those with histamine issues or who feel symptomatic leading up to ovulation)
- **Oat straw**, a mineral-rich herb that nourishes the nervous system
- **Peppermint** or **spearmint** to help with high androgen levels (great for PCOS or those who struggle with acne during this phase)

Herbal blend: ¾ teaspoon of each herb per serving

OVULATORY PHASE

- **Nettle** to continue to replenish minerals and nourish your maturing egg
- **Hibiscus,** loaded with vitamin C and minerals that support a healthy ovulation

Herbal blend: 1 teaspoon nettle plus 1 teaspoon hibiscus per serving

LUTEAL PHASE

- **Red raspberry leaf** to tonify the uterine muscles and reduce cramping, water retention, and bloat
- **Oat straw** to support and ground the nervous system
- **Cinnamon** to promote optimal circulation and blood flow, and reduce clotting

Herbal blend: 1 teaspoon red raspberry leaf plus ¾ teaspoon oat straw plus ½ teaspoon freshly ground cinnamon (or substitute 1 cinnamon stick)

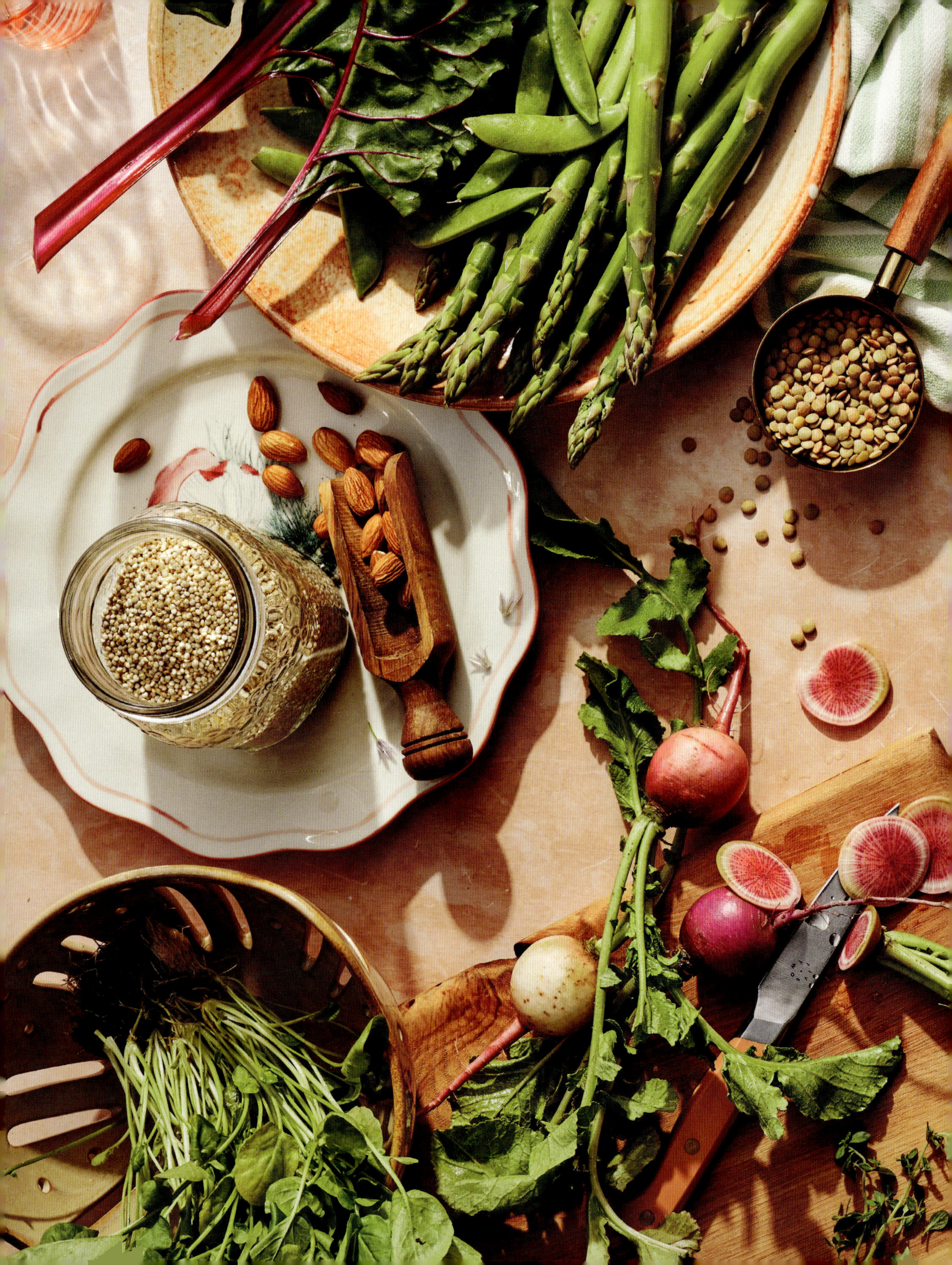

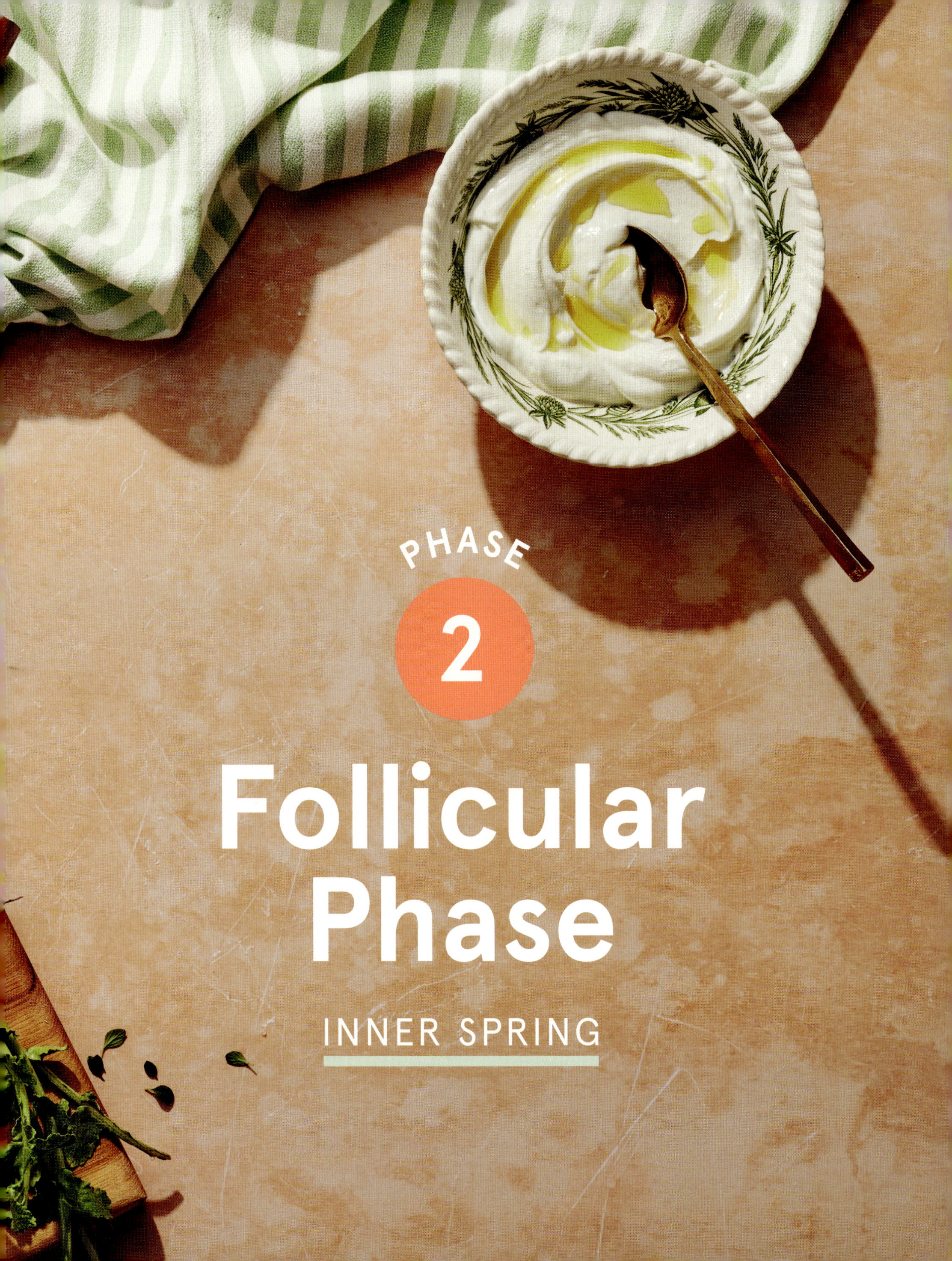

PHASE 2

Follicular Phase

INNER SPRING

RECIPES

WHAT'S HAPPENING

The follicular phase is a time of preparation, fresh starts, new beginnings, and major growth—in other words, peak spring vibes. This phase begins the day your period ends and lasts until ovulation, typically 7 to 10 days. At the start of the follicular phase, your pituitary gland releases a hormone called follicle stimulating hormone (FSH), which stimulates the follicles in one of the ovaries that contain your eggs to mature. Under normal circumstances, only one of these follicles will "ripen" and become mature. In response, the pituitary gland then starts to release luteinizing hormone, or LH, which is responsible for facilitating ovulation.

As the follicles grow, they produce increasing amounts of estrogen, a proliferative or "growth" hormone that signals to the endometrium to rebuild after menstruation, thickening it in preparation for a potential pregnancy. It also causes your cervix to soften, open, and produce wetter cervical fluid, designed to help sperm travel and survive the long journey to the egg.

Testosterone levels also rise, stimulating your libido to get you in the mood during your upcoming fertile window and bolstering your confidence. When hormones are balanced, this natural rise in estrogen and testosterone typically comes with a boost in energy, mood, and brain skills, helping you feel bolder, powerful, and willing to take more risks. On the flip side, if you're struggling with a hormonal imbalance, particularly excess estrogen in relation to progesterone, you might experience symptoms like pain or cramping during ovulation, as well as an influx of PMS-related symptoms during the latter half of your cycle.

Ultimately, you'll want to approach this phase as you would the spring season, by planting seeds (i.e., hormone-healthy habits) that will pay dividends during the rest of your cycle.

PILLARS OF EATING FOR YOUR FOLLICULAR PHASE

As mentioned above, this phase comes with a plethora of enjoyable benefits; however, it can also be a double-edged sword, particularly if estrogen levels remain too high in relation to progesterone levels. Thus, it's especially important to consume nutrients that support effective estrogen metabolism, along with optimized gut health, healthy liver function, egg maturation, and uterine lining growth.

Optimal Foods to Support Your Follicular Phase

HEALTHY FATS

During your follicular phase it's crucial to consume healthy fats as they play a direct role in ovarian hormone production, providing your body with the structural building blocks it needs to mature and release a follicle. These fats are also rich in micronutrients that support ovulatory function and overall menstrual cycle health. **They include:**

- Avocados and avocado oil
- Olives and olive oil
- Cod liver oil
- Nuts and seeds
- Full-fat dairy (grass-fed butter, ghee, yogurt, cream, etc.)
- Pasture-raised egg yolks
- Wild-caught fatty fish (salmon, sardines, mackerel, etc.)

CRUCIFEROUS VEGETABLES

During the follicular phase, estrogen levels naturally rise to thicken your uterine lining in preparation for a potential pregnancy. While estrogen production is important during this phase, excess levels can lead to uncomfortable symptoms later in your cycle, such as period pain, PMS, mood swings, weight gain, bloating, and depression. Cruciferous vegetables contain glucosinolates, sulfur-containing compounds rich in indole-3-carbinol, which helps your body safely remove harmful estrogen metabolites (i.e., excess estrogen) and works to keep symptoms at bay for the remainder of your cycle. **Optimal cruciferous vegetables to consume in your latter follicular phase and during ovulation include:**

- Broccoli
- Cauliflower
- Cabbage
- Kale
- Brussels sprouts
- Bok choy
- Arugula
- Watercress

LIVER-SUPPORTIVE FOODS

The liver plays a key role in detoxifying estrogen, as it is tasked with repackaging any leftover excess estrogen into an intestine-friendly form that can exit the body via the bowels. If you have a sluggish, overburdened liver, estrogen can sit in your intestines for too long and become reabsorbed, leading to excess estrogen. When you support liver function, you're also supporting estrogen metabolism and detoxification, which is essential during your follicular and ovulatory phases (when estrogen peaks). **Optimal liver-supportive foods include:**

- Raw carrots
- Cruciferous vegetables
- Broccoli sprouts
- Beets
- Green asparagus
- Dandelion greens
- Onion
- Garlic
- Leafy greens
- Turmeric
- Citrus

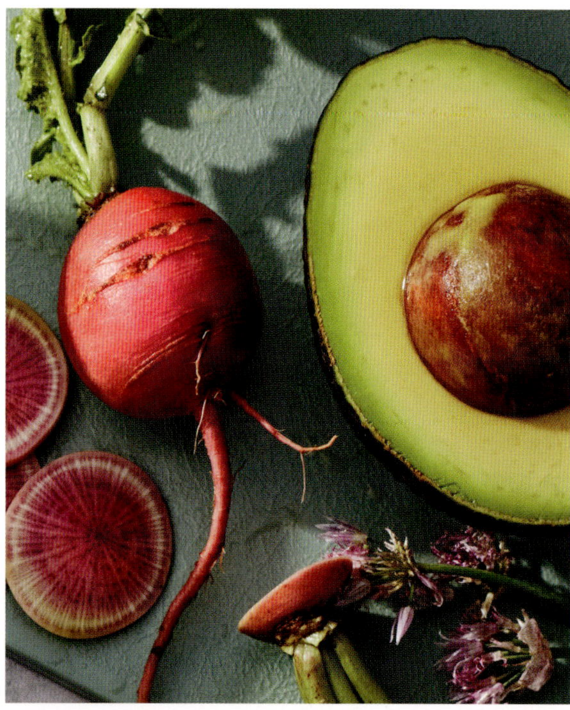

VITAMIN C–RICH FOODS

Eating a colorful, well-rounded diet rich in vitamin C–loaded raw fruits and vegetables helps to fight off free radicals and support liver detoxification, aiding in estrogen metabolism. **Optimal vitamin C–rich foods to incorporate into your follicular phase include:**

- Bell peppers
- Cruciferous vegetables
- Leafy greens
- Parsley
- Papaya and guava
- Dark-colored berries
- Citrus fruits

FERMENTED AND PROBIOTIC-RICH FOODS

Fermented and probiotic-rich foods support gut health, which also benefits our estrobolome, a unique set of bacteria in your gut that specifically works to break down estrogen and eliminate it safely via the bowels. **Fermented and probiotic-rich foods include:**

- Kimchi
- Sauerkraut
- Pickled vegetables
- Full-fat Greek or coconut yogurt
- Full-fat cottage cheese
- Kefir
- Organic non-GMO miso or tempeh
- Apple cider vinegar

FIBER-RICH FOODS

Another way to support estrogen elimination is by consuming enough dietary fiber, which helps flush excess estrogen safely via the bowels. Fiber helps draw water into the colon, adding bulk and softness to your stool, which helps it pass more smoothly through the digestive tract and increase transit time (byeeeee, constipation!). **Optimal fiber-rich foods to consume during your follicular and ovulatory phases include:**

- Avocado
- Cruciferous vegetables
- Artichokes
- Lentils/legumes
- Split peas
- Chia seeds and flaxseeds
- Leafy greens and green vegetables
- Gluten-free whole grains (quinoa, oats, millet, rice)
- Berries

PHYTOESTROGEN-RICH FOODS

Phytoestrogens are plant-based compounds that mimic the body's natural estrogen production. While you wouldn't want to consume these if you're experiencing symptoms of estrogen dominance, they can be beneficial to consume at the beginning of the follicular phase, when estrogen is lowest. *If you don't have problems with excess estrogen,* below are the **phytoestrogens I recommend consuming during the follicular phase:**

- Flaxseeds
- Pumpkin seeds
- Organic non-GMO soy products such as miso, tempeh, and soy in small amounts

HERBS AND SPICES

Herbs have long been used in traditional Chinese medicine (TCM) to help replenish the post-period body with minerals. Certain herbs like nettle can help to reduce high estrogen levels, while spearmint can regulate androgen levels, making these herbs especially beneficial if you struggle with symptoms like bloating, cramping or pain, and acne during this phase. **These herbs include:**

- Nettle
- Oat straw
- Spearmint and peppermint
- Schisandra
- Holy basil
- Dandelion
- Maca
- Turmeric

Cooking and Eating Tips to Support Your Follicular Phase

INCORPORATE MORE FRESH AND RAW FOODS

According to TCM, your follicular and ovulatory phases are "hot" phases of your cycle as your resting body temperature naturally rises. Opt for more raw fresh vegetables and fruits that have a natural cooling effect on the body during this phase—think foods you'd gravitate toward naturally in the spring such as leafy green salads, smoothies, crudités, and astringent and bitter vegetables. These foods are also loaded with antioxidants that promote optimal vascular support and egg quality.

USE LIGHTER COOKING METHODS

Following TCM guidelines (above), when cooking your food during this phase it's best to opt for lighter methods such as steaming, poaching, blanching, and sautéing. This helps to preserve the antioxidants and nutrients in most of the fruits and vegetables recommended for this phase. These foods tend to be lighter—as opposed to more grounding plants like potatoes and squash—and are easier to digest when cooked well at higher temperatures.

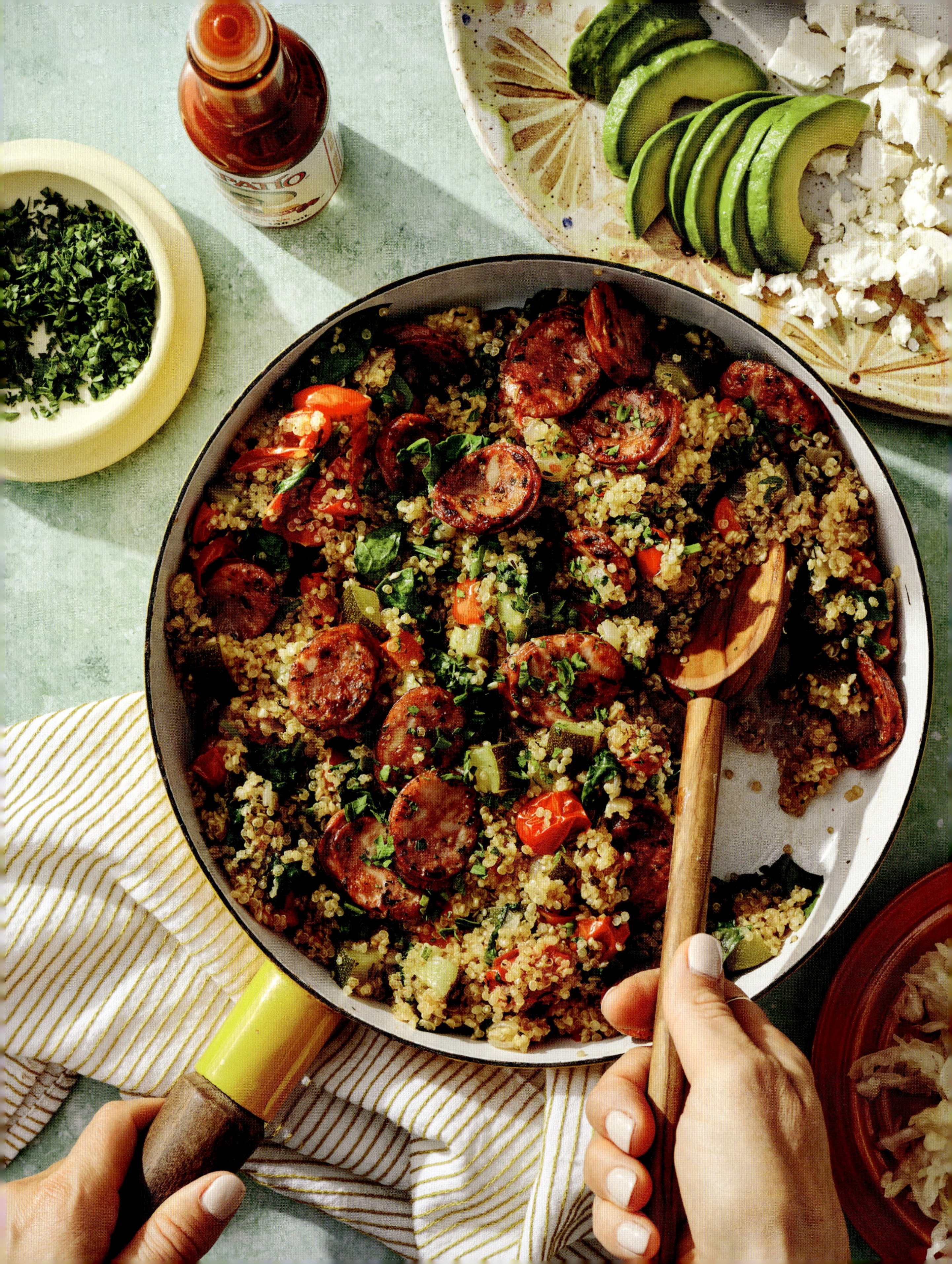

Savory Egg-Free Quinoa Breakfast Skillet

PREP: 15 MINUTES   COOK: 35 MINUTES   SERVES 4

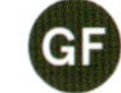
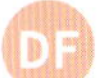
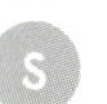
BF

It can be tough to find a savory breakfast option that doesn't have eggs, which even I need a break from every now and then. Enter this skillet meal, which is seriously satisfying, packed with protein, and incredibly delicious. It makes a huge portion, so it's great to feed a crowd, or to meal prep for quick heat-and-eat breakfasts throughout the week (see Note). It's also tasty for lunch or dinner.

- **2 tablespoons avocado oil**
- **½ yellow onion, diced**
- **4 cloves garlic, minced**
- **1 large zucchini, diced**
- **1 red bell pepper, seeded and diced**
- **1 cup cherry tomatoes, halved**
- **1 cup uncooked quinoa or millet**
- **1½ cups bone broth (use the Super Simple Homemade Bone Broth on page 109)**
- **1 tablespoon Italian seasoning**
- **1 teaspoon sea salt**
- **Black pepper to taste**
- **12 ounces fully cooked chicken sausage links, sliced into thin rounds**
- **2 cups spinach, chopped**
- **Sliced avocado, minced flat-leaf parsley, crumbled feta, sauerkraut, and hot sauce for topping (optional)**

1. Heat the avocado oil in a large skillet over medium heat. Add the onion and sauté for 3 to 5 minutes, until translucent. Add the garlic and sauté another minute, until fragrant. Stir in the zucchini and bell pepper and cook for 5 minutes, stirring frequently, until the vegetables have softened.

2. Add the tomatoes and quinoa, then pour in the bone broth and sprinkle with the Italian seasoning, salt, and pepper. Add the chicken sausage rounds and stir until everything is well mixed. Cover with a lid and bring to a boil. Reduce to a simmer and cook for 25 minutes, until the liquid is fully absorbed. Stir in the chopped spinach and cook for another 1 to 2 minutes, until wilted.

3. Spoon into bowls and finish with optional toppings of choice.

NOTE: If making this as a weekday breakfast option, I like to prepare it the night before or during the weekend as the cooking time up front is somewhat involved. However, the result is plenty of leftovers you can store in an airtight container for up to 5 days in the fridge and quickly reheat as needed.

FOLLICULAR PHASE BENEFITS

Supports estrogen detoxification • Rich in fiber • Rich in probiotics • High in protein • High in antioxidants

Protein PB&J Overnight Oats

PREP: 5 MINUTES, PLUS OVERNIGHT CHILLING COOK: 10 MINUTES SERVES 2

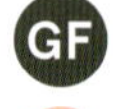
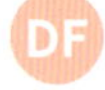

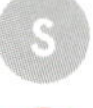

Overnight oats are one of my go-to breakfasts when I know I have an extra busy morning or day ahead of me. I love to sneak in plenty of protein to keep my blood sugar and energy stable, and this simple recipe packs in 30 grams per serving. It also contains plenty of probiotics and fiber to assist your gut in breaking down and eliminating excess estrogen, working to prevent PMS later in your cycle. No one would ever guess, based on taste alone (nostalgic! creamy! delicious!), that it's a nutritional powerhouse, and the kids love it too.

Overnight Oats

1¼ cups almond milk (or other nondairy milk, such as cashew)

½ cup full-fat unsweetened Greek yogurt (or coconut yogurt to make it dairy-free)

1 to 2 servings vanilla protein powder of choice

2 to 4 tablespoons pure maple syrup (start with 2, then add more if you find it still needs sweetener)

2 tablespoons chia seeds

1 teaspoon pure vanilla extract

¼ teaspoon sea salt

1 cup gluten-free protein oats (or sprouted oats)

2 to 4 tablespoons unsweetened creamy organic peanut butter

Fresh berries (strawberries, raspberries, or blueberries), for topping

Berry Chia Jam

2 cups fresh or frozen raspberries or strawberries

2 tablespoons chia seeds

2 tablespoons pure maple syrup

1 tablespoon fresh lemon juice (or water)

1. *For the oats:* Whisk together the almond milk, yogurt, protein powder, 2 tablespoons maple syrup, chia seeds, vanilla, and salt in a medium mixing bowl until combined. Stir in the oats, cover with a lid, and chill overnight in the fridge. This will create a thick and creamy texture as the oats absorb the liquid.

2. *For the jam:* While the oats are chilling, cook the berries in a small pot over medium-high heat, stirring and mashing until the fruit begins to break down and bubble, 3 to 5 minutes. Stir in the chia seeds, maple syrup, and lemon juice and bring to a simmer for another 3 to 5 minutes, until the mixture has thickened and reached a jammy consistency. Let cool, then store in an airtight glass jar in the fridge for up to 1 week.

3. Taste the oats and add more maple syrup if they need sweetening. Scoop the oats into two bowls or jars and layer on the peanut butter, berry chia jam, and fresh berries.

NOTES: If you're looking to save time, you can use store-bought jam in place of making your own, just make sure to avoid refined sugar and fillers if possible. Additionally, if you want to make overnight oats without the protein powder, you can leave it out but reduce the nondairy milk to 1 cup to achieve the perfect texture.

FOLLICULAR PHASE BENEFITS

Supports estrogen detoxification • High in healthy fats • Rich in fiber • Rich in probiotics • High in protein • High in antioxidants

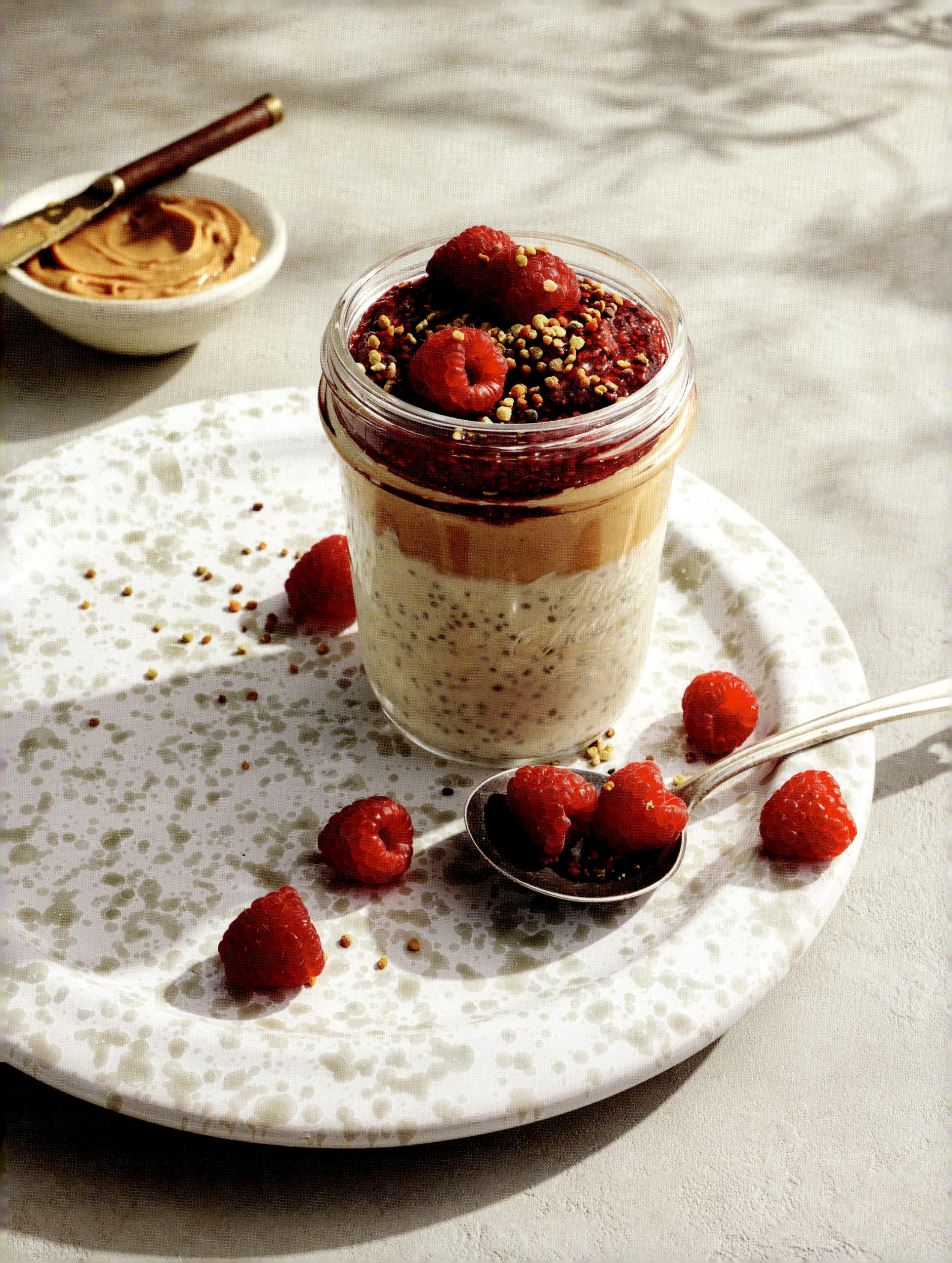

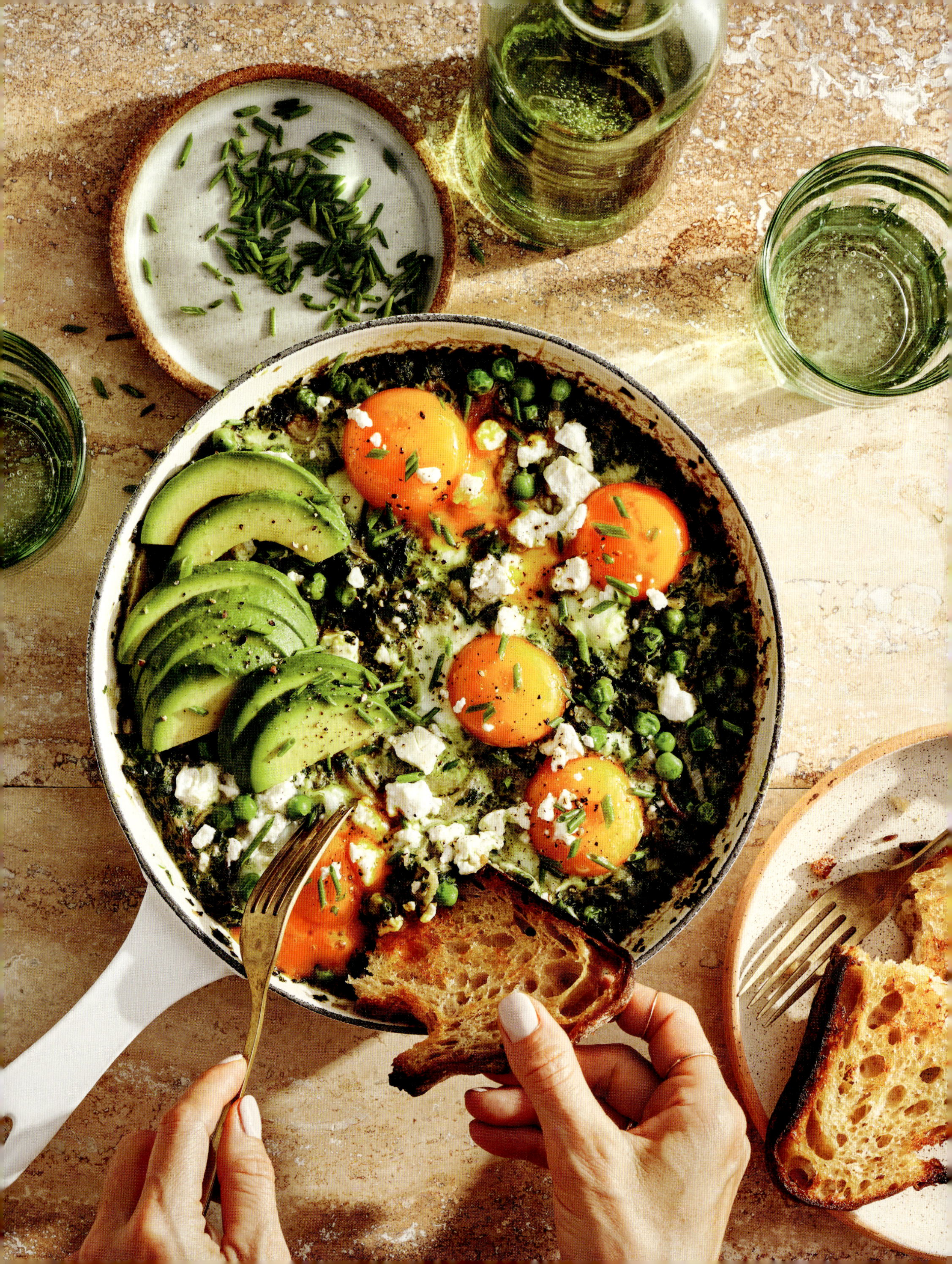

Dippy Spring Green Egg Skillet

PREP: 10 MINUTES   COOK: 15 MINUTES   SERVES 2–4

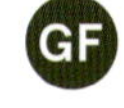

Many years ago, my hubby and I visited the Greek islands and discovered an adorable tiny cafe with the most delicious green shakshuka. It was my first time trying the dish, a Middle Eastern breakfast of eggs poached in a verdant, herby sauce, and it was unforgettable. This recipe is my attempt to pay homage, and while it's not quite a traditional shakshuka, it's seriously satisfying, with a bright and creamy green sauce (loaded with antioxidant-rich greens, alliums, and herbs that support liver detoxification), hunks of salty feta cheese, and yolky eggs (packed with nutrients required to develop a healthy follicle!)—perfect for dipping toast into.

- **4 tablespoons grass-fed ghee, divided**
- **1 large leek, white part only, thinly sliced into rounds (if not available, use 1 small shallot, minced)**
- **1 large bunch Swiss chard, leaves torn from stems and rinsed**
- **¼ cup fresh flat-leaf parsley leaves**
- **¼ cup nondairy milk or cream (almond, coconut, etc.)**
- **½ teaspoon sea salt, plus more for serving**
- **Black pepper to taste**
- **1 small fennel bulb or 2 green onions (white and green parts only, thinly sliced)**
- **1 cup frozen organic peas, thawed**
- **6 large pasture-raised eggs**
- **½ cup feta cheese, crumbled into large chunks**
- **2 tablespoons chopped fresh chives, for topping**
- **Sliced avocado, for serving**
- **Extra virgin olive oil, for serving**
- **Gluten-free toast, for serving**

1. Bring a medium pot of salted water to a boil.

2. Melt 2 tablespoons of the ghee in a large stovetop skillet over medium heat. Add the leek and sauté for 5 to 10 minutes, until softened. Remove from the heat and let cool.

3. While the leek is cooking, add the Swiss chard and parsley to the boiling water and blanch for 10 seconds, then immediately transfer to ice water to cool.

4. In a food processor, combine the cooked leeks, blanched greens, nondairy milk or cream, salt, and pepper. Pulse until a thick and creamy paste has formed.

5. Melt 1 tablespoon of the ghee in the skillet over medium heat. Add the fennel or green onions and sauté until softened, 5 or so minutes. Add the remaining 1 tablespoon ghee and spread the vegetables around the bottom of the pan. Pour in the green sauce, stir in the peas, and spread the sauce evenly over the pan.

6. Use a large spoon or spatula to make six small divots in the sauce. One at a time, crack the eggs and add them to the divots. Crumble the feta cheese on top and sprinkle with more salt. Cover and cook for 4 to 5 minutes. The egg whites should be opaque, and the yolks should still be runny. Remove from the heat, sprinkle with the chives, top with sliced avocado, and drizzle with extra virgin olive oil.

7. To serve, either dish individual portions onto the toast on serving plates, or simply dip the toast directly into the skillet, soaking up the sauce and egg yolks—my favorite way to eat, plus so fun as a family-style dish!

FOLLICULAR PHASE BENEFITS

Supports liver function • Supports estrogen detoxification • High in healthy fats • High in antioxidants

Creamy Chia Pudding 3 Ways

PREP: 5 MINUTES, PLUS OVERNIGHT CHILLING   COOK: NONE   SERVES 3

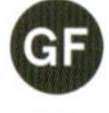
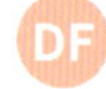

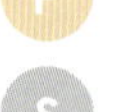

Chia pudding is a legit breakfast staple of mine. This prep-ahead breakfast option is light but filling, nutrient-packed, and creamy and delicious, especially with a good topping situation. It's ideal during the follicular phase thanks to the high amount of dietary fiber (10 grams per 2 tablespoons!), which helps flush out excess estrogen that could negatively affect the latter half of your cycle. I rotate between all three flavors outlined below, and you really can't go wrong with any of them. Note that you need to prepare the pudding the night before (or a minimum of 8 hours) to give it enough time to gel in the fridge and achieve an ideal creamy, pudding-like texture.

Chia Pudding Base

1 (13.5-ounce) can full-fat unsweetened coconut milk (or 1¾ cups other creamy nondairy milk, like cashew)

2 to 4 tablespoons pure maple syrup

½ teaspoon sea salt

1 to 2 servings protein powder of choice (if sweetened you may want less maple syrup), optional

½ cup chia seeds

Classic Vanilla Chia Pudding

1 teaspoon pure vanilla extract

Super Chocolatey Chia Pudding

¼ cup cacao powder

Bright Berry Chia Pudding

1 cup organic blueberries, raspberries, or strawberries, rinsed and drained

Seed-Cycle Maple Cinnamon Granola (page 65), creamy nut butter, chopped nuts and seeds, fresh berries, sliced banana, bee pollen, cacao nibs, drizzle of honey, etc., for topping (optional)

1. *For the pudding base:* Combine the coconut milk, 2 tablespoons of the maple syrup, salt, and protein powder (if using) in a medium bowl and whisk until completely smooth. Test for sweetness and add more maple syrup if preferred.

2. *For the classic vanilla or super chocolatey pudding:* Add the vanilla extract *or* cacao powder, then stir in the chia seeds. Pour into an airtight glass jar and let sit for 10 minutes. Give it another stir (this helps to prevent clumping). Refrigerate to let gel overnight.

3. *For the bright berry pudding:* Transfer the coconut milk mixture to a blender, add the berries, and mix until creamy and smooth (or use an immersion blender directly in the bowl). Stir in the chia seeds, then pour into glass jars with airtight lids and refrigerate to let gel overnight.

4. When ready to serve, scoop a large portion (about ½ cup) into a bowl and top with desired toppings. For the chocolate pudding, I especially love peanut butter, banana, and cacao nibs. For the vanilla, I go for granola, fresh berries, and coconut shavings. And for the berries, I like bee pollen, chopped pistachios, and almond butter.

NOTE: If you need a quick breakfast or snack on the go, try pre-portioning into individual glass jars with airtight lids.

FOLLICULAR PHASE BENEFITS

Supports estrogen detoxification • High in healthy fats • Rich in fiber • High in antioxidants

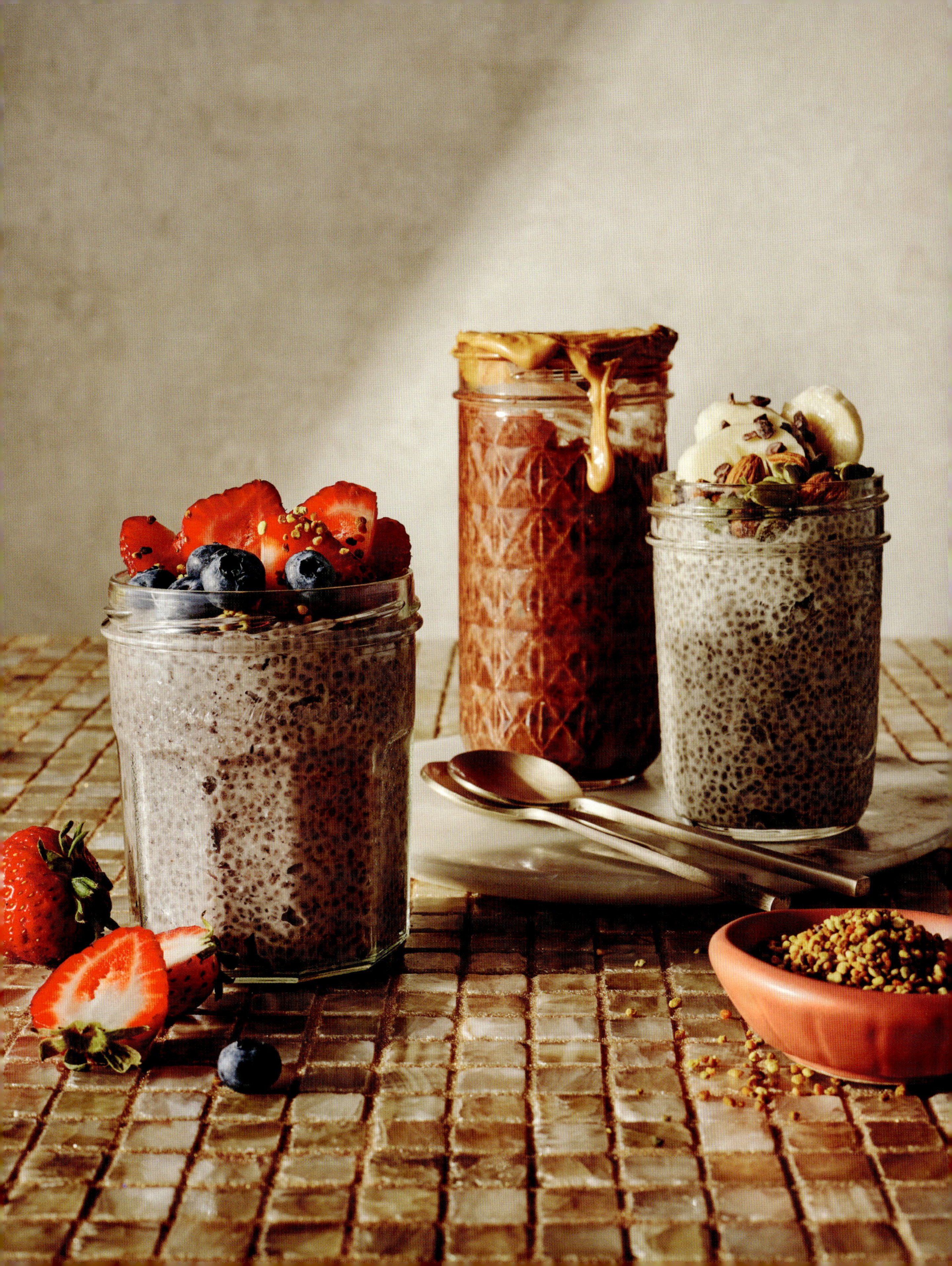

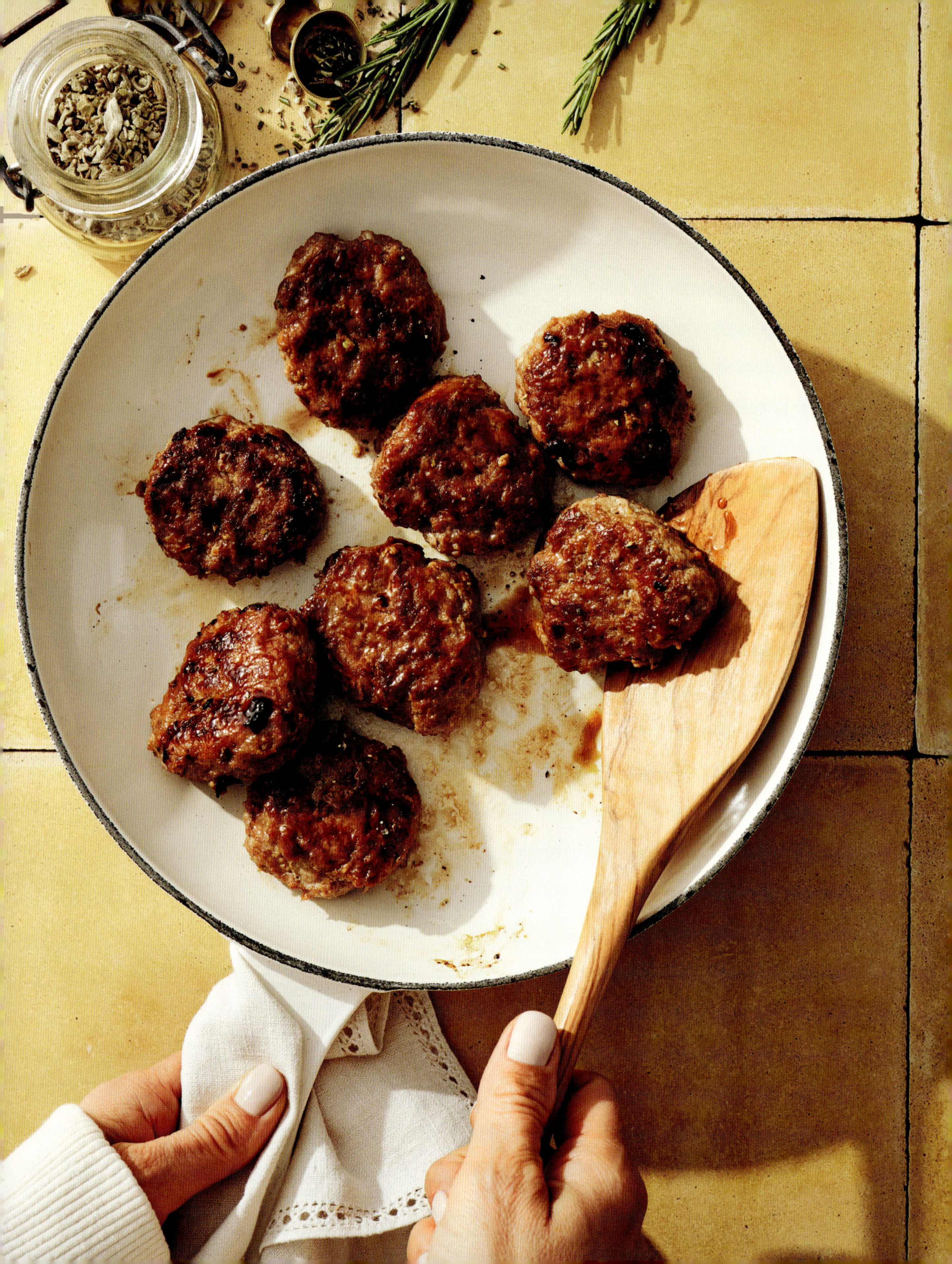

Sticky Maple Turkey Breakfast Sausage

PREP: 10 MINUTES COOK: 15 MINUTES SERVES 10–12

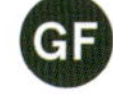

DF

One of my go-to hacks to sneak in more protein is breakfast sausage. This recipe is incredibly flavorful (savory with the perfect hint of sweet) and naturally high in protein (about 20 grams in two or three small patties), which supports everything from optimal blood sugar to the facilitation of tissue and muscle growth (key for rebuilding your uterine lining post-period and firing up your metabolism!). I love to make a big batch of patties and store them in the freezer for 2 to 3 months for a quick reheat-and-eat option on busy mornings.

- **1 pound organic ground turkey thighs (you can substitute ground turkey breast, but it tends to be drier)**
- **¼ cup pure maple syrup**
- **1 teaspoon poultry seasoning**
- **1 teaspoon sea salt**
- **1 teaspoon smoked paprika**
- **1 teaspoon garlic powder**
- **½ teaspoon cinnamon**
- **½ teaspoon dried sage**
- **3 sprigs fresh rosemary, needles minced**
- **2 tablespoons grass-fed ghee or avocado oil, for frying**

1. Combine all the ingredients except the ghee or avocado oil in a medium mixing bowl using your hands (I like to wear gloves for this). Form into 10 to 12 balls (a little larger than the size of a golf ball).

2. Heat the ghee in a large stovetop pan over medium heat until the pan is hot and the ghee is melted. In batches if necessary, add the sausage balls and use a spatula to mash each ball to form more of a patty. Cook for 2 to 3 minutes on each side, until the internal temperature reaches 165°F. Remove from the pan, then serve or let cool to room temperature and store in an airtight container in the fridge for up to 5 days or in the freezer for 2 to 3 months.

FOLLICULAR PHASE BENEFITS

Protein-rich

Herby Egg Salad Bagel Sandwich

PREP: 5 MINUTES COOK: 10 MINUTES SERVES 1

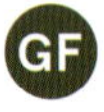

V

Egg salad isn't for everyone, but if you love it, then you're going to *love* this herby version. The pickles add crunch and probiotics that work to boost gut health and support estrogen elimination, while the eggs themselves are rich in both macro- and micronutrients that support follicle maturation and ovulatory function. This recipe is on our regular lunch rotation, and while I prefer the egg salad on a toasted everything bagel, it's also delicious on bread, in lettuce wraps, or served in a bowl with crackers and crudités for dipping.

3 large pasture-raised eggs

1 tablespoon apple cider vinegar

1 medium dill pickle, *fermented if possible,* diced (about ¼ cup)

1 tablespoon minced fresh chives

1 tablespoon minced fresh dill

2 tablespoons avocado oil mayonnaise (or ½ small avocado, mashed)

1 teaspoon Dijon mustard

¼ teaspoon sea salt

Black pepper to taste

Red pepper flakes to taste

Gluten-free everything bagel, halved

Extra virgin olive oil or ghee

Sliced avocado, thinly sliced radish, microgreens, and hemp seeds, for topping

1. Add water to a small pot and use a large slotted spoon to gently add the eggs (you don't want the shells to break). Cover and bring to a boil, then immediately remove from the heat. Let sit in the hot water for 5 to 6 minutes. Remove with the slotted spoon and place in a bowl of ice water combined with the apple cider vinegar to cool (the vinegar will help with the peeling process).

2. Remove the shells from the eggs and chop into pieces. In a small bowl, combine the eggs, pickle, chives, dill, mayonnaise, mustard, salt, black pepper, and red pepper, stirring well with a spoon.

3. Toast the bagel and smooth on some olive oil or ghee, then place the sliced avocado on one side of the toasted bagel. Add the egg salad to the other half of the bagel and top with sliced radish and microgreens, sprinkle with hemp seeds, then sandwich the two halves together.

FOLLICULAR PHASE BENEFITS

High in healthy fats • Rich in probiotics • Supports estrogen elimination

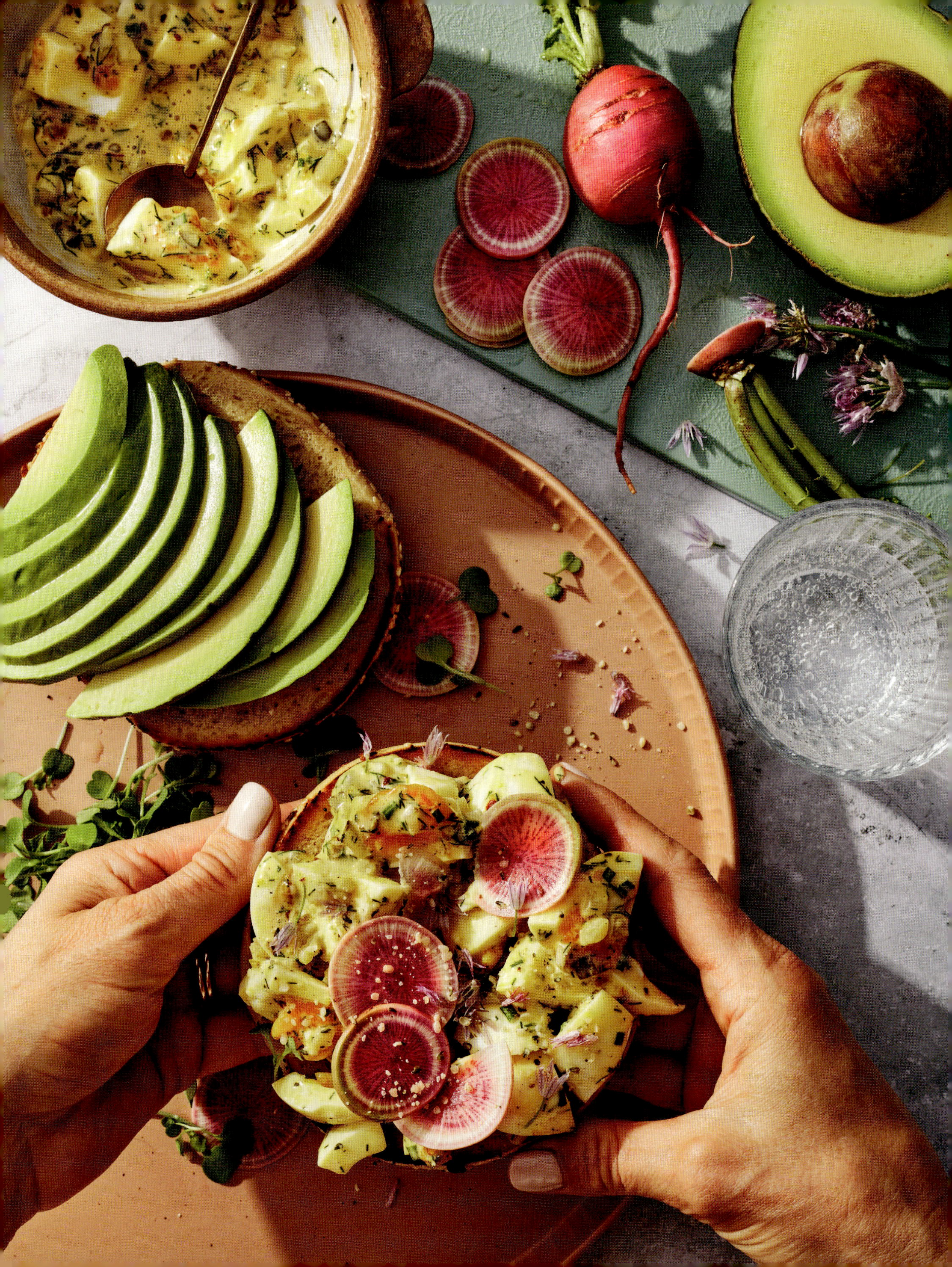

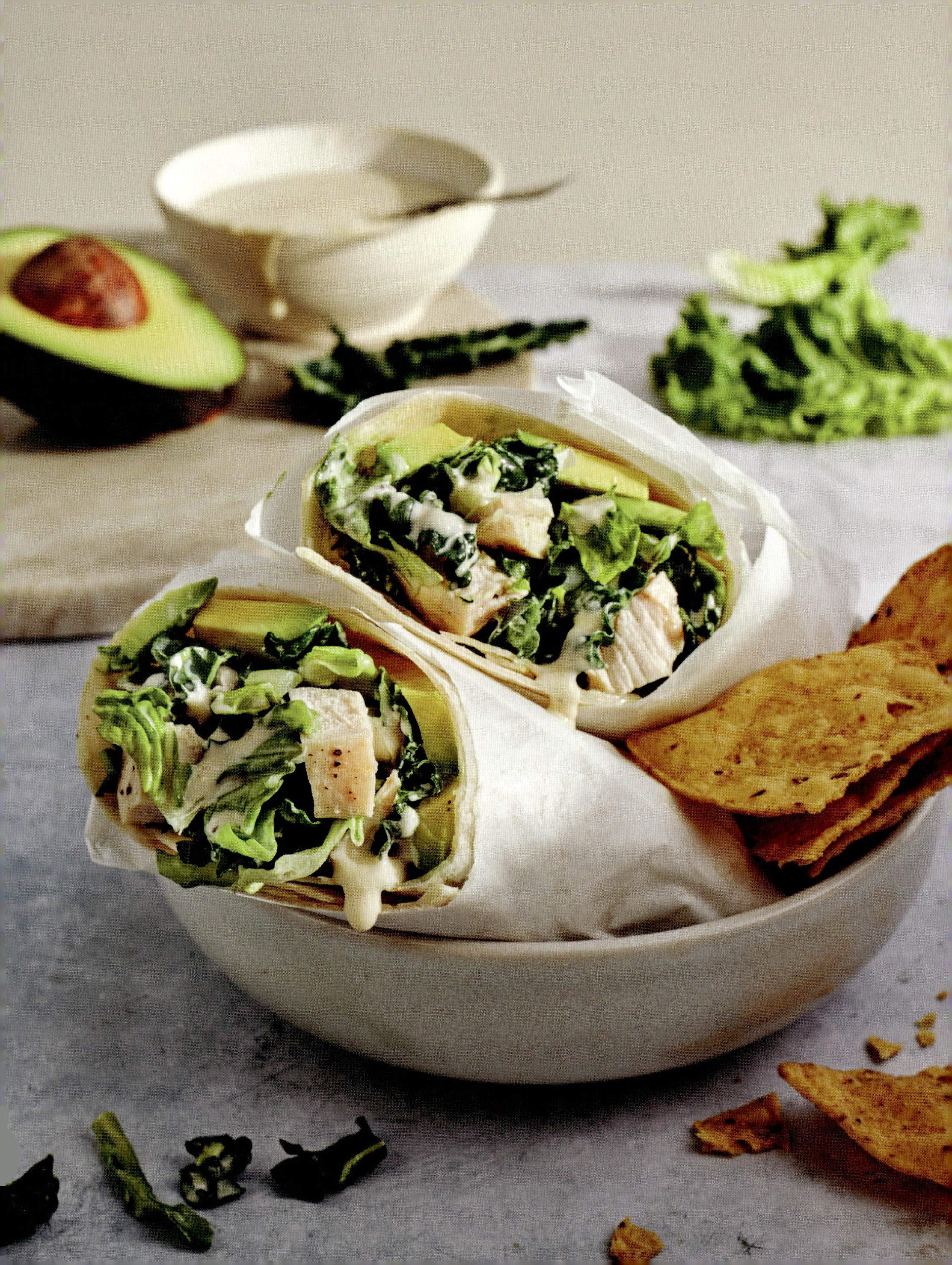

Speedy Chicken Caesar Salad Wraps

PREP: 15 MINUTES   COOK: 5 MINUTES   SERVES 2

I combined two of my ultimate lunch loves (chicken Caesar salad and wraps) to create this wrap, and I have zero regrets. It's incredibly tasty and satisfying thanks to the creamy, tangy miso dressing, which sneaks in probiotics that support your gut in breaking down and eliminating excess estrogen. This is the ideal quick meal on the go, making it great for busy weekdays or the weekend adventures (hikes! road trips!) you may feel like embarking on in your follicular phase.

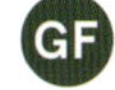

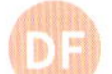

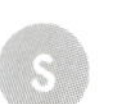

BF

Miso Caesar Dressing

- **½ cup avocado oil mayonnaise (or full-fat Greek yogurt)**
- **2 tablespoons miso**
- **2 tablespoons extra virgin olive oil**
- **Juice of 1 large lemon (about 3 tablespoons)**
- **2 cloves garlic, minced**
- **1 teaspoon anchovy paste**
- **¼ teaspoon sea salt**
- **Black pepper to taste**

Wraps

- **½ small head romaine lettuce, rinsed, drained, and chopped**
- **4 leaves dinosaur kale, torn from the stems, rinsed, drained, and chopped**
- **1 large rotisserie chicken breast, diced**
- **Grated Parmesan or vegan Parmesan for topping (optional)**
- **2 large burrito-sized gluten-free tortillas of choice (I like wraps made from cassava or sprouted brown rice)**
- **½ avocado, pitted, peeled, and sliced**

1. *For the dressing:* Whisk together all the ingredients in a small bowl until creamy and well combined and set aside.

2. *For the wraps:* Combine the romaine, kale, chicken, and Parmesan (if using) in a bowl, pour the dressing over, and toss to combine well.

3. Warm the tortillas on the stove, either briefly over an open flame or in a dry skillet (this makes them more pliable and easier to wrap). Place each tortilla on a piece of parchment paper and mash the avocado slices in the centers. Divide the kale/romaine/chicken mixture between the two wraps, adding it in the center on top of the avocado.

4. Fold the right and left sides of one tortilla inward, 1 to 2 inches over the salad filling. Fold the bottom of the tortilla over the filling, keeping the sides tucked in and pulling the bottom flap taut as you roll one or two more times until the wrap is secured. Then, roll the wrap in the parchment paper until covered, tucking in the sides. Repeat with the second wrap. Slice each in half and enjoy.

NOTE: While the parchment paper isn't mandatory, I find it helps to keep the wrap intact while you're enjoying it.

FOLLICULAR PHASE BENEFITS

Supports estrogen detoxification • High in healthy fats • Rich in probiotics • High in antioxidants

Blackened Fish Tacos and Cabbage Slaw + Avocado Lime Crema

PREP: 30 MINUTES COOK: 10 MINUTES SERVES 4

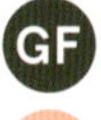
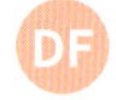
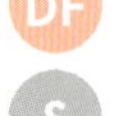

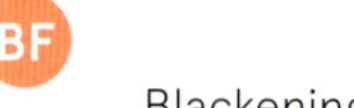

Taco night is a weekly occurrence in our house, and I'm always making this festive and flavorful version during my follicular phase, when I'm craving light, fresh, nutrient-rich foods. The crunchy cabbage slaw contains compounds that support estrogen and liver detoxification, while the avocado crema adds tang and healthy fats to support follicle growth and ovulation. I like to pan-sear the fish in the winter and grill it in the summer—either way you can't go wrong!

Blackening Spice Mix and Fish

- **1 tablespoon smoked paprika**
- **2 teaspoons ancho chile powder**
- **1 teaspoon cumin**
- **1 teaspoon coriander**
- **1 teaspoon garlic powder**
- **1 teaspoon onion powder**
- **1 teaspoon sea salt**
- **1 teaspoon oregano**
- **½ teaspoon cayenne pepper**
- **1½ pounds wild-caught cod fillets or other flaky white fish**

Avocado Lime Crema

- **1 large ripe avocado, pitted, peeled, and chopped**
- **½ cup full-fat organic sour cream (or coconut yogurt or lactose-free yogurt)**
- **¼ cup cilantro leaves, roughly chopped**
- **Juice of 1 large lime (about 2 tablespoons)**
- **1 teaspoon sea salt**

Slaw

- **½ red cabbage, cored and shredded**
- **1 large carrot, peeled and shredded**
- **½ cup cilantro leaves, chopped**
- **2 tablespoons extra virgin olive oil**
- **Juice of 1 large lime (about 2 tablespoons)**
- **Sea salt and black pepper to taste**

- **2 tablespoons grass-fed ghee or avocado oil**
- **8 organic corn or grain-free tortillas (such as almond flour, cassava, etc.)**
- **Cotija cheese and limes for serving (optional)**

1. *For the blackening spice mix and fish:* Mix all the spices together in a small bowl until well combined. Slice the fish into 1-inch-thick fillets and generously rub the blackening spice all over. Let the fish sit for 30 minutes in the spice mixture in the fridge while you prep the rest of the ingredients.

2. *For the avocado lime crema:* Combine all the ingredients in a blender or food processor and mix until creamy and smooth. Set aside in the fridge until ready to serve.

3. *For the slaw:* In a bowl, toss the cabbage, carrot, and cilantro together. Drizzle with the olive oil and lime juice and season with salt and pepper. Toss with spoons or salad tongs until well combined. Set aside.

4. *To cook the fish:* Heat the ghee or avocado oil in a large skillet over medium-high heat, tilting the pan evenly to coat. Add the seasoned cod fillets and cook for 3 minutes, then gently flip and cook for another 2 to 3 minutes, until they are cooked through and the internal temperature reaches 145°F. Remove from the heat.

5. *For the tacos:* Warm the tortillas (I like to do this over an open stovetop flame on medium heat, warming about 1 minute per side, but you can also do it in a pan, microwave, etc.). Generously spread the avocado crema on top of each warmed tortilla, then add the blackened fillets and top with the slaw and optional cotija cheese. Serve with more crema and lime wedges.

NOTE: You can save time by buying a packaged taco spice mix (I like the ones from Siete) as well as a shredded cabbage slaw.

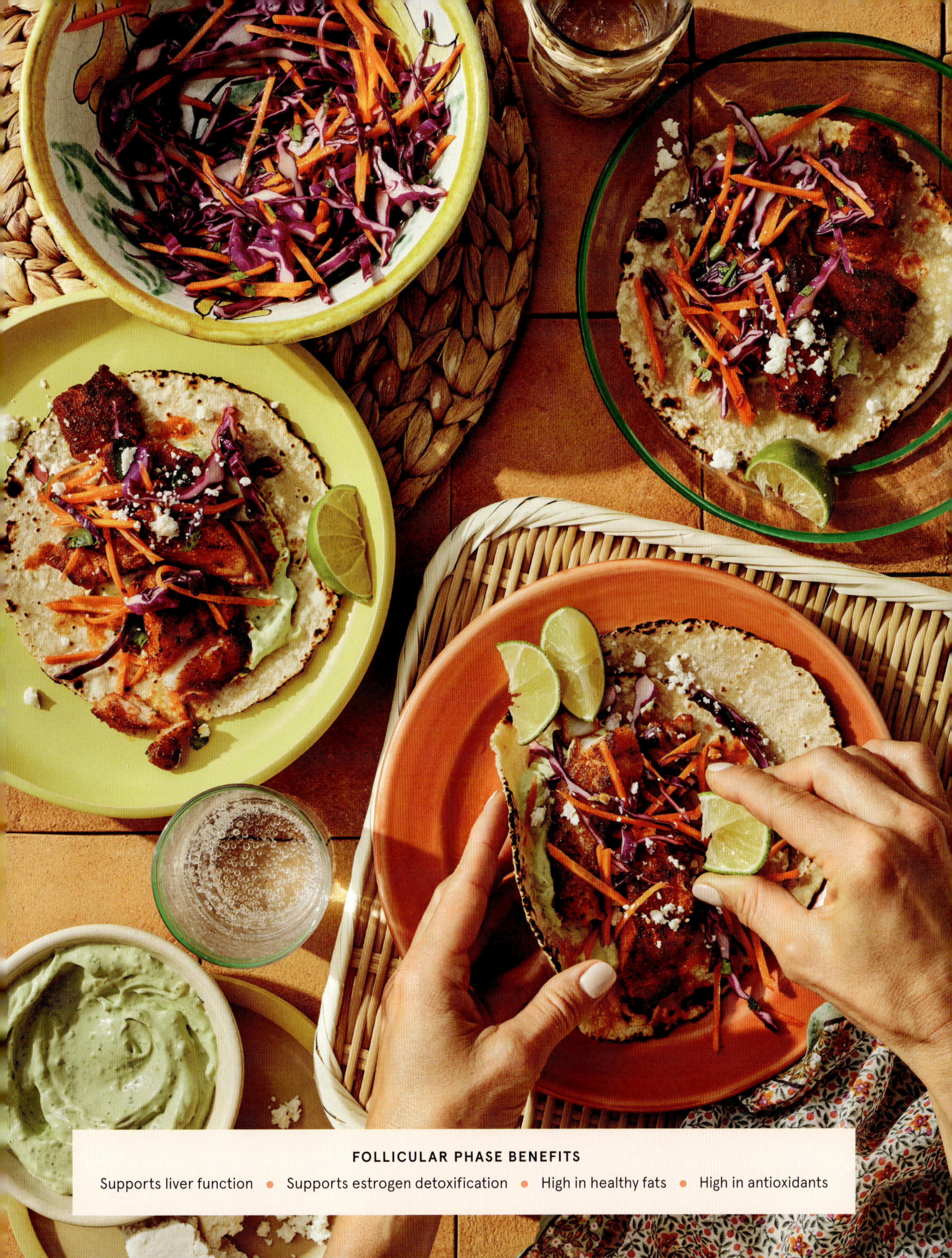

FOLLICULAR PHASE BENEFITS

Supports liver function • Supports estrogen detoxification • High in healthy fats • High in antioxidants

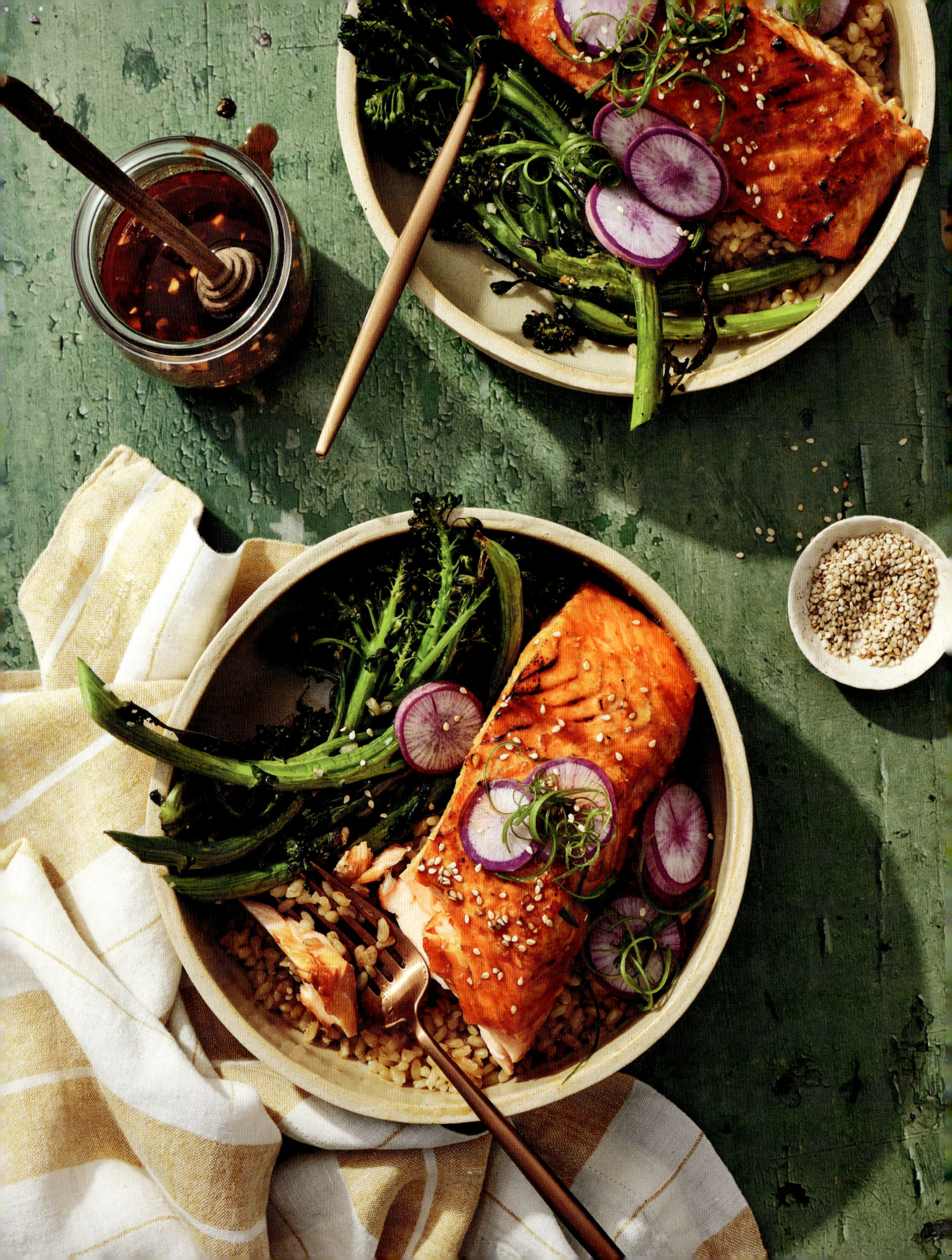

Honey-Chipotle Glazed Salmon Bowls

PREP: 15 MINUTES COOK: 12 MINUTES SERVES 2

This delicious bowl satisfies so many nutrient needs during your energy-intensive follicular phase! I love serving salmon with broccolini, a cruciferous vegetable that assists our body in safely eliminating any excess estrogen (which if left unchecked can lead to PMS), but any cruciferous or liver-supportive vegetable (such as bok choy, carrots, beets, and Brussels sprouts) would also be tasty and functional.

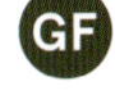

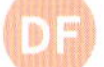

Rice

- **1 cup brown rice, rinsed three times in cold water and drained**
- **2 cups bone broth (try using the Super Simple Homemade Bone Broth on page 109)**

Honey-Chipotle Marinade

- **2 tablespoons raw honey**
- **1 to 2 tablespoons chipotle in adobo sauce (to taste, depending on spice tolerance/ preference)**
- **1 tablespoon coconut aminos**
- **Juice of ½ medium lime (1½ teaspoons)**
- **1½ teaspoons unseasoned rice vinegar**
- **1 teaspoon toasted sesame oil**
- **1 teaspoon minced fresh ginger**

Salmon Bowls

- **2 (6-ounce) fillets wild-caught center-cut salmon (such as Atlantic or king)**
- **1 large bunch broccolini, ends trimmed**
- **2 tablespoons avocado oil**
- **4 cloves garlic, minced**
- **Sea salt and black pepper to taste**
- **Sliced avocado; sliced radish; handful of microgreens, watercress or arugula; sesame seeds; green onions sliced on the bias, for topping (optional)**

1. *For the rice:* Cook the brown rice according to package instructions, using the bone broth for the liquid.

2. *For the marinade:* Combine all the marinade ingredients in a medium bowl.

3. *For the bowls:* Place the salmon in a shallow dish and cover with half the marinade. Cover and marinate for a minimum of 10 minutes or up to 1 hour. Preheat the oven to broil. Line a large baking sheet with parchment paper.

4. Coat the broccolini in the avocado oil, garlic, salt, and pepper and arrange evenly on one side of the baking sheet. Remove the salmon from the marinade and place on the other side of the baking sheet. Broil on the top rack for 10 to 12 minutes, until the broccolini is charred and the salmon has an opaque center or registers an internal temperature of 135°F.

5. Divide the rice among serving bowls, top each with a salmon fillet and broccolini, and add the toppings of your choice. Drizzle with the reserved marinade and serve.

FOLLICULAR PHASE BENEFITS

Supports estrogen detoxification • High in healthy fats • High in antioxidants

Life-Saving Burrito Bowls

PREP: 10 MINUTES COOK: 30 MINUTES SERVES 4

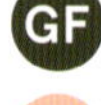

This is my go-to meal whenever I don't feel like cooking/have no idea what to make/need something quick and easy that the whole family will eat. It's rich in protein, amino acids, and healthy fats, which provide our bodies with adequate energy to develop and release a follicle (necessary for ovulation to occur). Don't forget the tortilla chips, which add crunch and make this a winner with kiddos. I highly recommend saving leftovers for fantastic breakfast burritos or tacos!

- 1½ cups basmati rice, rinsed in cold water three times and drained
- 3¼ cups bone broth, divided (try using the Super Simple Homemade Bone Broth on page 109)
- 1 tablespoon grass-fed ghee (or olive oil, avocado oil, or butter)
- ½ teaspoon sea salt, plus more to taste
- 2 tablespoons avocado oil
- ½ white or yellow onion, diced
- 4 cloves garlic, minced
- 1 pound ground grass-fed beef
- 1 (15-ounce) can black beans, rinsed and drained
- 1 tablespoon arrowroot starch
- 1 teaspoon chili powder
- 1 teaspoon cumin
- 1 teaspoon coriander
- 1 teaspoon garlic powder
- ½ teaspoon chipotle powder
- 2 tablespoons tomato paste
- Grated zest and juice of 1 lime
- ½ cup cilantro, minced
- 2 red bell peppers, seeded and diced
- 2 small to medium Roma or plum tomatoes, chopped
- 2 avocados, pitted, peeled, and sliced
- ½ head romaine lettuce, rinsed, drained, and chopped
- Full-fat or nondairy sour cream, grated cheese, and salsa for topping (optional)
- 2 cups tortilla chips for serving (optional)

1. In a medium pot, combine the rinsed rice, 2¾ cups of the bone broth, the ghee, and salt and bring to a boil. Cover, reduce the heat to low, and simmer for 20 minutes, until the liquid is absorbed. Remove from the heat and let rest for 5 minutes covered.

2. While the rice is cooking, heat the avocado oil in a large skillet over medium-high heat. Add the onion and sauté until softened, about 5 minutes. Stir in the garlic and sauté for 1 more minute. Add the ground meat and cook until no longer pink, breaking up any large chunks with a spatula. Add the beans and arrowroot and sprinkle in all the spices. Stir in the tomato paste and the remaining ½ cup bone broth, mixing it all together. Reduce the heat to low and simmer until the mixture is very thick, about 10 minutes.

3. After the rice has rested, gently fold in the lime zest and juice and the cilantro. Taste and season with a bit more salt if needed.

4. For each serving, scoop a generous portion of rice into a bowl, top with the ground meat and bean mixture, followed by bell peppers, tomatoes, avocado, and romaine. Top with sour cream, shredded cheese, or salsa and serve with tortilla chips if you like.

NOTE: This bowl is extremely versatile, so feel free to customize any way you like. You can swap out the ground beef for ground turkey or chicken and the rice for cauliflower rice or more shredded romaine. Or serve all the elements in burrito wraps, tortillas, or taco shells.

FOLLICULAR PHASE BENEFITS

Supports liver function • High in healthy fats • High in antioxidants

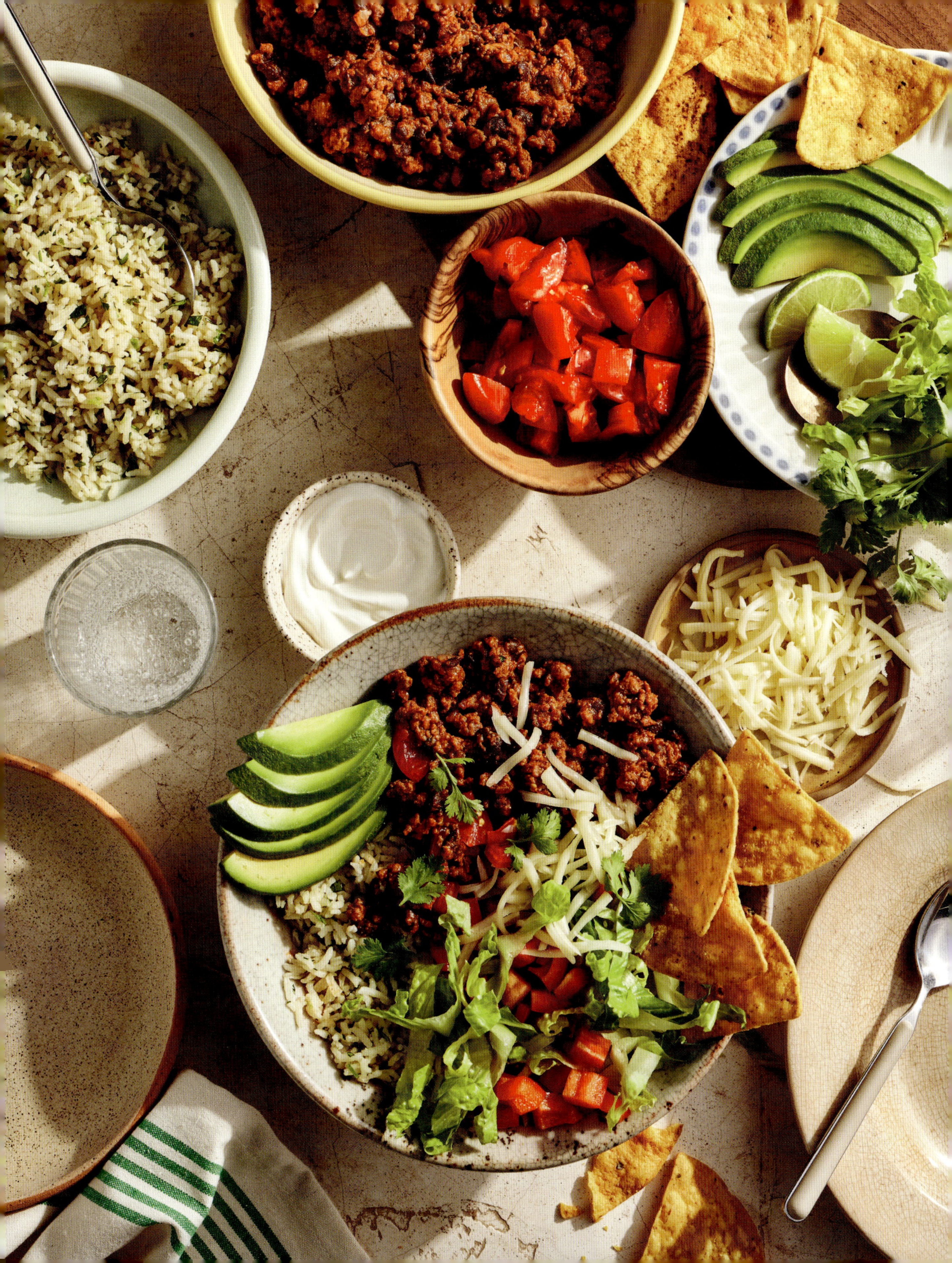

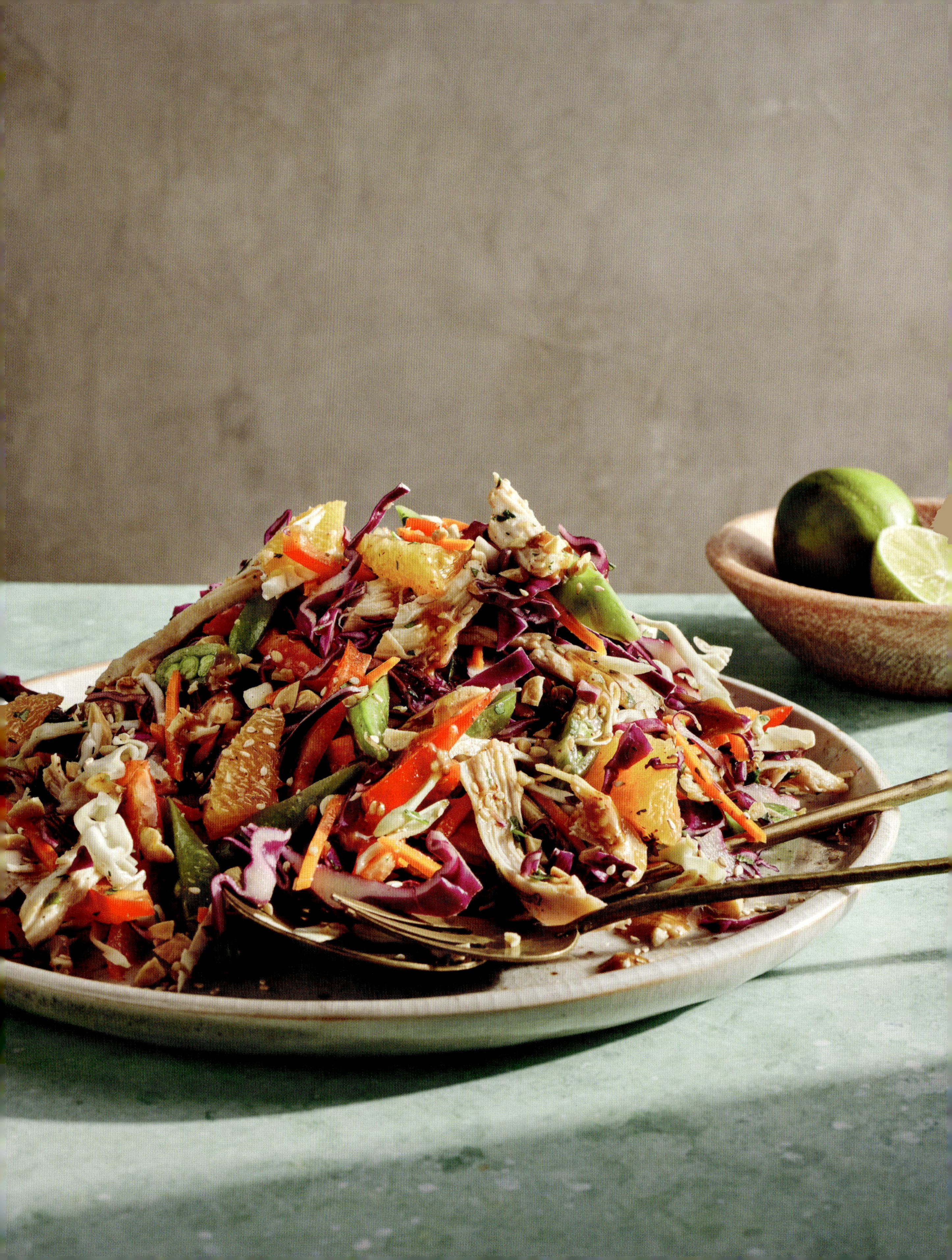

Crave-Worthy Chinese Chicken Salad + Almond Butter Dressing

PREP: 15 MINUTES COOK: NONE SERVES 2

One of the most crave-worthy (hence the name) and functional salads, this recipe is abundant in fiber and compounds that support liver function and estrogen detoxification, helping to keep PMS at bay during the latter half of your cycle. It's also rich in bright, colorful fruits and vegetables that are loaded with vitamin C and antioxidants that work to fight off oxidative stress, which tends to peak right before ovulation occurs. But I'd be lying if I said the almond butter dressing wasn't my favorite part.

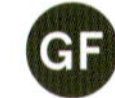

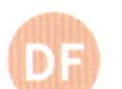

BF

Almond Butter Dressing

- ⅓ cup avocado oil
- ¼ cup coconut aminos (or gluten-free soy sauce)
- ¼ cup creamy almond butter
- 3 tablespoons rice vinegar
- 2 tablespoons raw honey
- 1 tablespoon toasted sesame oil
- 1 teaspoon minced fresh ginger
- 2 cloves garlic, minced
- ¼ teaspoon sea salt
- 1 tablespoon sesame seeds

Salad

- 2 large cooked organic chicken breasts, chopped (I like to use rotisserie chicken for convenience)
- ½ small red cabbage, shredded (about 2 cups)
- ½ small green cabbage, shredded (about 2 cups)
- 1 large red bell pepper, seeded and thinly sliced
- 2 large carrots, peeled and shredded
- 1 large orange or 2 mandarin oranges, peeled and chopped
- 1 cup sugar snap peas, chopped
- ¼ cup fresh cilantro, minced
- ½ cup toasted peanuts

1. Whisk together all the dressing ingredients in a small bowl or mix in a blender or food processor until creamy and well combined.
2. Toss all the salad ingredients together in a large bowl.
3. Drizzle the dressing on top and enjoy!

NOTE: The dressed salad holds up well for another day in the fridge. But to extend its shelf life, store the salad ingredients and dressing separately (they'll both last up to 3 to 5 days on their own), then toss together when you're ready to eat.

FOLLICULAR PHASE BENEFITS

Supports liver function • Supports estrogen detoxification • Rich in fiber • High in antioxidants

Viral Raw Carrot Salad

PREP: 5 MINUTES COOK: 5 MINUTES SERVES 1

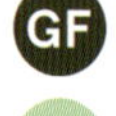

Raw carrot salad had a serious moment on social media, but it remains a steadfast staple in my monthly rotation thanks to its effectiveness at binding to endotoxins and excess estrogen to safely eliminate them from the body. While most of the benefits reported are anecdotal, I personally notice a reduction in bloat and improvement in digestion and transit time, not to mention I love how easy and delicious it is! I especially enjoy it during my follicular and ovulatory phases, when estrogen is peaking, helping to pave the way for a smoother, symptom-free second half of the cycle. I've included both the original recipe (OG Raw Carrot Salad), developed by Dr. Ray Peat, as well as my go-to version, featuring my honey-lime dressing.

OG Raw Carrot Salad

- **1 or 2 large organic raw carrots, peeled and cut into long ribbons with a vegetable peeler**
- **1 teaspoon extra virgin olive oil or melted unrefined organic coconut oil**
- **1 teaspoon apple cider vinegar**
- **Sprinkle of sea salt**

My Go-to Raw Carrot Salad

- **¼ cup extra virgin olive oil**
- **2 tablespoons white vinegar or apple cider vinegar**
- **2 tablespoons raw honey**
- **1 tablespoon lime juice (or lemon juice)**
- **1 tablespoon Dijon mustard**
- **½ teaspoon sea salt**
- **1 or 2 large raw organic carrots, peeled and cut into long ribbons with a vegetable peeler**
- **1 to 2 tablespoons crunchy nuts or seeds (pistachios, peanuts, or sesame seeds)**
- **Chopped fresh herbs (cilantro, mint, or basil)**
- **Lime wedges for garnish**

1. *For the OG raw carrot salad:* In a bowl, toss the carrot ribbons with the oil, vinegar, and salt.

2. *For my go-to carrot salad:* In a small bowl, whisk together the olive oil, vinegar, honey, lime juice, mustard, and salt. Combine the carrot ribbons, nuts or seeds, and herbs in a serving bowl. Drizzle about 2 tablespoons of the dressing over the salad, toss, and serve with a lime wedge.

NOTE: The dressing makes 2 to 4 servings, so I recommend storing the remainder in an airtight glass jar in the fridge for up to 1 week.

FOLLICULAR PHASE BENEFITS

Supports liver function • Supports estrogen detoxification • High in healthy fats • Rich in fiber • Rich in probiotics • High in antioxidants

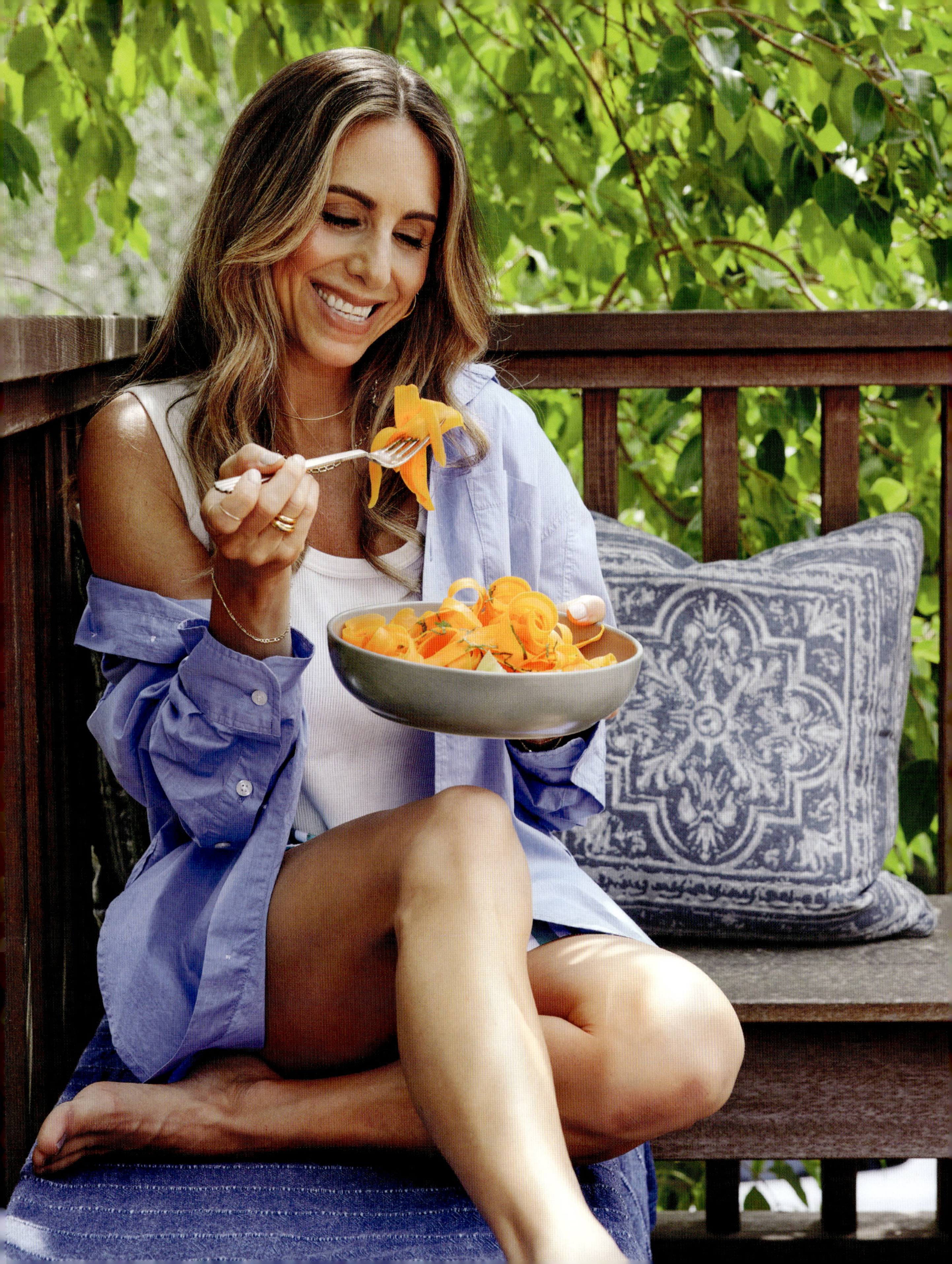

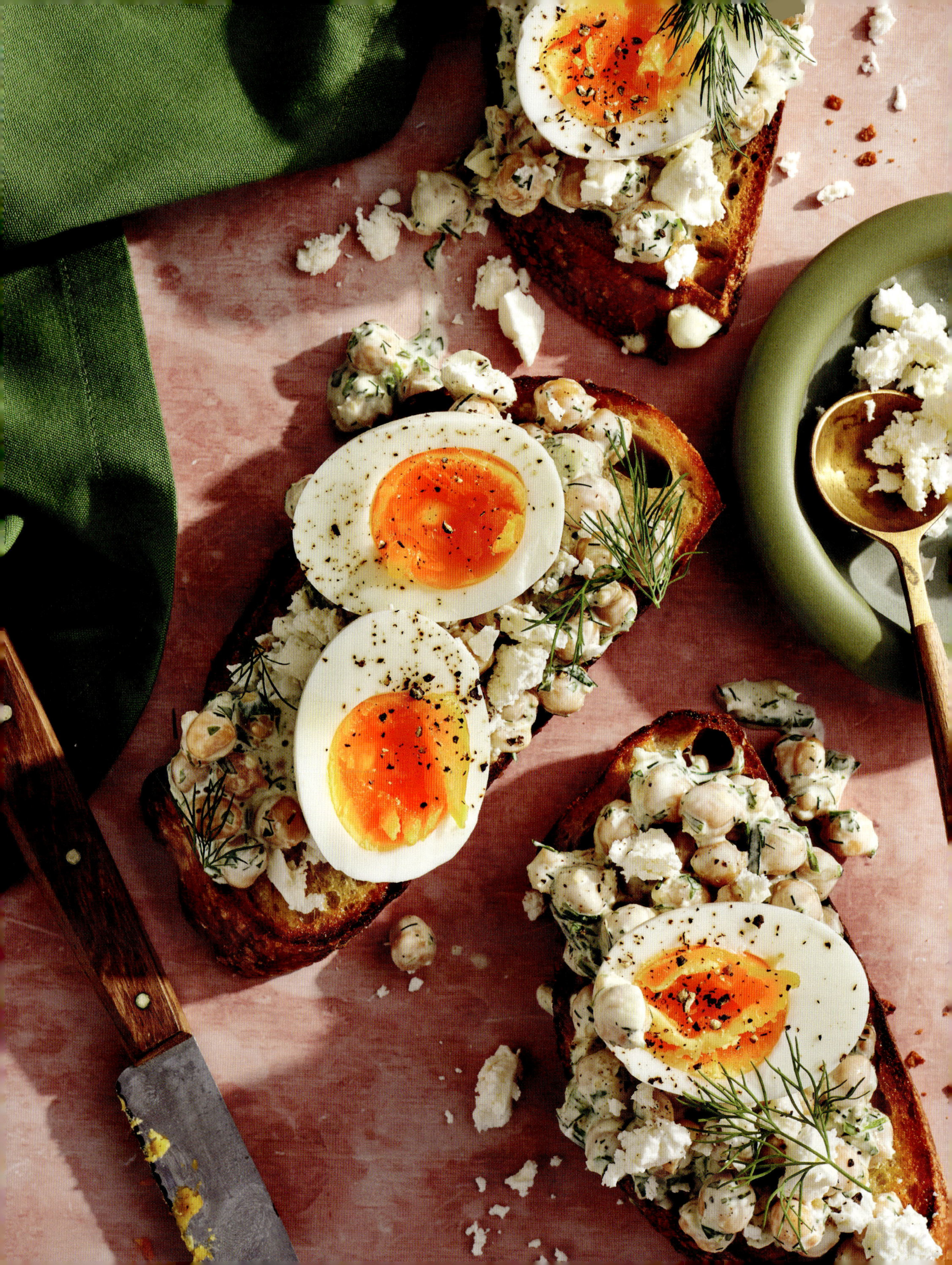

Green Goddess Chickpea Smash Toast

PREP: 5 MINUTES   COOK: 10 MINUTES   SERVES 1

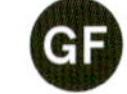

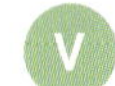

BF

If I'm ever in a lunch rut, this toast always helps me bust right out of it. It's quick to whip up, packed with fiber to help flush out excess estrogen (12 grams per 1 cup!), and loaded with gut-boosting probiotics and flavor—thanks to the herby green goddess dressing. It's also great for make-ahead meals on busy days, as it holds up well for several days in the fridge. Note: As long as you use 1 full cup of fresh herbs, you can mix and match depending on what's available.

Green Goddess Dressing

½ cup unsweetened full-fat Greek or coconut yogurt

½ cup avocado oil mayonnaise

¼ cup fresh basil leaves

¼ cup fresh dill leaves

¼ cup fresh parsley leaves

¼ cup chopped fresh chives

2 tablespoons fresh tarragon leaves

1 tablespoon fresh lemon juice

2 cloves garlic, minced

1 teaspoon sea salt

Black pepper to taste

Toast

1 can organic chickpeas, rinsed and drained

2 slices gluten-free sourdough (or Sweet Potato Toast slices, page 232, or lettuce wraps)

2 tablespoons feta cheese

Extra virgin olive oil

Flaky sea salt for topping

1 or 2 soft-boiled eggs, halved, for topping (optional)

1. *For the dressing:* Combine all the dressing ingredients in a food processor and pulse until mostly smooth (it should have a somewhat chunky texture).

2. *For the toast:* In a small bowl, combine the chickpeas and about one-half of the green goddess dressing, until the chickpeas are evenly coated.

3. Spread the chickpea mixture evenly on top of the toasts, using a fork to lightly mash it down. Sprinkle the feta cheese on top and drizzle with olive oil. Top with flaky sea salt and optional soft-boiled eggs.

NOTE: This recipe makes a double portion of dressing. Store the remainder in the fridge for up to 5 days. It's amazing on salads, drizzled over bowls, as a dip for veggies, and more.

FOLLICULAR PHASE BENEFITS

Supports estrogen detoxification • Rich in fiber • Rich in probiotics

Maple-Roasted Carrots + Goat Cheese, Candied Pistachios, and Mint

PREP: 5 MINUTES   COOK: 30 MINUTES   SERVES 4

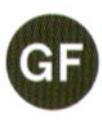

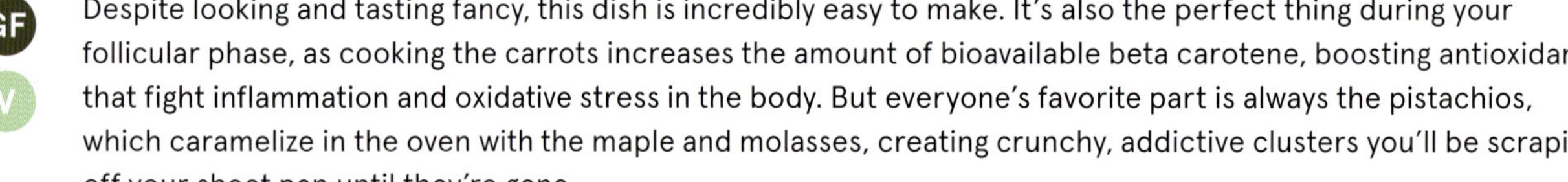

Despite looking and tasting fancy, this dish is incredibly easy to make. It's also the perfect thing during your follicular phase, as cooking the carrots increases the amount of bioavailable beta carotene, boosting antioxidants that fight inflammation and oxidative stress in the body. But everyone's favorite part is always the pistachios, which caramelize in the oven with the maple and molasses, creating crunchy, addictive clusters you'll be scraping off your sheet pan until they're gone.

- 2 to 3 bunches organic stem-on carrots (about 1 pound), stems trimmed, thoroughly scrubbed and rinsed, and halved lengthwise
- 2 tablespoons grass-fed ghee, melted (or avocado oil or grass-fed butter)
- Sea salt and black pepper to taste
- 2 tablespoons pure maple syrup
- 1 tablespoon blackstrap molasses
- ½ cup shelled pistachios, roughly chopped
- ¼ cup goat cheese, crumbled
- ¼ cup fresh mint leaves, torn
- ¼ cup fresh pomegranate seeds, for topping (optional)

1. Preheat the oven to 425°F and line a large baking sheet with parchment paper.

2. Add the halved carrots to the pan and drizzle with the ghee, then sprinkle with salt and pepper to taste. Roast for 20 minutes, then remove from the oven. Drizzle the carrots with the maple syrup and molasses and sprinkle with the pistachios. Stir everything with a spatula until the carrots and pistachios are evenly coated. Return to the oven and roast for 10 minutes, until the carrots and pistachios are caramelized.

3. Let cool for 1 to 2 minutes, then sprinkle with the goat cheese, fresh mint, and optional pomegranate seeds.

NOTE: If you can't find or just don't like molasses, you can leave it out or substitute 1 tablespoon freshly squeezed orange juice.

FOLLICULAR PHASE BENEFITS

Rich in fiber • High in antioxidants

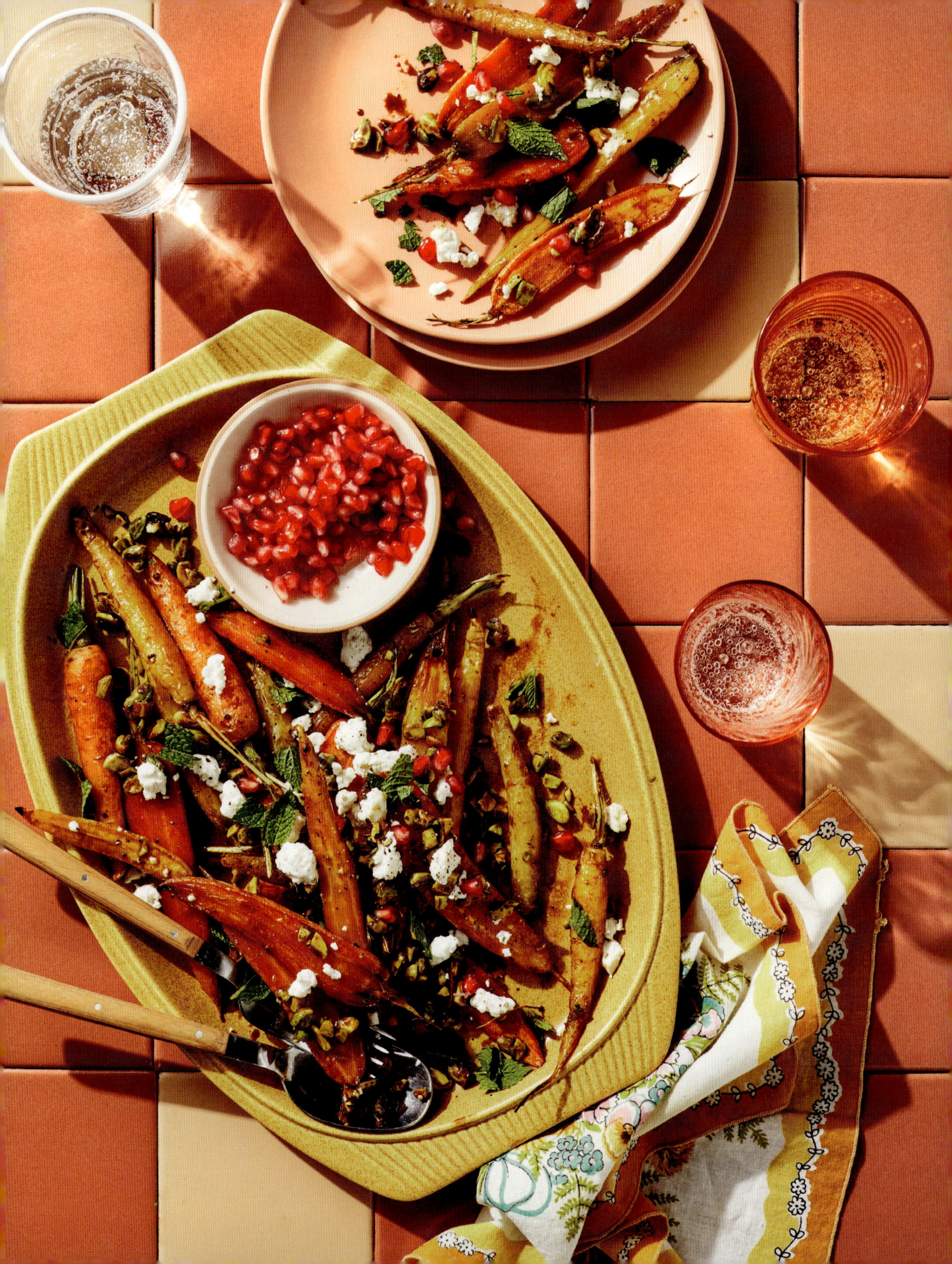

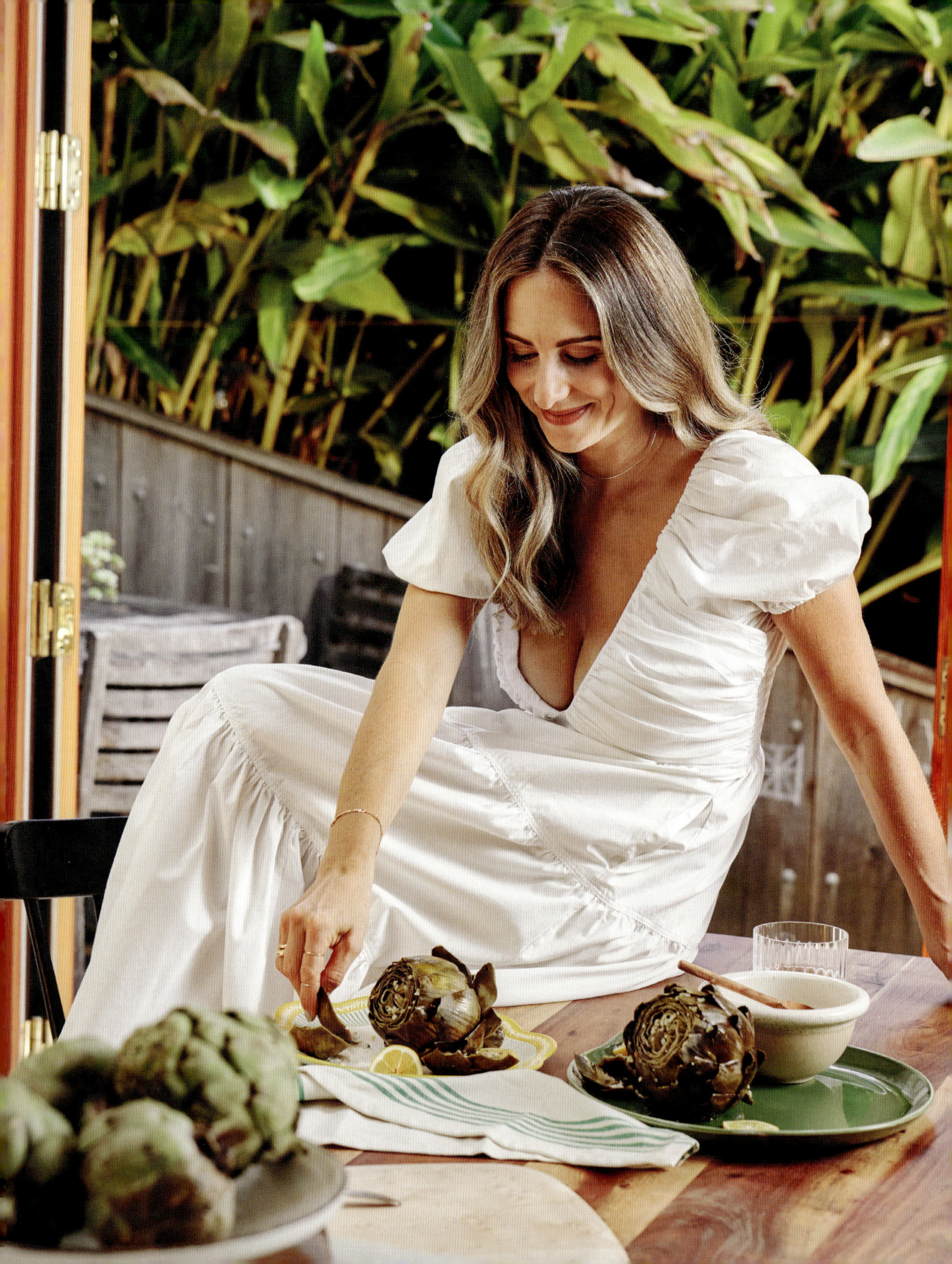

Whole Roasted Lemony Artichokes + Caper Aioli

PREP: 15 MINUTES COOK: 1½ HOURS SERVES 4

This is an OG recipe, one of the first I posted on my blog back when I started it in 2016. I've brought these roasted artichokes to so many parties and gatherings, and the enthusiastic consensus is always the same, especially when the tender leaves are dipped in the addictive aioli. The artichokes are loaded with both inulin and insoluble fiber (10 to 14 grams per cup!), working to increase regularity and transit time, which is important for the safe removal of excess estrogen. While there's a healthy online debate regarding the best method to cook artichokes, roasting them whole is my favorite easy, no-fail approach.

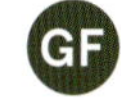

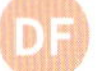

Artichokes

- **2 whole globe artichokes (jumbo preferred)**
- **1 lemon**
- **4 cloves garlic, minced**
- **Avocado oil for drizzling**
- **Sea salt and black pepper to taste**

Caper Aioli

- **1 cup avocado oil mayonnaise**
- **Grated zest and juice of 1 lemon (about 1 tablespoon zest and 2 tablespoons juice)**
- **2 tablespoons capers**
- **1 tablespoon Italian seasoning**
- **3 cloves garlic, minced**
- **½ teaspoon sea salt**

1. Preheat the oven to 425°F.

2. *For the artichokes:* Rinse the artichokes and pat dry. Using a sharp knife, slice about ¼ to ½ inch off the top of each artichoke, then use the knife to slice an X into the bottom stems (this helps with the cooking). Next use a pair of sharp scissors to trim the pointy edges off all of the leaves. The top and leaves of the artichoke should be flat across.

3. Slice a few rounds off the lemon and use the rest of the lemon to drizzle juice all over the artichokes. Rub each with the minced garlic and a drizzle of avocado oil, then sprinkle with salt and pepper. Place a lemon slice or two on the top of each artichoke.

4. Place two large pieces of foil (big enough to completely cover each artichoke) on the counter, then layer with a large piece of parchment paper. Place an artichoke in the center of one, then pull up the sides of the parchment paper and foil to enclose the artichoke, twisting and sealing at the top, essentially creating a foil packet. Repeat with the second artichoke. (This method keeps in all of the juices, so the artichokes turn out tender, juicy, and flavorful. I use the parchment paper to keep the foil from touching the food when cooking to be safe.) Put the wrapped artichokes directly on the oven rack and bake for 1 hour for regular-sized artichokes, or 1¼ to 1½ hours for jumbo artichokes. The artichokes should be completely cooked through and browned when finished. Let the artichokes rest until cool enough to handle.

5. *For the aioli:* While the artichokes are roasting, combine all the aioli ingredients in a small bowl and whisk until well mixed. Keep in the fridge until the artichokes are ready to serve.

6. Unwrap the artichokes and place on a platter with the aioli. To enjoy, use your hand to pull off a leaf and dip the meaty part into the aioli, then scrape off the meat with your teeth. When you get to the heart (the *best* part), use a knife or a spoon to scrape off the fuzzy part (called the "choke") and discard. Cut the heart into pieces and dip in the aioli. Pure heaven.

FOLLICULAR PHASE BENEFITS

Supports liver function • Supports estrogen detoxification • Rich in fiber • Rich in probiotics

Weeknight Chicken Cashew Stir-Fry

PREP: 10 MINUTES   COOK: 30 MINUTES   SERVES 4

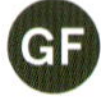
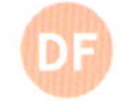
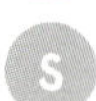
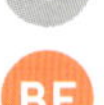

Another weeknight staple I turn to whenever I want something quick, healthy, protein-packed, and satisfying! It's also loaded with a variety of colorful vegetables, adding a hefty dose of fiber to assist in estrogen elimination, along with vitamin C, working to reduce inflammation and support detoxification. This is one of those meals I make so often I know them by heart, and I have a sneaking suspicion it might become a part of your regular rotation too.

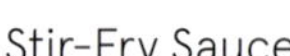

Stir-Fry Sauce

- ⅓ cup coconut aminos or gluten-free soy sauce
- ⅓ cup bone broth (or water)
- 2 to 3 tablespoons raw honey (or coconut sugar), to taste
- 2 tablespoons unseasoned rice vinegar
- 1 tablespoon toasted sesame oil
- 1 tablespoon minced ginger
- 2 cloves garlic, minced
- ½ teaspoon sea salt
- 1 tablespoon arrowroot starch
- Sriracha or chili oil, for spice (optional)

Stir-Fry

- ¾ cup raw organic cashews
- 2 tablespoons high-heat cooking oil (such as coconut or avocado oil), divided
- 1 pound organic skinless boneless chicken thighs, trimmed of fat and cubed
- Sea salt and black pepper to taste
- 4 cloves garlic, minced
- ½ white onion, chopped
- 1 red bell pepper, seeded and thinly sliced
- 1 cup fresh green beans, ends trimmed
- 1 cup sugar snap peas (can substitute additional green beans)
- 1 large carrot, peeled and sliced into rounds

- Cooked rice, sesame seeds, and sliced green onions, for serving (optional)

1. Preheat the oven to 350°F.
2. *For the sauce:* Mix all the sauce ingredients together in a small bowl and set aside.
3. *For the stir-fry:* Spread the cashews evenly on a small baking sheet and roast for 10 minutes, until toasted and golden brown. Set aside.
4. Heat a large skillet over medium-high heat and add 1 tablespoon of the cooking oil. Add the cubed chicken, sprinkle with salt and pepper, and sear until golden brown, 3 to 5 minutes. Flip and cook the other sides, until the chicken is just barely cooked through. Transfer the chicken with a slotted spoon to a plate and set aside.
5. Reduce the heat to medium, add the remaining 1 tablespoon cooking oil to the skillet, and stir in the garlic. Add the onion and cook for 1 to 2 minutes, until softened. Add the bell pepper, green beans, sugar snaps, and carrot and stir-fry for 10 to 12 minutes, stirring occasionally, until cooked through. Stir in the cashews and the chicken, then add the sauce, continuing to stir until well mixed. Cover the skillet and reduce the heat to medium-low. Cook for 3 to 5 minutes, until the sauce has thickened and the mixture looks glazed.
6. If serving with rice, add it as the base to large bowls, then scoop the chicken cashew mixture on top. Top with optional sesame seeds and green onions if you like.

NOTE: This is such a versatile dish: You could easily swap out the chicken for another protein of choice and play around with different veggie combos based on what you have on hand.

FOLLICULAR PHASE BENEFITS

Supports liver function • Supports estrogen detoxification • Rich in fiber • High in antioxidants

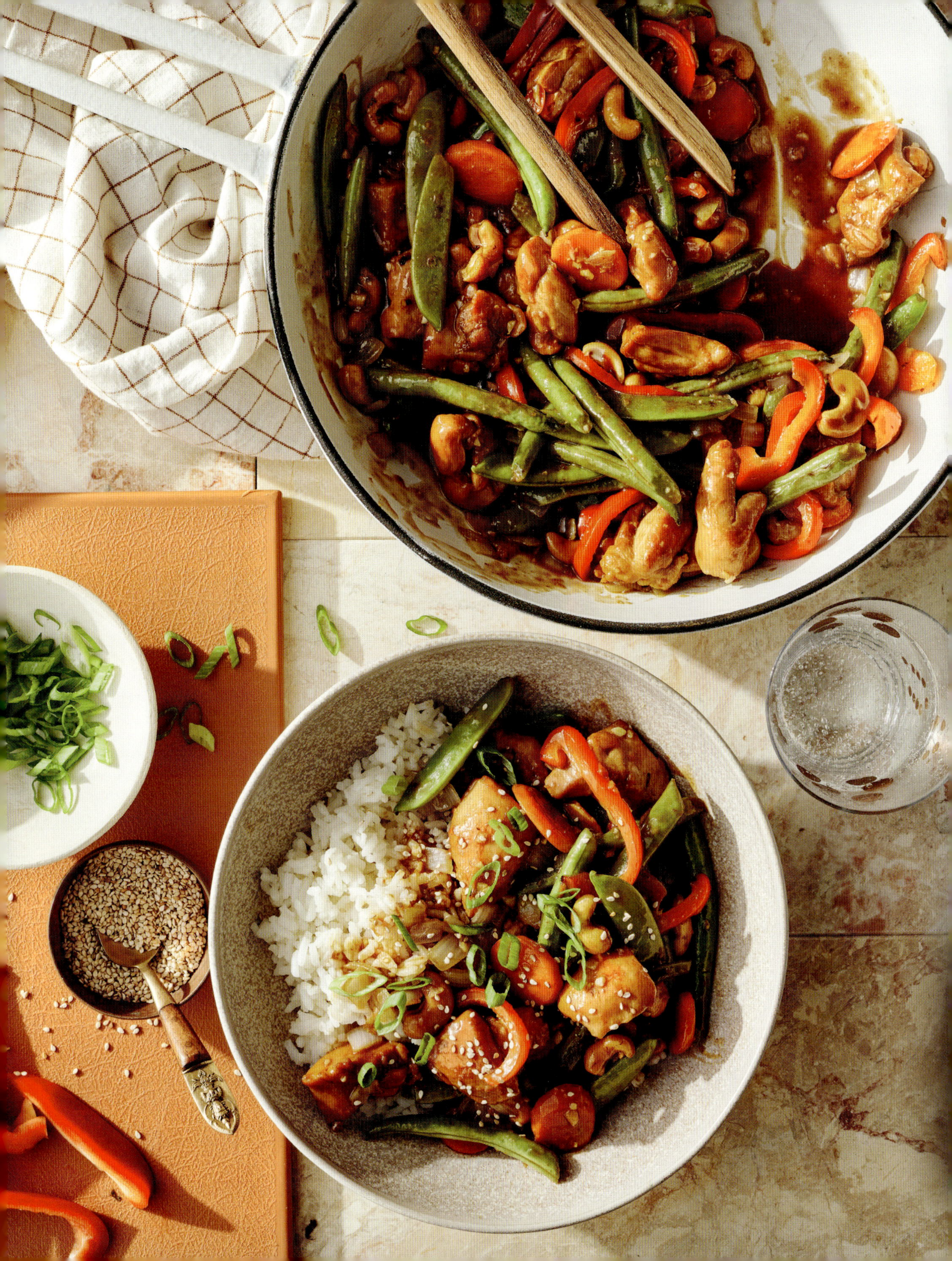

Thai Pork Lettuce Wraps + Sriracha Aioli

PREP: 10 MINUTES   COOK: 10 MINUTES   SERVES 2–4

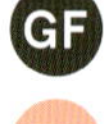
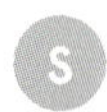
GF DF S BF

This fresh, delicious, and protein-packed meal takes very little time to put together. It also contains a variety of liver-supportive foods that help our main detox organ repackage excess estrogen and safely eliminate it. Soaking the carrots in vinegar quickly pickles them, adding a tangy taste that balances out the pork. Don't skimp on the herbs, which add loads of flavor!

Pickled Carrots

- **2 large carrots, peeled and shredded**
- **2 tablespoons rice vinegar**

Thai Pork

- **1 tablespoon unrefined organic coconut oil**
- **1 large shallot, diced**
- **4 cloves garlic, minced**
- **1½ pounds organic ground pork (or ground turkey or chicken)**
- **2 tablespoons coconut aminos or gluten-free soy sauce**
- **1 tablespoon rice vinegar**
- **1 tablespoon fish sauce**
- **1 tablespoon fresh lime juice**
- **1 tablespoon coconut sugar**
- **1 teaspoon sriracha**

Sriracha Aioli

- **½ cup avocado oil mayonnaise**
- **1 to 2 tablespoons sriracha (add more if you like it spicy!)**
- **½ teaspoon sea salt**
- **Sea salt and black pepper to taste**

Wraps

- **6 to 8 large lettuce leaves, such as romaine, bibb, or green-leaf, individually rinsed and patted dry**
- **¼ cup each fresh cilantro, Thai basil, and mint leaves**
- **Chopped peanuts for topping**

1. *For the pickled carrots:* Place the carrots in a small bowl, drizzle with the rice vinegar, and let sit at room temperature to pickle while you prepare the rest of the meal.

2. *For the pork:* Heat the coconut oil in a large skillet over medium-high heat. Add the shallot and cook for 1 to 2 minutes, until softened. Add the garlic and cook for 1 additional minute. Add the ground pork and cook, breaking it up with a spoon, for 3 to 4 minutes, until almost cooked through.

3. Whisk together the coconut aminos, rice vinegar, fish sauce, lime juice, coconut sugar, and sriracha and pour evenly over the pork. Let the pork cook an additional 2 to 3 minutes, until completely cooked and the sauce is mostly absorbed.

4. *For the aioli:* While the pork is cooking, whisk together the aioli ingredients in a small bowl.

5. *To assemble the wraps:* Arrange the lettuce leaves on plates, drizzle with sriracha aioli, and top with the ground pork mixture, followed by the pickled carrots and fresh herbs and peanuts. Enjoy immediately.

FOLLICULAR PHASE BENEFITS

Supports liver function • Supports estrogen detoxification • Rich in fiber • High in antioxidants

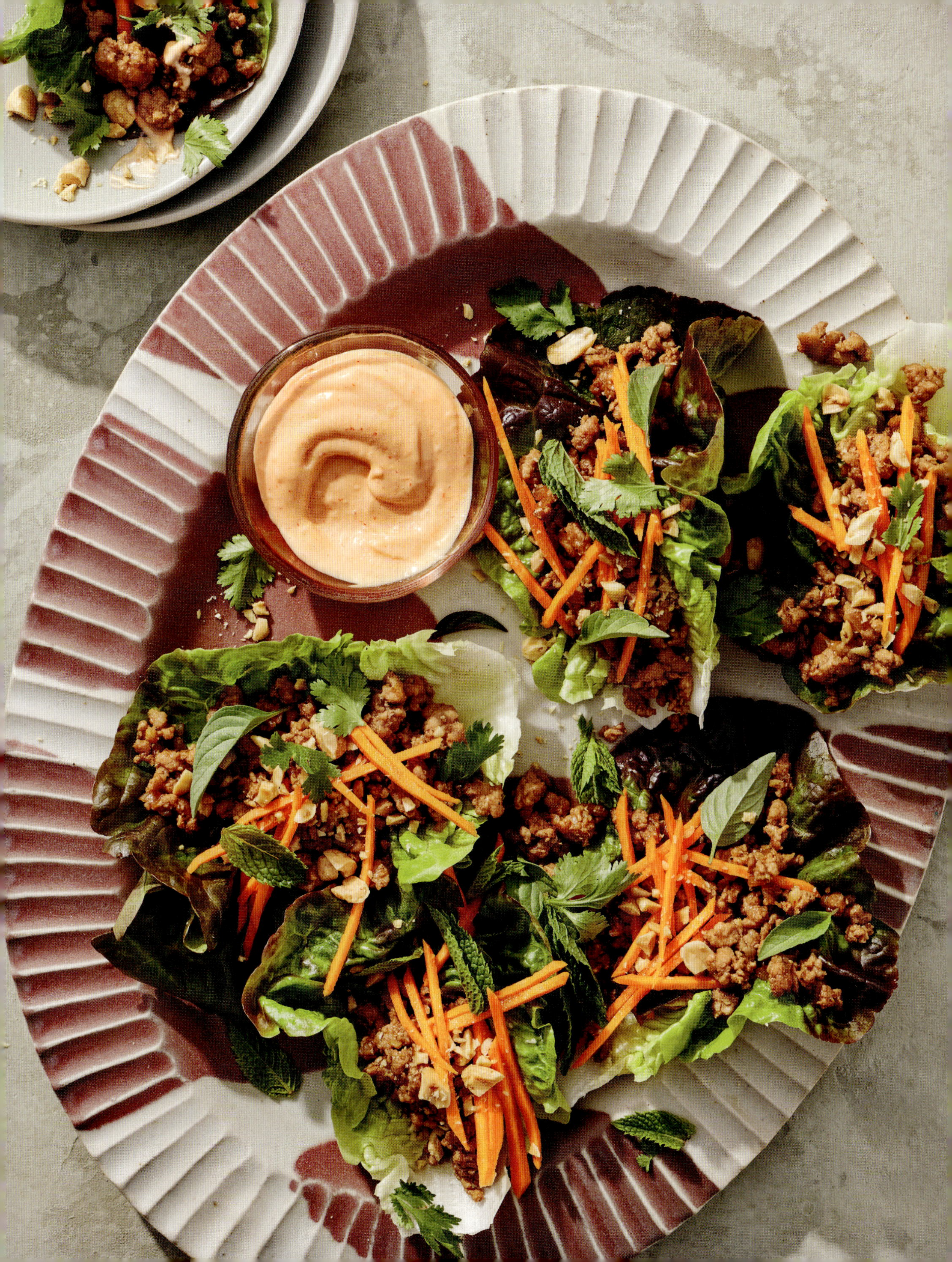

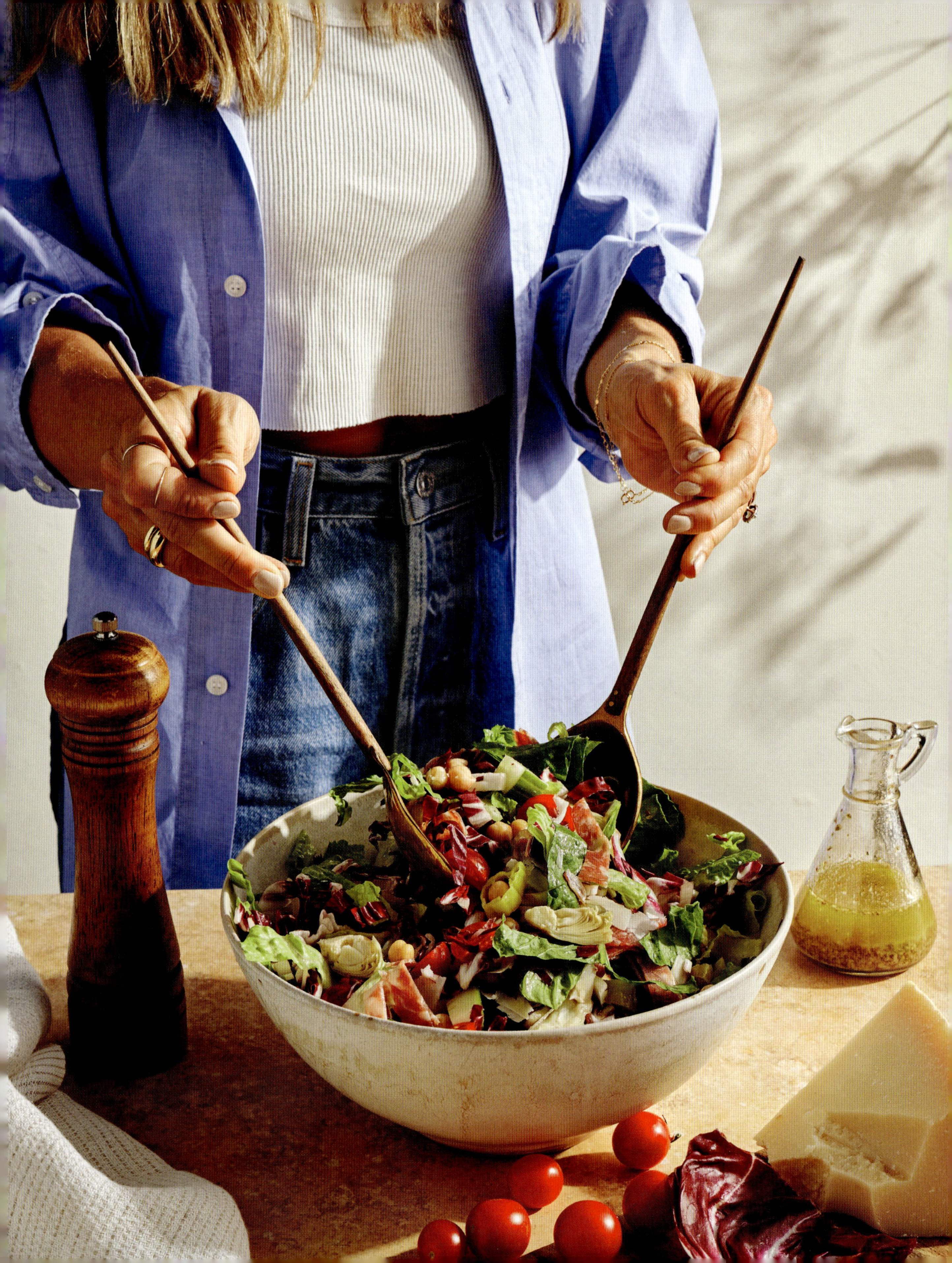

Chopped Italian Sub Salad

PREP: 20 MINUTES   COOK: NONE   SERVES 4–6

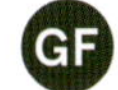

BF

This salad is like enjoying the inside of one giant chopped Italian sub from a bowl—need I say more? Not only is it huge, filling, and loaded with quintessential pizza salad flavors, it's incredibly rich in dietary fiber thanks to the artichoke hearts and chickpeas, which add a whopping 40 grams! The radicchio (a type of bitter chicory) has been reported to improve regularity thanks to its inulin fiber, which is also great for blood sugar stabilization. The salad is large and feeds a crowd, making it the perfect side when hosting a large gathering, which you're more wont to do during your social follicular phase. (Or see the Note for tips on storing the salad.)

Dressing

- **¼ cup red wine vinegar**
- **1 tablespoon dried oregano**
- **1 teaspoon Dijon mustard**
- **1 teaspoon garlic powder**
- **1 teaspoon sea salt**
- **Black pepper to taste**
- **½ cup extra virgin olive oil**

Salad

- **1 head romaine lettuce, rinsed and patted dry**
- **1 head radicchio, rinsed and patted dry**
- **1 (15-ounce) can chickpeas, rinsed and drained**
- **1 (15-ounce) can artichoke hearts or hearts of palm, rinsed, drained, and diced**
- **1 large English cucumber, diced**
- **1 cup cherry tomatoes, chopped**
- **½ cup chopped Genoa salami**
- **½ cup kalamata olives, chopped**
- **½ cup pepperoncini, diced (optional)**
- **½ cup grated Parmesan or feta cheese, plus more for topping**

1. Whisk together all the dressing ingredients in a small bowl.

2. Combine all the salad ingredients in a very large salad bowl, pour the dressing on top, and toss until well combined.

NOTE: This recipe makes a huge portion, so if you're just making it for yourself, I recommend tossing all of the salad ingredients together, then adding a portion to a bowl and drizzling with some of the dressing. Save the remaining dressing in a small glass jar and the chopped salad ingredients in a bowl with an airtight lid in the fridge, then enjoy for 1 to 2 more days.

FOLLICULAR PHASE BENEFITS

Supports liver function • Supports estrogen detoxification • Rich in fiber • High in healthy fats • High in antioxidants

Hot Honey Halloumi Spring Bowls

PREP: 10 MINUTES   COOK: 30 MINUTES   SERVES 2

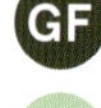

V

This bowl offers an abundance of bright spring flavors and antioxidant-rich bitter greens to help fight off rising oxidative stress. It's also rich in probiotics and prebiotic fiber to support a healthy gut microbiome and estrogen detoxification. But the best part—without a doubt—is the hot honey halloumi (a semi-hard cheese made from sheep's and goat's milk), which is slightly sweet, salty, spicy, creamy, and savory. It seamlessly balances out all of the other astringent components of the bowl.

- 1 cup brown lentils
- 1 bunch organic asparagus, ends trimmed
- 4 tablespoons avocado oil, divided
- 2 cloves garlic, minced
- Sea salt and black pepper to taste
- 1 cup thinly sliced red onion
- ¼ cup red wine vinegar
- 1 teaspoon coconut sugar
- ½ teaspoon sea salt
- 1 (8.8-ounce) package halloumi, sliced into 1-inch pieces
- 2 to 4 tablespoons hot honey (or regular honey), to taste
- 2 cups arugula or other leafy greens
- ½ cup thinly sliced radishes
- Sliced avocado and fresh herbs (like dill and basil), for topping (optional)

Tzatziki Sauce

- 1 cup plain unsweetened coconut yogurt or Greek yogurt
- ½ organic cucumber, peeled, shredded, and drained
- Juice of 1 lemon (about 2 tablespoons)
- 2 tablespoons minced garlic
- 2 tablespoons fresh dill leaves, minced
- ½ teaspoon sea salt

1. Cook the lentils according to package instructions, as this will most likely take the longest time.

2. Preheat the oven to 400°F. Line a small baking sheet with parchment paper.

3. Arrange the asparagus on the baking sheet, drizzle with 2 tablespoons of the avocado oil, and sprinkle with the garlic and salt and pepper to taste. Use your hands to coat the asparagus evenly. Roast for about 15 minutes, flipping halfway through, until the asparagus is tender and slightly charred.

4. While the asparagus is cooking, quickly pickle the red onion by mixing the sliced red onion, vinegar, coconut sugar, and ½ teaspoon sea salt together in a small bowl. Use your hands to massage the onion (this helps it break down and better absorb the liquid), then set aside until ready to use. (You can store any leftovers in a jar in the fridge for up to 1 week.)

5. Add the remaining 2 tablespoons avocado oil to a skillet and heat over medium heat. Add the sliced halloumi and drizzle a little bit of hot honey on the top of each piece, then flip. Cook for 3 to 4 minutes, until the bottom sides with the honey are golden brown. Drizzle hot honey on the top side, then flip and cook for another 3 to 4 minutes, until golden brown on the bottoms.

6. *For the tzatziki:* While the halloumi is cooking, whisk together all the tzatziki ingredients in a small mixing bowl.

7. To serve, spoon the lentils into large bowls, then top with the arugula, roasted asparagus, hot honey halloumi, pickled onion, sliced radishes, and avocado (if using). Drizzle with the tzatziki sauce and sprinkle with fresh herbs, plus more salt and pepper to taste.

FOLLICULAR PHASE BENEFITS

Supports liver function • Supports estrogen detoxification • Rich in fiber • Rich in probiotics • High in antioxidants

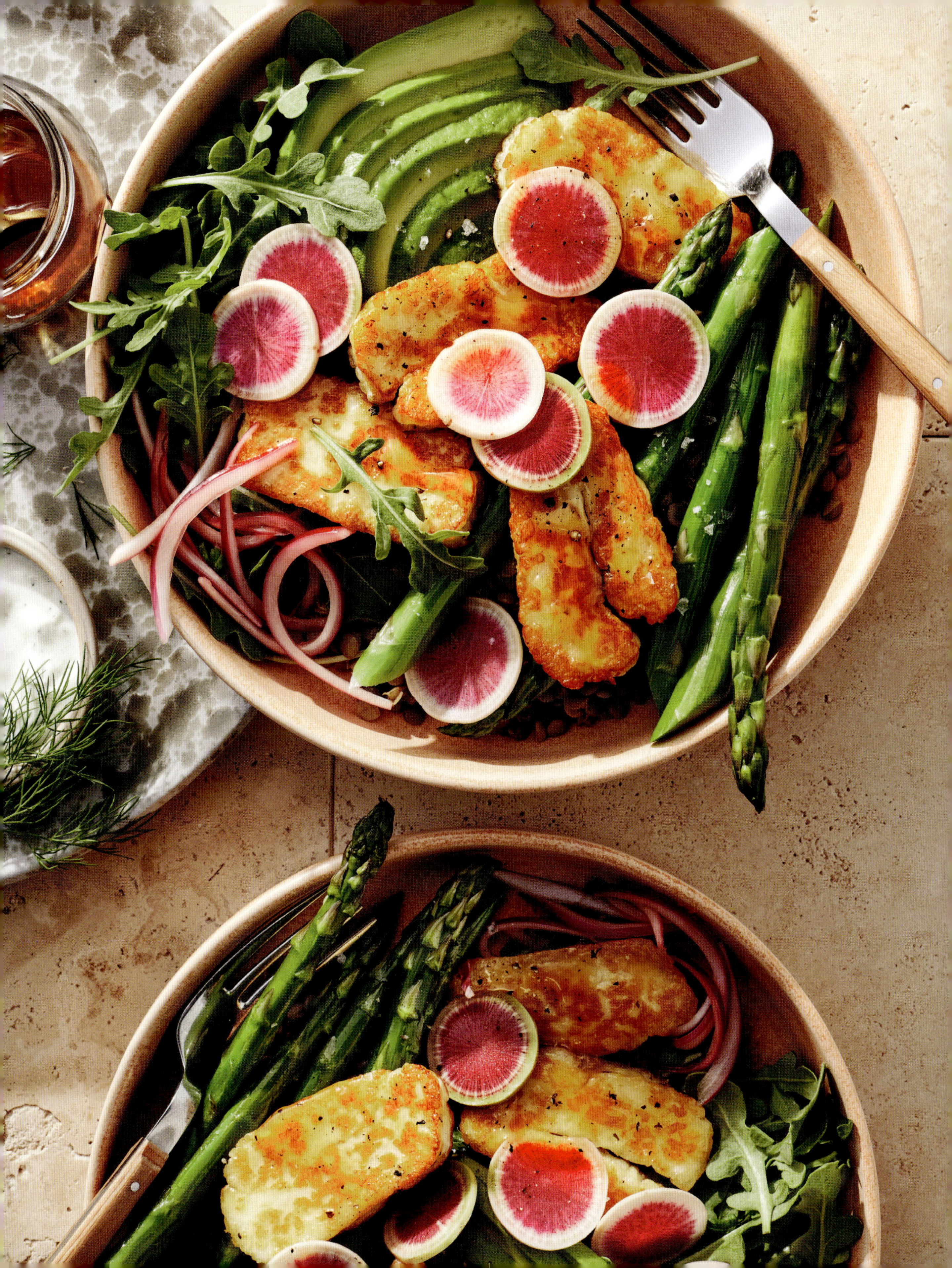

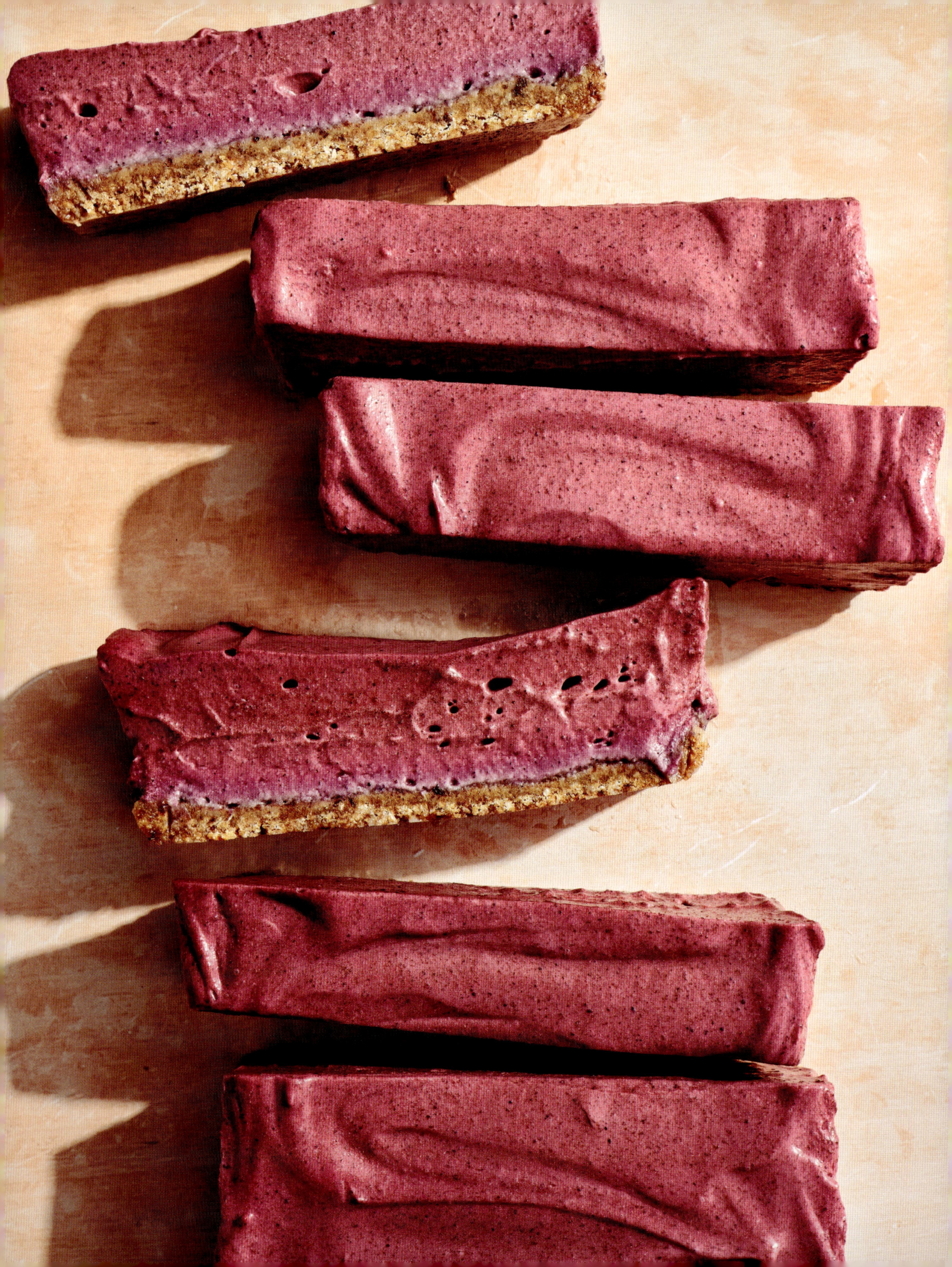

No-Bake Wild Blueberry Cheesecake Bars

PREP: 20 MINUTES, PLUS 5 HOURS FREEZING | COOK: NONE | SERVES 8

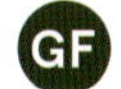
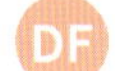
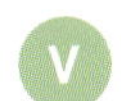
BF

While I tend to gravitate toward chocolate desserts, these bars are *so* creamy, refreshing, and delicious I would choose them anytime. I especially love them in my follicular and ovulatory phases, when I naturally crave cooler treats. The wild blueberries are loaded with polyphenols, an antioxidant that helps to lower inflammation, regulate cortisol levels, and protect your cells from stress—which is especially important leading up to ovulation, as too much cortisol can delay or prevent ovulation, the main event of your cycle. I highly recommend keeping a batch of these in the freezer so you can have one whenever your sweet tooth strikes (see Note).

- **1 cup gluten-free graham-style crackers of choice (look for a brand with minimal ingredients)**
- **4 dates, pitted**
- **¼ cup unrefined organic coconut oil, melted**
- **¾ teaspoon sea salt, divided**
- **2 cups vegan or full-fat organic cream cheese**
- **½ cup pure maple syrup**
- **1 teaspoon pure vanilla extract**
- **1½ cups frozen wild blueberries**
- **1 teaspoon grated lemon zest, plus more for topping**
- **Fresh blueberries for topping (optional)**

1. Line a 5 by 9-inch loaf pan with parchment paper. In a food processor, pulse together the crackers, dates, coconut oil, and ¼ teaspoon of the salt until well combined and no large chunks remain (it should be moist and crumbly). Pat the mixture evenly into the bottom of the lined loaf pan and place in the freezer while you make the filling.

2. Combine the cream cheese, maple syrup, vanilla extract, frozen blueberries, lemon zest, and remaining ½ teaspoon salt in a high-speed blender and mix on high until creamy and smooth.

3. Pour the filling over the cracker crust, spreading it evenly with a spatula if needed. Freeze for a minimum of 5 hours to set.

4. Remove the bars from the freezer 30 to 60 minutes before serving and let sit at room temperature. Use a sharp knife to slice into eight pieces, then top with lemon zest and optional fresh blueberries.

NOTE: These bars get very soft once defrosted, which makes them extra delicious but also very messy! That's why I recommend storing them in the freezer and removing them 30 to 60 minutes before consuming to let them defrost at room temperature and keep their shape and texture. You can also individually wrap and freeze them for 1 to 2 months, providing you with a quick single-serving option whenever a craving strikes.

FOLLICULAR PHASE BENEFITS

Rich in probiotics • High in antioxidants

Dreamy High-Protein Chocolate Pudding

PREP: 10 MINUTES, PLUS 4 HOURS CHILLING COOK: NONE SERVES 4

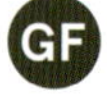

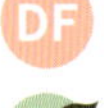

I've been obsessed with pudding since I was little (hello, Jell-O Snack Packs!) so this recipe is both nutrient-dense *and* nostalgic for me. The texture is thick and creamy and the taste is decadent, all while being naturally vegan, gluten-free, and protein-packed to boot! Tofu adds a good amount of protein (10 grams per serving) and also contains phytoestrogens, which are plant compounds that can be helpful when estrogen is low, like at the beginning of your follicular phase, to support rising levels.

- 1 cup dark chocolate chunks or chips
- 1 (16-ounce) package organic, non-GMO-certified silken tofu, drained and patted dry
- ¼ cup pure maple syrup
- ¼ cup cacao powder
- 1 teaspoon pure vanilla extract
- 1 teaspoon instant espresso (try decaf if sensitive to caffeine)
- ½ teaspoon sea salt, plus more for topping
- 1 to 2 servings chocolate protein powder, optional
- Coconut Whipped Cream (see page 110), optional
- Dark chocolate shavings, optional

1. Add the chocolate chunks or chips to a microwave-safe bowl and heat in 30-second increments until melted. Set aside.

2. Combine the tofu, maple syrup, cacao powder, vanilla, espresso, and salt in a high-speed blender. Pour in the melted chocolate, cover the blender, and start mixing on the lowest setting. Slowly increase the speed until the mixture is completely combined. It should be thick, creamy, and uniformly chocolatey throughout.

3. Use a spatula to spoon the pudding into four ramekins or glass jars and cover with lids. Refrigerate for 4 hours or up to overnight before serving. When ready to enjoy, feel free to add more flaky sea salt, coconut whipped cream, and chocolate shavings.

NOTE: These puddings freeze well (and last for 1 to 2 months), so I like to always have a batch in the freezer. Just defrost for 1 to 2 hours before serving!

FOLLICULAR PHASE BENEFITS

High in antioxidants • Source of phytoestrogens

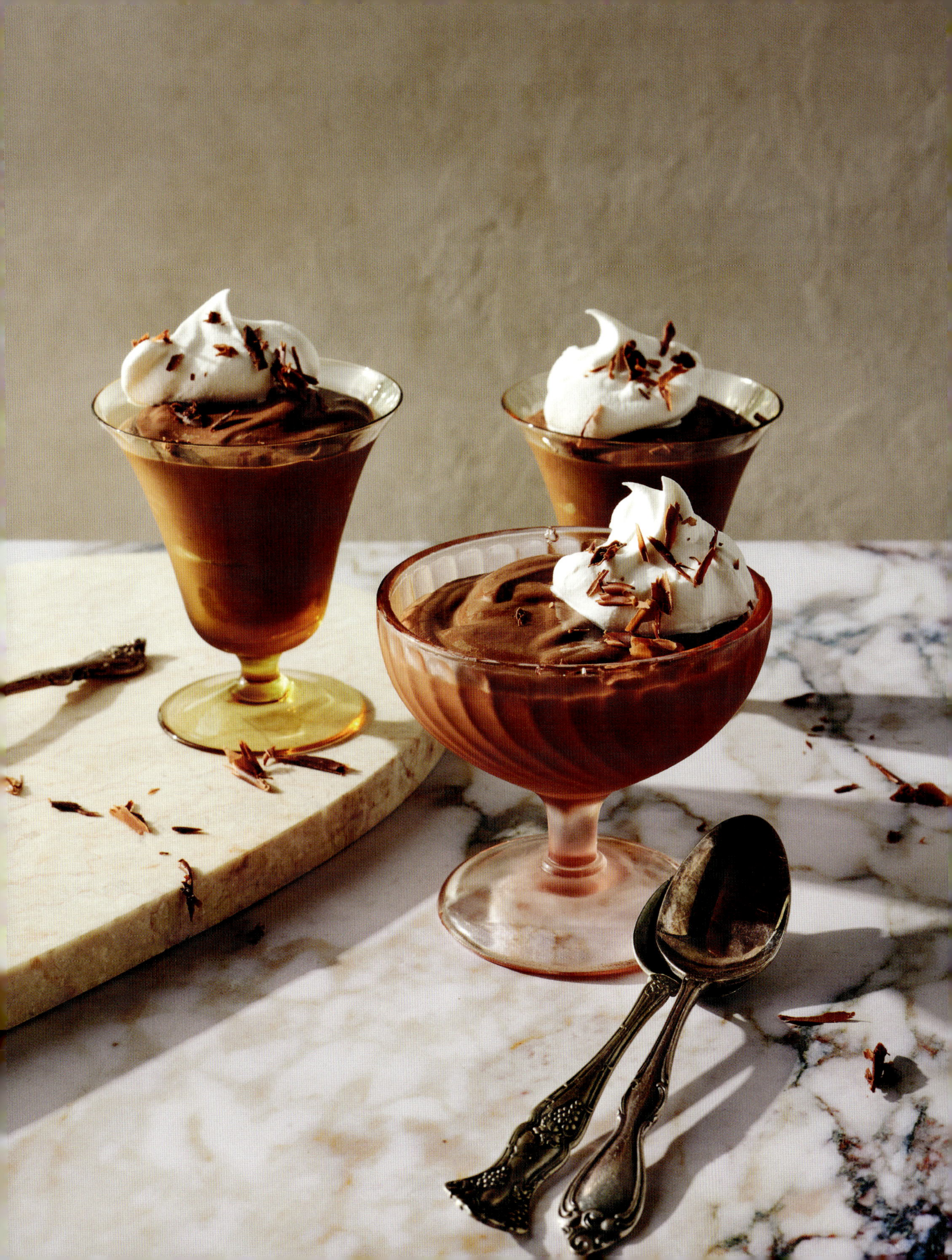

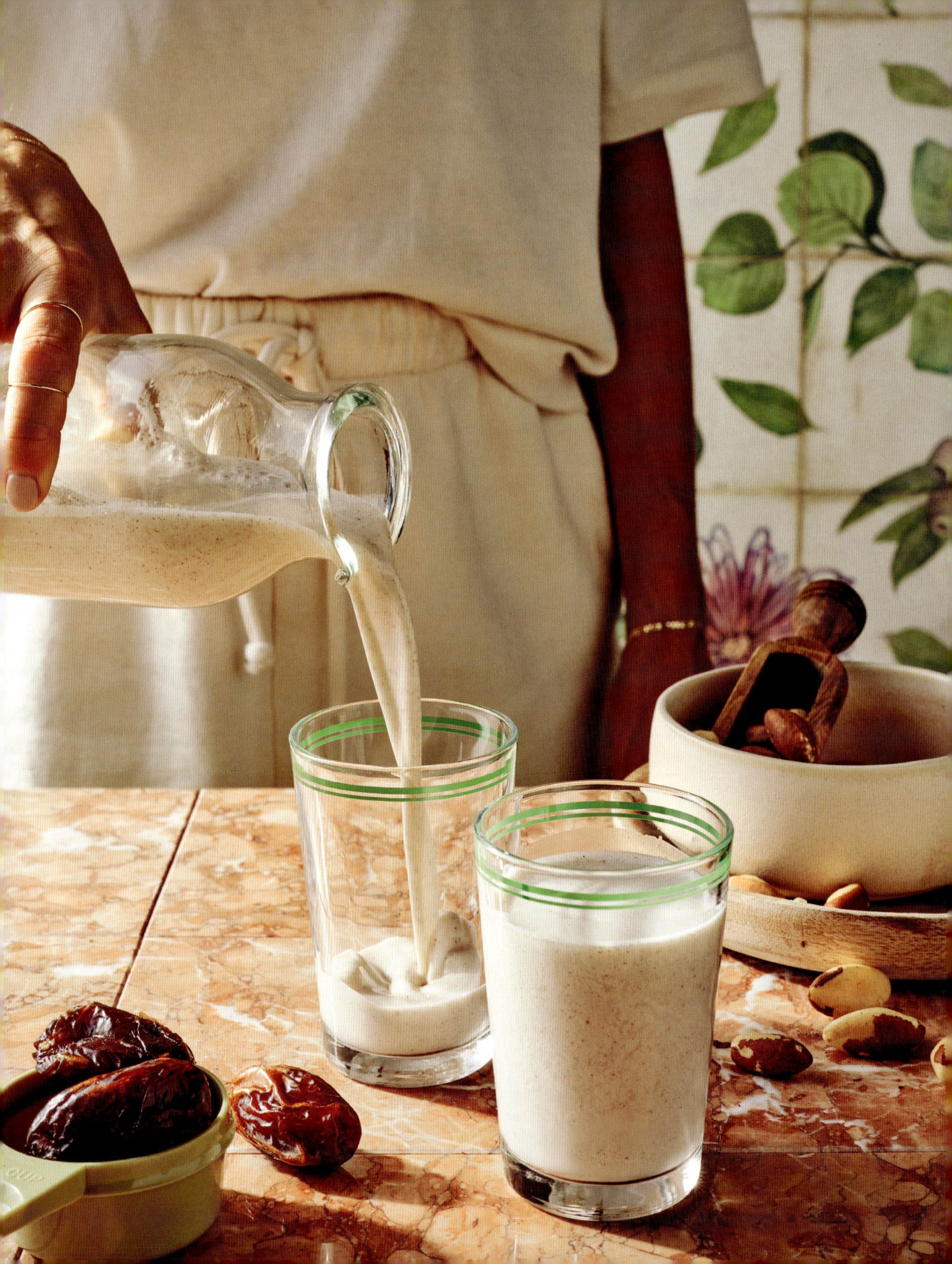
CUP

Thyroid-Lovin' Vanilla-Date Brazil Nut Milk

PREP: 30 MINUTES   COOK: NONE   SERVES 4

One thing I make without fail every single week is a fresh batch of Brazil nut milk. The concept might seem intimidating at first (it was to me), but once you start, I can almost guarantee you'll get hooked, as the subtly sweet flavor and creamy texture can't be beat! If you're a beverage girlie like me, it's also a simple habit that can yield impactful results, as most store-bought nondairy milks contain refined sugar, inflammatory seed oils, and shelf-stabilizing chemicals that disrupt hormones and gut health. I especially love this recipe because Brazil nuts provide plenty of selenium, an essential mineral needed for optimal thyroid and ovulatory function.

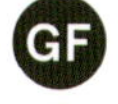

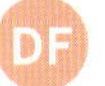

S

1 cup unsalted raw Brazil nuts

4 cups filtered water

2 dates, pitted

1 teaspoon vanilla bean paste (or the seeds scraped from 1 halved vanilla bean pod, or 2 teaspoons pure vanilla extract)

½ teaspoon Himalayan pink salt

1. *If you have the time, soak the Brazil nuts:* Place in a small bowl and pour boiling water over until completely covered, then soak for 30 minutes. Drain. (You can skip this step if short on time, but it does help to soften the nuts for a better texture.)

2. Combine the drained nuts, filtered water, dates, vanilla bean paste, and sea salt in a blender and blend until smooth. Strain through a fine-mesh strainer or nut milk bag (my personal preference), squeezing to release all the liquid into a large bowl. Discard the pulp. Transfer the milk to glass jars and store in the fridge for 5 to 6 days.

NOTE: Try using this as a base for the Snickers Smoothie (page 215) or Better-Than-Botox Smoothie (page 164)—it's absolutely divine!

FOLLICULAR PHASE BENEFITS

High in healthy fats • High in antioxidants

Better-Than-Botox Green Smoothie

PREP: 10 MINUTES COOK: NONE SERVES 1 (24 OUNCES)

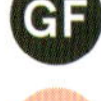

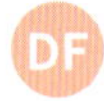

BF

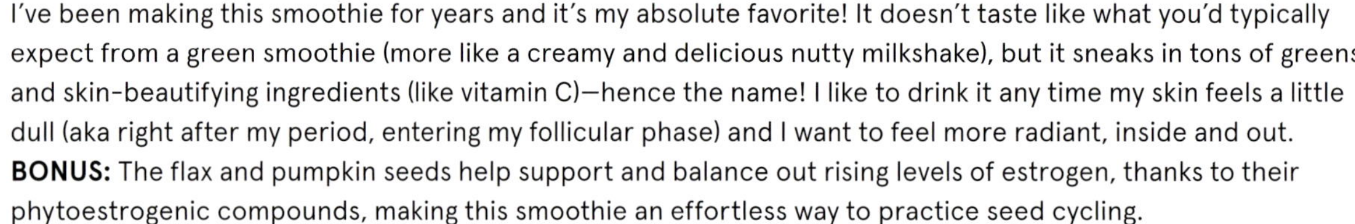

I've been making this smoothie for years and it's my absolute favorite! It doesn't taste like what you'd typically expect from a green smoothie (more like a creamy and delicious nutty milkshake), but it sneaks in tons of greens and skin-beautifying ingredients (like vitamin C)—hence the name! I like to drink it any time my skin feels a little dull (aka right after my period, entering my follicular phase) and I want to feel more radiant, inside and out. **BONUS:** The flax and pumpkin seeds help support and balance out rising levels of estrogen, thanks to their phytoestrogenic compounds, making this smoothie an effortless way to practice seed cycling.

- 1 cup organic unsweetened almond milk (add more for a thinner consistency if preferred) or Thyroid Lovin' Vanilla-Date Brazil Nut Milk (page 163)
- 1 serving vanilla protein powder
- 1 serving collagen peptides (optional)
- 2 tablespoons creamy almond butter
- 1 tablespoon raw pumpkin seeds
- 1 tablespoon organic flaxseeds
- 1 to 2 dates, pitted
- 1 teaspoon cinnamon
- ¼ teaspoon sea salt
- 1 cup frozen spinach
- ½ cup kale leaves, stems removed
- ½ cup frozen organic strawberries
- ½ frozen banana, optional
- ¼ cup broccoli sprouts or other microgreens, optional

Add the almond milk to a high-speed blender, followed by all the remaining ingredients. Turn the blender on low and slowly increase the speed until it's running on high and the smoothie is completely mixed and smooth. If it becomes too thick, try scraping down the sides or adding more almond milk.

FOLLICULAR PHASE BENEFITS

Supports liver function • Supports estrogen detoxification • High in healthy fats • Rich in fiber • High in antioxidants • Source of phytoestrogens

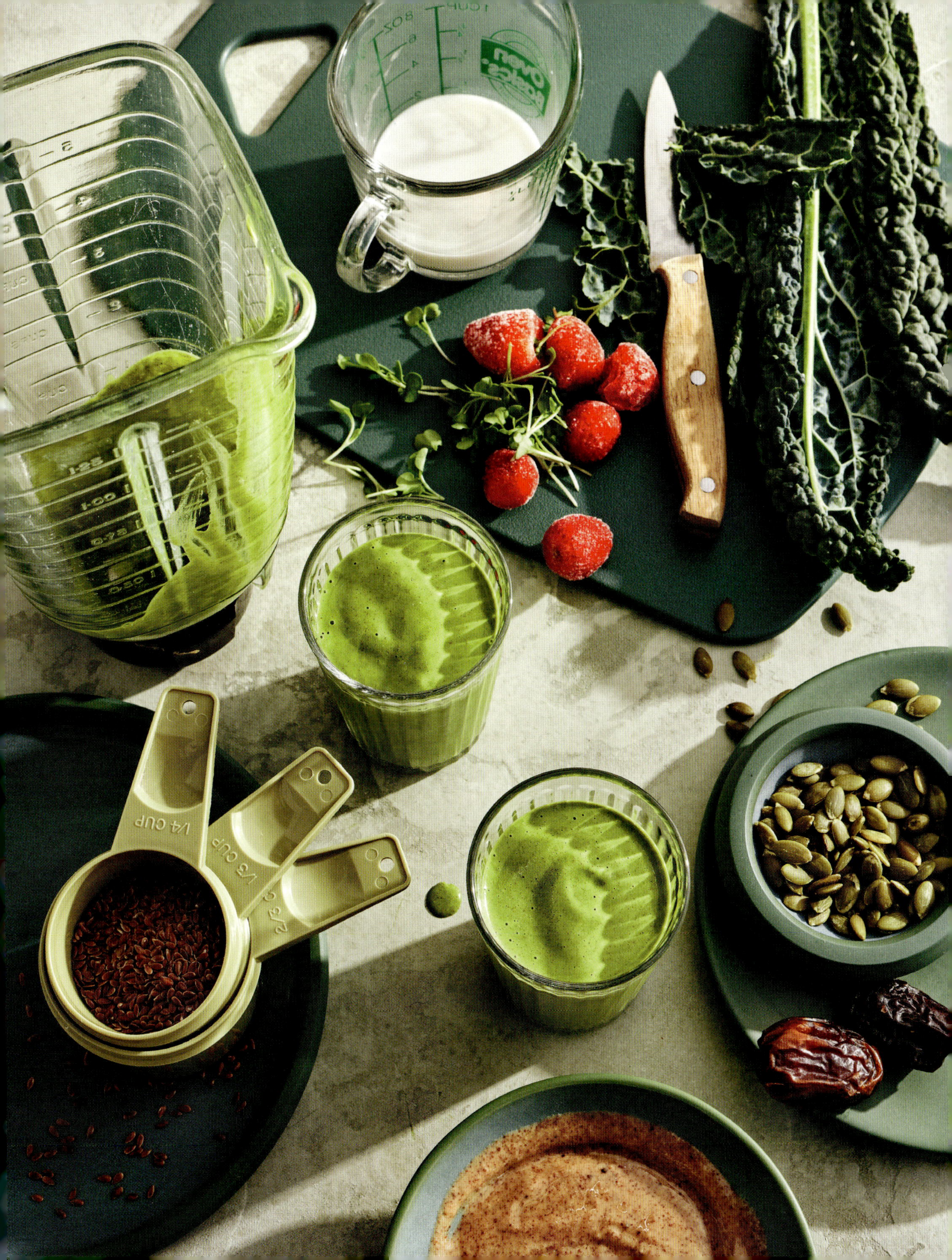
1/4 CUP
1/3 CUP

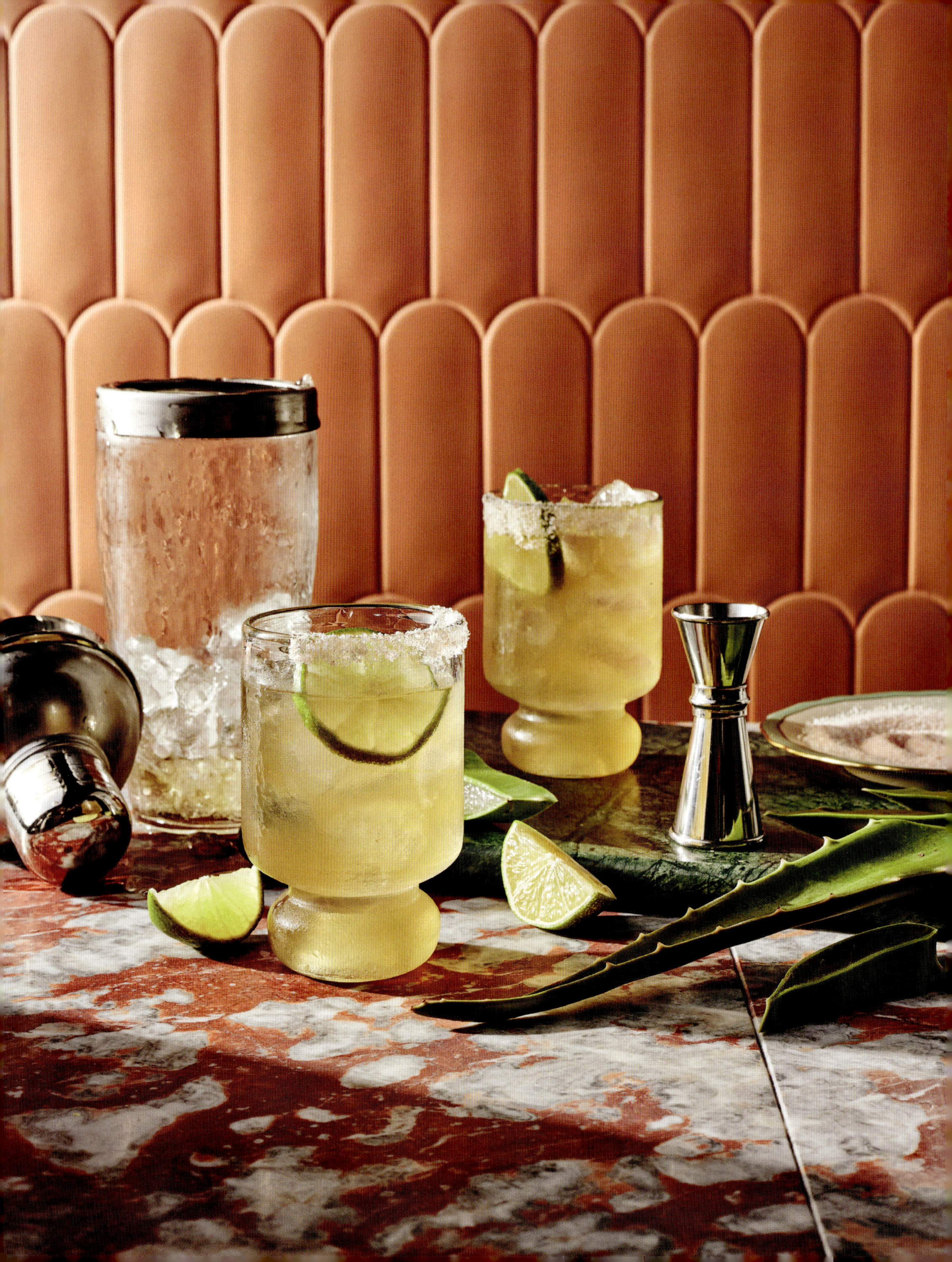

Refreshing Nettle + Aloe Margarita Mocktail

PREP: 15 MINUTES   COOK: NONE   SERVES 1–2

This herb-infused mocktail might sound a bit strange, but it tastes like a citrusy margarita sans alcohol thanks to the inclusion of freshly squeezed lime juice, a touch of honey, and a salted rim. It's also loaded with potassium, vitamin C, and sodium, a trifecta of minerals that supports your adrenal glands and combats stress, not to mention nettle is a powerhouse herb that helps restore nutrients post-period. This is functional imbibing at its finest.

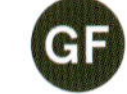

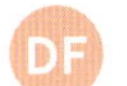

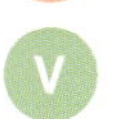

P

⅔ cup steaming-hot water

1 teaspoon dried loose-leaf nettle leaves

1 tablespoon raw honey

1 tablespoon hot water

½ cup inner-leaf aloe vera juice (avoid whole leaf, which can have a laxative-like effect)

¼ cup fresh lime juice

Ice cubes

Lime wedge

Sea salt

1. In a strainer, filter, or tea infuser, pour the ⅔ cup hot water over the nettle leaves and let sit for 10 minutes. Discard the herbs and place the tea in the fridge to chill for a minimum of 10 minutes.

2. Whisk together the honey and the 1 tablespoon hot water in a cocktail shaker until well combined (you can do this in a glass or small bowl as well). The hot water will help the honey mix with the rest of the drink. Add the chilled nettle tea, aloe vera juice, lime juice, and ice, then shake until the drink is chilled and well mixed.

3. Rub the lime wedge around the rim of a large glass, then dip the glass rim in a shallow plate of sea salt. Add ice cubes to the glass and pour the mixed mocktail over it until full.

NOTE: If you want to save time, you can prepare a pot of tea 1 day before and keep it in the fridge until ready to make the mocktail.

FOLLICULAR PHASE BENEFITS

Supports liver function • High in antioxidants

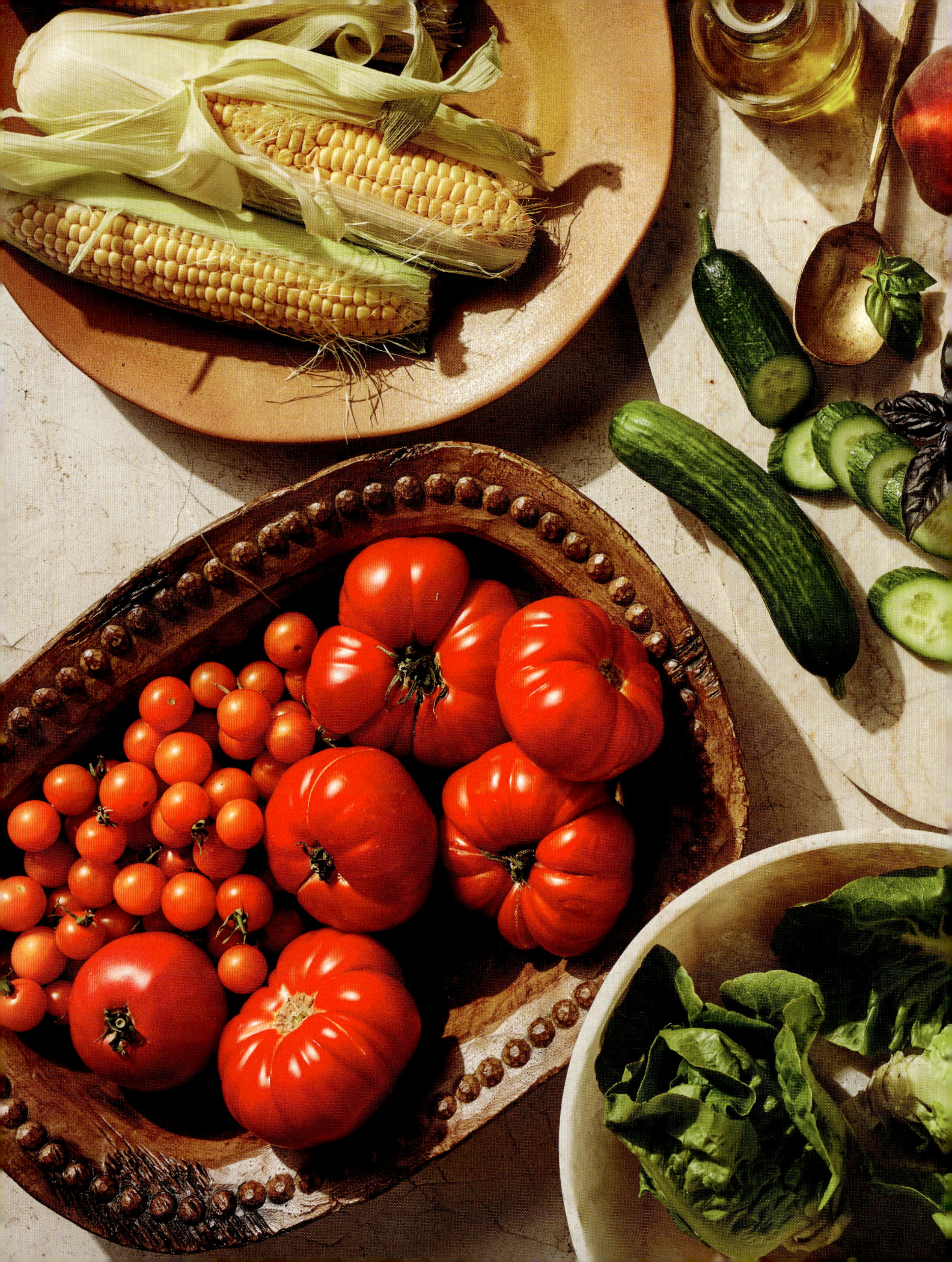

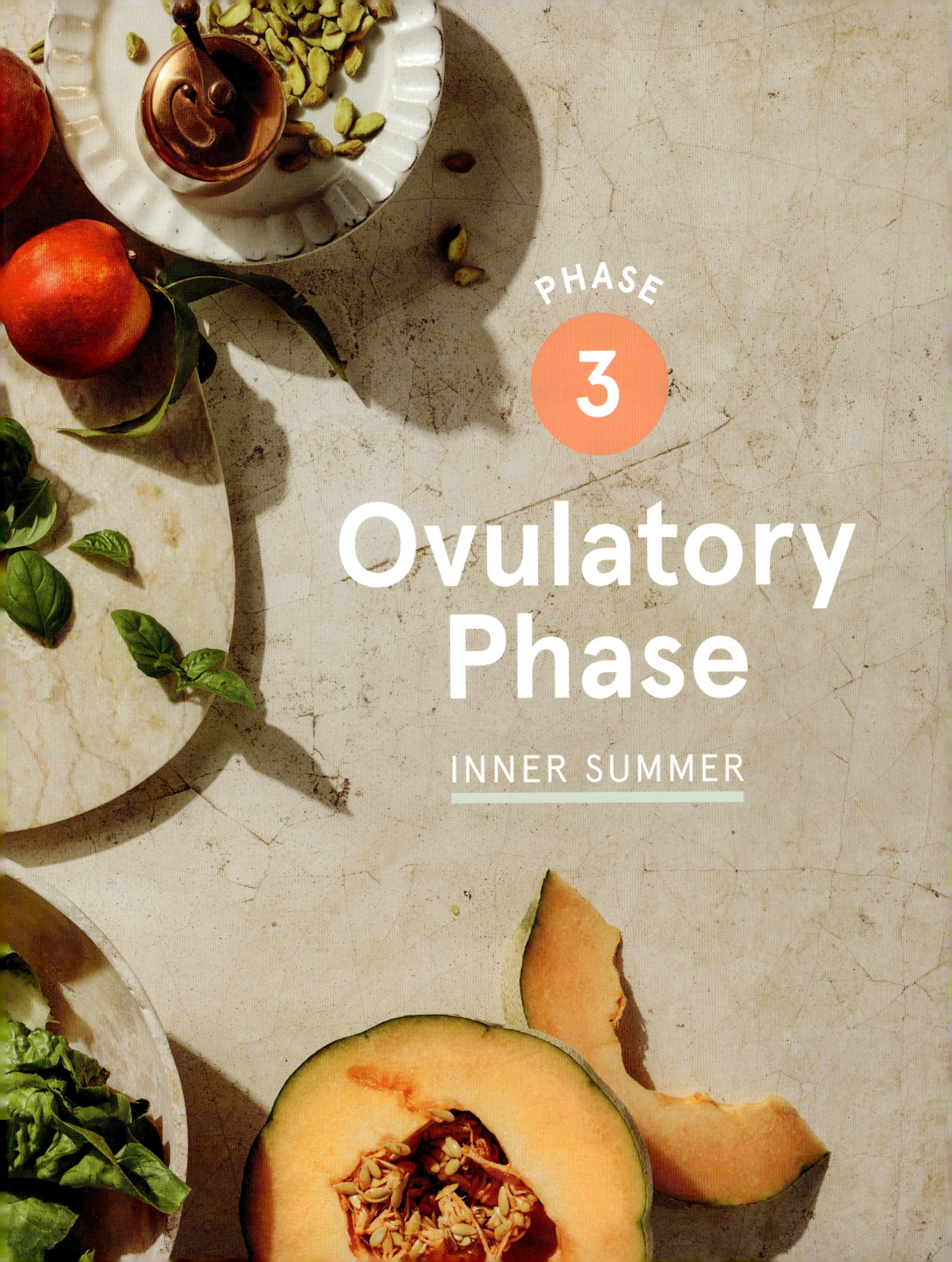

PHASE

3

Ovulatory Phase

INNER SUMMER

RECIPES

WHAT'S HAPPENING

Right before ovulation, peaking estrogen levels prompt your pituitary gland to release luteinizing hormone (LH), causing the dominant follicle to rupture and release an egg into the fallopian tube. This egg will be viable for roughly 12 to 24 hours, and if not fertilized by sperm (which can live up to five days in the female body), it will disintegrate.

Ovulation typically occurs somewhere between days 12 and 17 of your cycle, but you'll need to use the fertility awareness methods outlined on page 30 to determine when exactly it happens for you. While this phase is short, you will feel the hormonal effects in the days leading up to and following ovulation, which is great news for most women, as a majority report looking and feeling their most attractive during this phase.

This can be attributed to surging levels of estrogen and testosterone, helping you *feel* yourself, with a rise in energy, mood, magnetism, confidence, creativity, and communication skills, inclining you to get out, connect, see, and be seen (i.e., peak summer vibes). Your libido is also running high to naturally get you in the mood during your fertile window and attract a mate with "genetic potential." While this phase brings with it an abundance of fun and fabulous characteristics, it's especially important to focus on keeping peaking estrogen levels in check, as an excess can lead to pain during ovulation, as well as many of the symptoms we often dread in the upcoming phase (including PMS, heavy periods, weight gain, mood swings, and cramping).

Physically, your uterine lining continues to thicken in preparation for a potential pregnancy, while your cervix opens and starts producing wetter quality cervical fluid (similar to the consistency of egg whites), designed to help sperm travel and survive the long journey to the egg in order to fertilize it.

PILLARS OF EATING FOR OVULATION

Consuming specific macro- and micronutrients during your ovulatory phase works to support cyclical hormonal fluctuations, helping your body keep surging estrogen levels in check and providing it with the energy it needs to release an egg. But not only that: Because ovulation is often considered the most vital part of your cycle, it lays the foundation to optimize your biology for the phases that follow, mitigating uncomfortable symptoms and empowering you to feel your best the rest of your menstrual cycle.

Optimal Foods to Support Ovulation

FOODS THAT SUPPORT VASCULAR HEALTH

A healthy vascular system (also known as your circulatory system) is key to healthy ovarian function and egg quality, as well as ensuring that once you ovulate your ruptured follicle seamlessly transitions into a corpus luteum that produces enough progesterone to sustain your menstrual cycle (and a healthy uterine lining if trying to conceive!). **Optimal foods to incorporate during ovulation for vascular support include:**

- Olives and olive oil
- Wild-caught fatty fish
- Oats
- Beets
- Tomatoes
- Spinach and leafy greens
- Pomegranates
- Berries (especially blueberries)
- Citrus
- Ginger

CRUCIFEROUS VEGETABLES

The emphasis on cruciferous vegetables begins in your follicular phase and continues during ovulation, as they contain sulfur compounds that assist in safely eliminating excess estrogen that could otherwise lead to PMS and other uncomfortable symptoms. **These include:**

- Broccoli
- Cauliflower
- Brussels sprouts
- Bok choy
- Cabbage
- Kale
- Watercress
- Arugula

LIVER-SUPPORTIVE FOODS

You'll also want to continue to focus on liver-supportive foods that assist in estrogen metabolism and detoxification. **These include:**

- Cruciferous veggies
- Raw carrots
- Beets
- Green asparagus
- Onion
- Garlic
- Broccoli sprouts
- Dandelion greens
- Leafy greens
- Citrus
- Turmeric

GLUTATHIONE- AND ANTIOXIDANT-RICH FOODS

Eating a colorful, well-rounded diet rich in antioxidant-loaded foods helps to enhance mitochondrial function, fight off free radicals, and mitigate oxidative damage, all of which improve egg quality. It also supports the liver in estrogen detoxification (glutathione is especially vital in this process). **Optimal glutathione- and antioxidant-rich foods to incorporate into your ovulatory phase include:**

- Cruciferous veggies
- Bell peppers
- Tomatoes
- Avocado
- Asparagus
- Okra
- Berries (especially strawberries)
- Citrus
- Papaya

SELENIUM-RICH FOODS

Selenium is an essential mineral (especially important for thyroid health!) and a glutathione cofactor, meaning it's vital in reducing oxidative stress levels, supporting liver detoxification, and eliminating excess estrogen. **Selenium-rich foods to incorporate during ovulation include:**

- Organ meats
- Lamb
- Grass-fed beef
- Poultry
- Wild-caught fish
- Organic full-fat cottage cheese
- Brazil nuts
- Brown rice

FERMENTED AND PROBIOTIC-RICH FOODS

You'll want to continue to emphasize fermented and probiotic-rich foods that positively influence our gut flora, particularly our estrobolome, a collection of gut bacteria and fungi that metabolizes and regulates estrogen levels. **These sources include:**

- Organic non-GMO miso or tempeh
- Kimchi
- Sauerkraut
- Pickled vegetables
- Full-fat Greek or coconut yogurt
- Full-fat cottage cheese
- Kefir
- Apple cider vinegar

FIBER-RICH FOODS

Keep up consumption of fiber (as recommended in the follicular phase), which also supports your gut microbiome, digestive tract, and the elimination of excess estrogen. **Optimal fiber-rich sources include:**

- Gluten-free whole grains (quinoa, oats, millet, rice)
- Lentils/legumes
- Cruciferous veggies
- Artichokes
- Avocado
- Split peas
- Leafy greens and green vegetables
- Berries
- Chia and flaxseeds

HERBS AND SPICES

Incorporating herbal teas, digestive bitters, and adaptogens into your ovulatory phase routine can be an extremely effective way to support optimal hormonal balance and reduce or reverse menstrual cycle symptoms. The "whole food supplements" below contain vitamins and minerals that work to support liver detox and excess estrogen elimination, naturally balance out estrogen levels, enhance energy and libido, and overall support healthy ovulation. I recommend purchasing most in loose-leaf form to drink as a daily tea or herbal infusion. **These include:**

- Maca
- Turmeric
- Dandelion root
- Burdock root
- Nettle tea
- Hibiscus tea
- Bee pollen
- Digestive bitters

Cooking and Eating Tips to Support Ovulation

INCORPORATE MORE FRESH AND RAW FOODS

According to traditional Chinese medicine (TCM) your follicular and ovulatory phases are "hot" phases of your cycle due to the physiological changes happening, such as estrogen rising—a heating force. During this phase, opt for more fresh raw vegetables and fruits that have a natural cooling effect on the body—think foods you'd gravitate toward naturally in the summer such as ripe, juicy produce, smoothies, crudités, and fermented veggies. These foods are also loaded with antioxidants that promote optimal vascular support and egg quality.

USE LIGHTER COOKING METHODS

Following TCM guidelines (above), when cooking your food during this phase it's best to opt for lighter methods such as steaming, poaching, blanching, and sautéing. This helps to preserve the antioxidants and nutrients in most of the fruits and vegetables recommended for this phase (they tend to be lighter vs. more grounding plants like potatoes and squash, which are easier to digest when cooked well at higher temperatures).

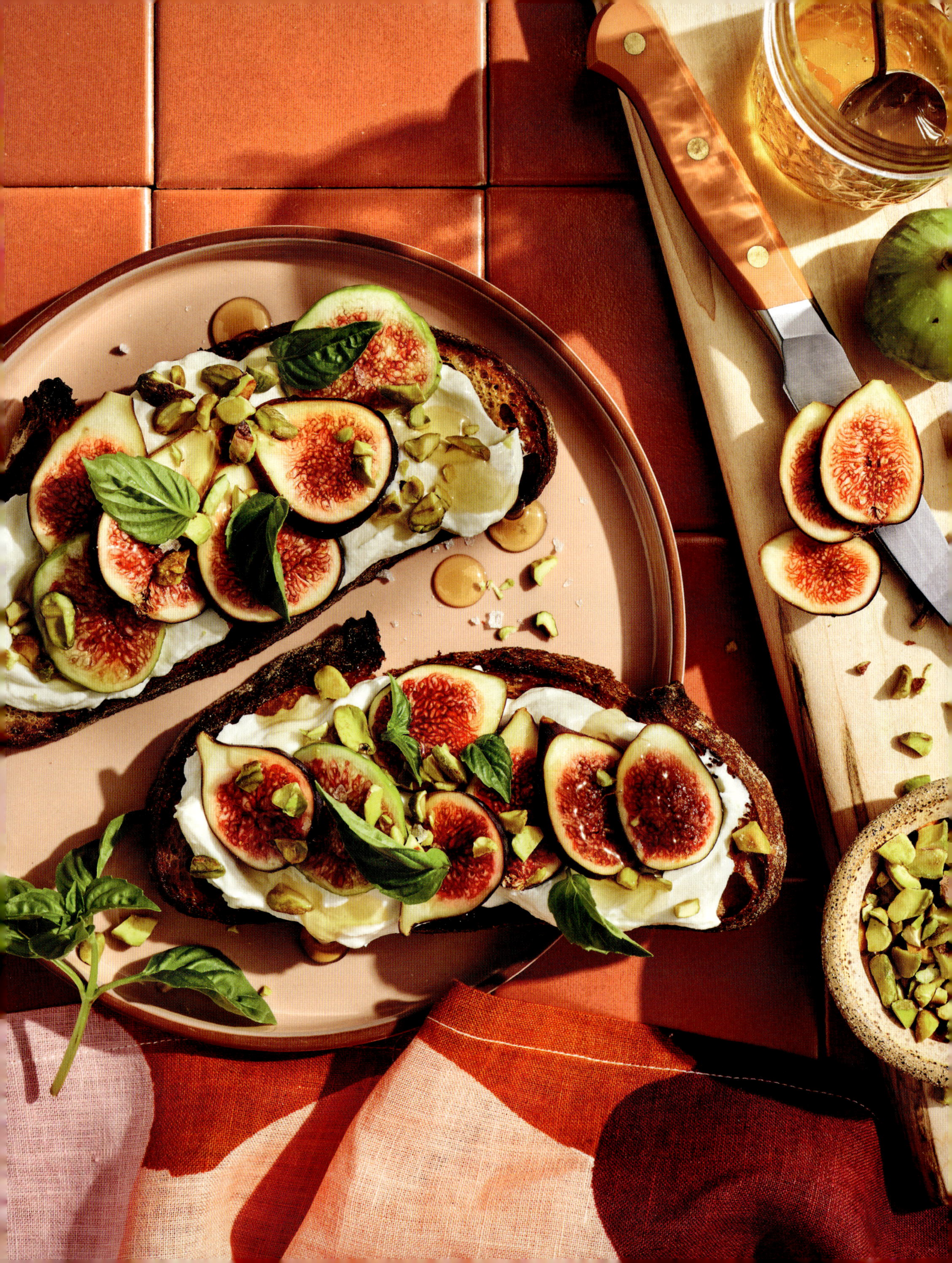

Whipped Ricotta Toast + Figs, Pistachios, and Honey

PREP: 5 MINUTES COOK: 5 MINUTES SERVES 4 (MAKES ABOUT 2 CUPS WHIPPED RICOTTA)

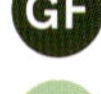

During my pregnancy with my third baby girl, Frankie, I had terrible first-trimester nausea. I knew if I wanted to feel better, I needed to eat more protein, but the mere thought of meat was just too much...So I started experimenting with different toppings on my daily toast, and I soon discovered that whipping ricotta cheese transforms it into the creamiest silky-smooth spread that also happens to be loaded with protein (28 grams per cup!) as well as minerals like selenium and calcium, which optimize thyroid function and protect against oxidative stress. I especially love this combo during ovulation for its juicy, decadent flavor, fertility-boosting nutrient profile, and overall feminine vibe. Note that I include both savory and sweet options for versatility; I lean toward the honey ricotta for this fig-centric toast.

Whipped Ricotta Cheese

- **1 (15-ounce) container (about 2 cups) whole-milk ricotta cheese**
- **2 tablespoons extra virgin olive oil**
- **1 tablespoon fresh lemon juice**
- **½ teaspoon sea salt**
- **2 tablespoons raw honey (to make sweet) or 1 small garlic clove, minced (to make savory), optional**

Toast

- **2 pieces gluten-free sourdough bread, lightly toasted**
- **½ cup ripe figs (or another fruit like apricot, peach, etc.), thinly sliced**
- **2 tablespoons torn fresh basil or mint**
- **2 tablespoons pistachios, roughly chopped**
- **1 to 2 tablespoons raw honey**
- **Handful of dark berries or cherries (optional)**
- **Sprinkle of flaky sea salt**

1. *For the whipped ricotta cheese:* Combine all the ricotta ingredients in a food processor and mix until creamy and mostly smooth.

2. Spread 2 to 4 tablespoons whipped ricotta on each slice of toasted bread. Top with the figs, basil or mint, pistachios, honey, and optional berries, and sprinkle with salt. Enjoy immediately.

NOTE: The whipped ricotta cheese will make a large portion (about 2 cups or 4 servings), so you can store the rest in an airtight container in the fridge for up to 5 days. Use as a topping for toast, pancakes, bowls, etc., or as a high-protein dip for fruits or veggies.

OVULATORY PHASE BENEFITS

Supports vascular health • Rich in probiotics • High in glutathione and antioxidants

Debloat Papaya Boat

PREP: 5 MINUTES, PLUS OVERNIGHT IF MAKING CHIA PUDDING | COOK: NONE | SERVES 2

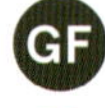

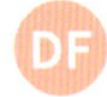

This recipe elevates your basic breakfast bowl, both flavor- and nutrient-wise. I especially love it anytime I'm feeling bloated (which can be a common symptom during ovulation due to the surge in LH), thanks to the digestive enzymes in the papaya. It's also loaded with vitamin C and antioxidants that naturally boost glutathione production, supporting detoxification and combating oxidative stress. Try to get fresh, organic papaya if possible, which comes into season in early summer. You'll *almost* feel like you're on vacation. If making the chia pudding filling, make sure to prepare it the night before to gel in the fridge.

1 ripe organic papaya

1 cup Classic Vanilla Chia Pudding (page 126), unsweetened full-fat Greek yogurt, or cottage cheese

Organic berries, chopped nuts or seeds, creamy nut butter, bee pollen, cacao nibs, drizzle of raw honey, or fresh mint, for topping (optional)

1. Slice the papaya in half lengthwise and scoop out all of the seeds with a spoon to make two shallow bowls.

2. Spoon the chia pudding filling, yogurt, or cottage cheese into the two papaya bowls. Add your desired toppings of choice. Use a spoon to scoop up the papaya flesh with big bites of filling (just don't eat the papaya skin).

OVULATORY PHASE BENEFITS

Supports liver function • Rich in fiber • Rich in probiotics • High in glutathione and antioxidants

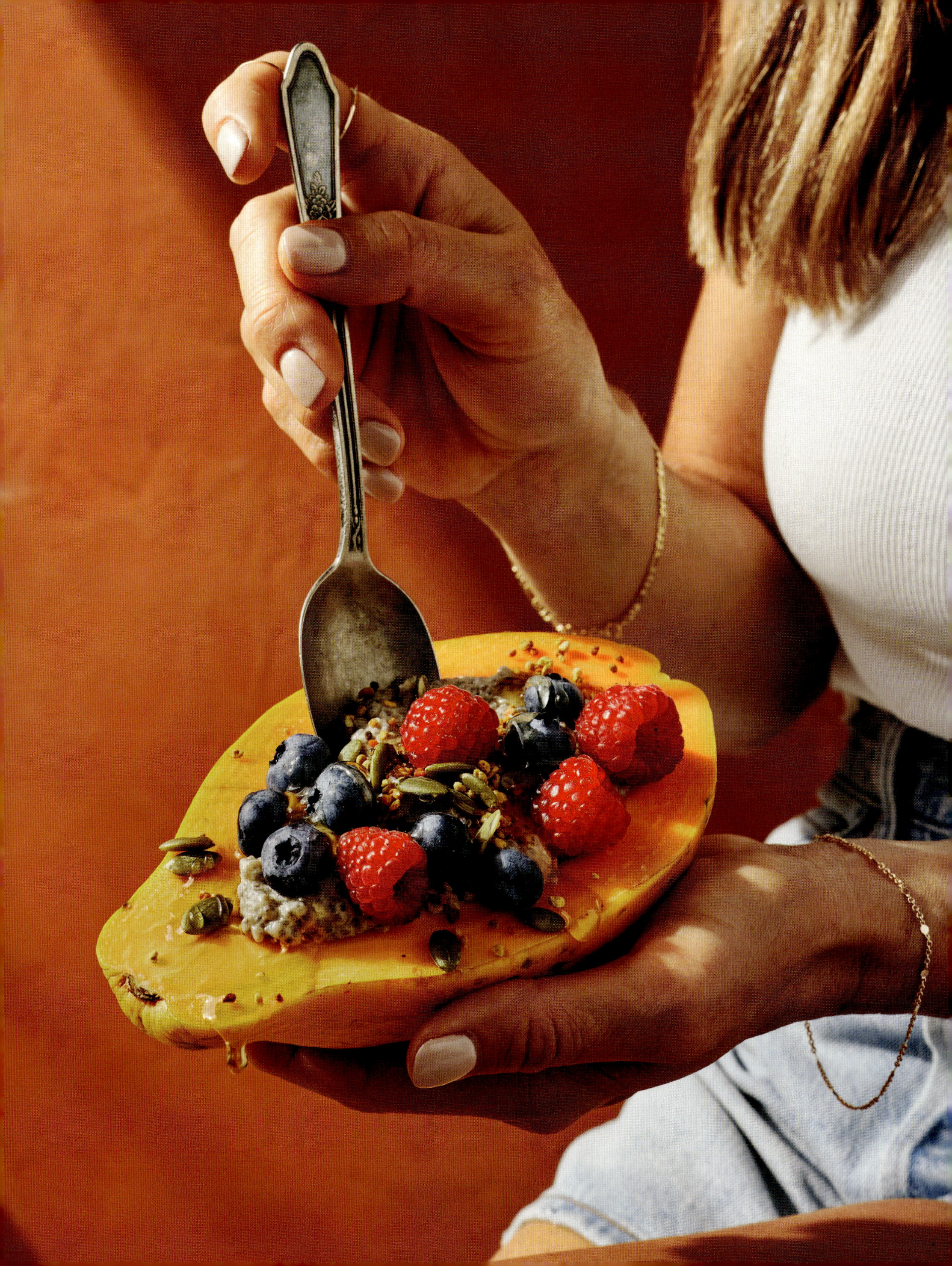

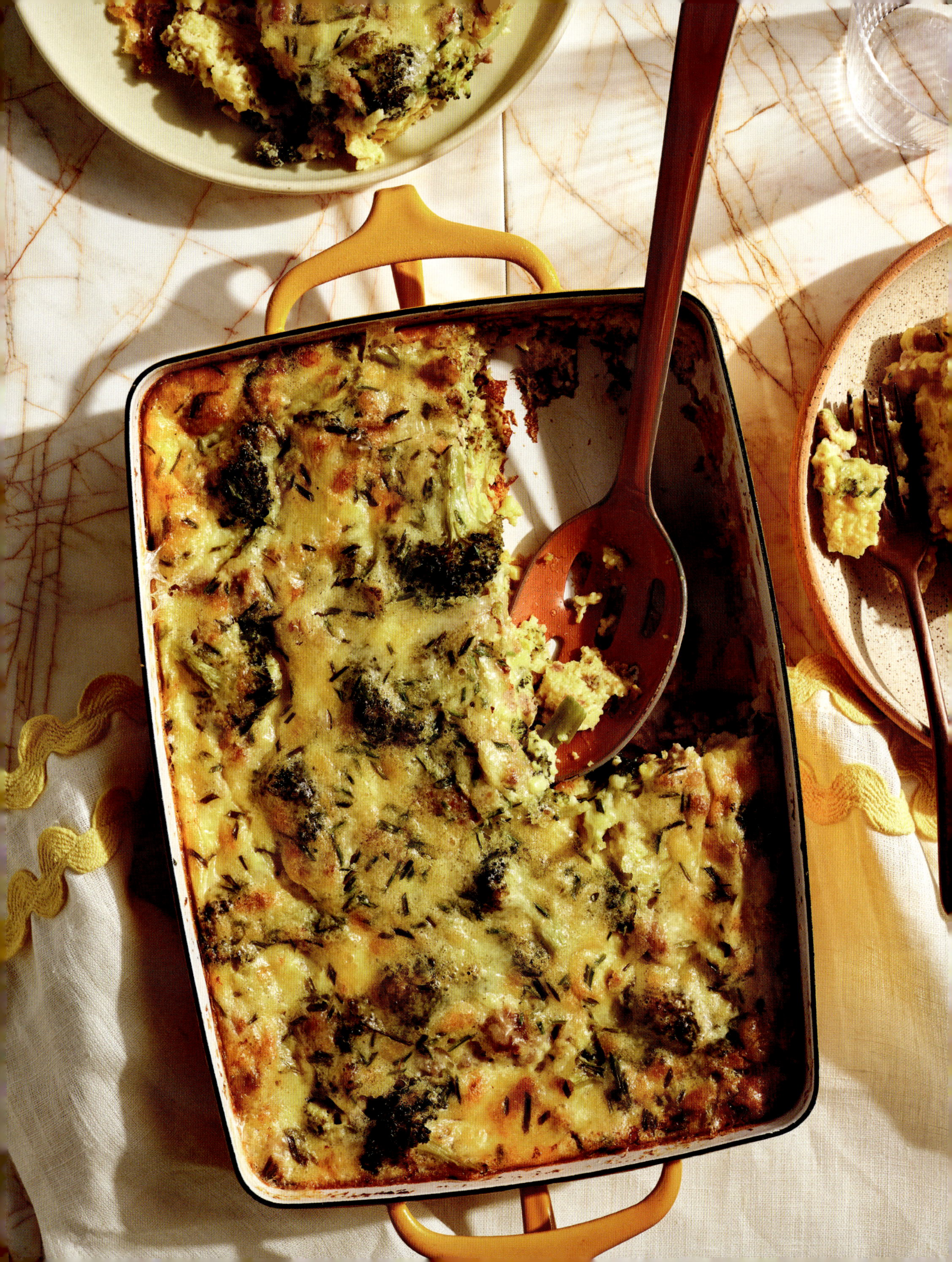

High-Protein Broccoli-Cheddar Breakfast Casserole

PREP: 10 MINUTES COOK: 35 MINUTES SERVES 4–6

This protein-packed savory breakfast can be prepped ahead of time *and* feed a crowd. Blending cottage cheese with eggs not only lends a delicious fluffy texture but adds a whopping 30 grams of protein and boosts minerals like selenium that support glutathione production. I prefer incorporating ground sausage meat for more protein and flavor, but you can leave it out if you're looking for a vegetarian option. This breakfast always keeps me feeling energized and on my A game, which is especially helpful when I'm in my ovulatory phase and tend to be in go-go-go mode.

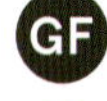

- 1 head organic broccoli, chopped into small florets
- Avocado oil or spray
- 2 cloves garlic, minced
- Sea salt and black pepper
- 1 pound organic ground breakfast sausage or chorizo (optional)
- 10 large pasture-raised eggs
- 1 cup organic full-fat cottage cheese
- 1 teaspoon garlic powder
- ¼ cup diced chives
- 1 cup shredded raw organic cheddar cheese

1. Preheat the oven to 400°F. Place the broccoli in a 9 by 13-inch baking pan or casserole dish and generously coat or spray with avocado oil. Mix in the garlic and sprinkle with salt and pepper. Roast for 10 minutes, until the broccoli is cooked through. Set aside. Immediately reduce the oven temperature to 350°F.

2. Meanwhile, if using breakfast sausage or chorizo, cook in a separate skillet over medium heat until cooked through (follow package instructions). Set aside until ready to use.

3. Combine the eggs, cottage cheese, garlic powder, and ½ teaspoon salt in a blender and mix until creamy and well combined.

4. Distribute the sausage or chorizo evenly over the broccoli in the baking pan, then pour the egg mixture evenly over the top. Sprinkle with the chives and cheddar. Bake for 25 to 30 minutes, until the center of the casserole is firm and the cheese is melted. Store in an airtight glass container in the fridge for 3 to 5 days, or cut into individual servings, wrap, and store in the freezer for up to 2 months.

NOTE: If you want to make this dish dairy-free, swap out the cottage cheese for ⅔ cup dairy-free unsweetened milk (like almond milk) and use a vegan cheddar for topping (or simply omit). Just note that this will reduce the amount of protein in the dish.

OVULATORY PHASE BENEFITS

Supports vascular health • Supports liver function • Supports estrogen detoxification • High in glutathione and antioxidants

Mineral-Rich Prosciutto-Wrapped Melon

PREP: 5 MINUTES | COOK: 20 MINUTES | SERVES 4

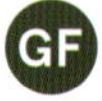
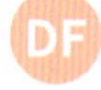

The MVP of summer apps and snacks! Melon wrapped in prosciutto is nothing new or novel (you can thank the Italians for this one), but you might not have guessed how nutrient-dense it is, thanks to high amounts of electrolytes or intracellular minerals like potassium and sodium that regulate blood sugar, cell hydration, and thyroid and bowel function—to name just a few. We need to consume these minerals daily, but it can be especially beneficial during ovulation to combat common symptoms like bloat and ensure you're eliminating excess estrogen efficiently.

Balsamic Glaze

2 cups balsamic vinegar

½ cup coconut sugar

Prosciutto-Wrapped Melon

1 ripe cantaloupe or honeydew melon

1 (4-ounce) package very thinly sliced prosciutto di Parma

High-quality extra virgin olive oil

Flaky Maldon sea salt

¼ cup freshly torn basil leaves, for garnish

1. *For the balsamic glaze:* Combine the vinegar and coconut sugar in a small pot over medium heat and cook, stirring occasionally, until it comes to a boil. Reduce the heat to low and let the mixture simmer for 20 minutes, until it's reduced by half and has a thick, slightly sticky texture. Let cool, then pour into an airtight glass jar (see Note).

2. *For the melon:* Use a sharp knife to remove half an inch off the top and bottom of the melon. Stand the melon up on one of the flat, cut sides. Starting from the top and following the contour of the melon, carefully slice the rind off with a knife, cutting off about ¼ inch (the entire green inner rind). Repeat this process until you've peeled the entire melon. Slice in half and scoop out the seeds with a spoon. Lay each half flat and slice into wedges.

3. Wrap one slice of prosciutto around each melon wedge and arrange on a plate. Top with just a drizzle of olive oil and balsamic glaze. Sprinkle with Maldon sea salt and garnish with fresh basil. Serve immediately or chill in the fridge in an airtight container until ready, up to 3 hours.

NOTE: To help this dish come together quickly, you can use store-bought balsamic glaze (or raw honey). Or make your own glaze well ahead of time and store in the fridge for up to 2 weeks. The leftovers are terrific on the Cottage Cheese Caprese with Heirloom Tomatoes + Stone Fruit (page 183) or drizzled over ripe summer produce like heirloom tomatoes and stone fruit.

OVULATORY PHASE BENEFITS

Supports vascular health • Supports estrogen detoxification • High in glutathione and antioxidants

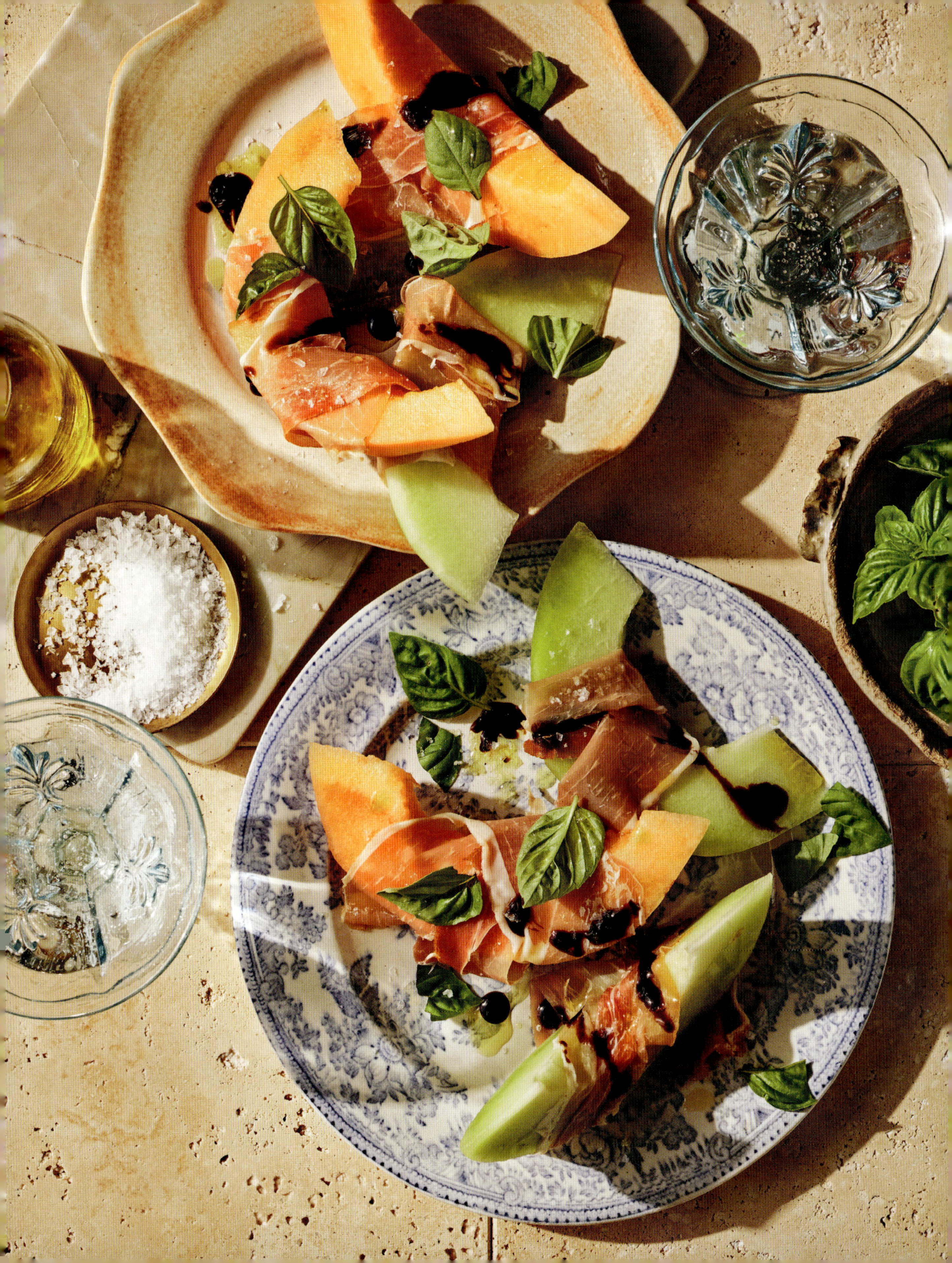

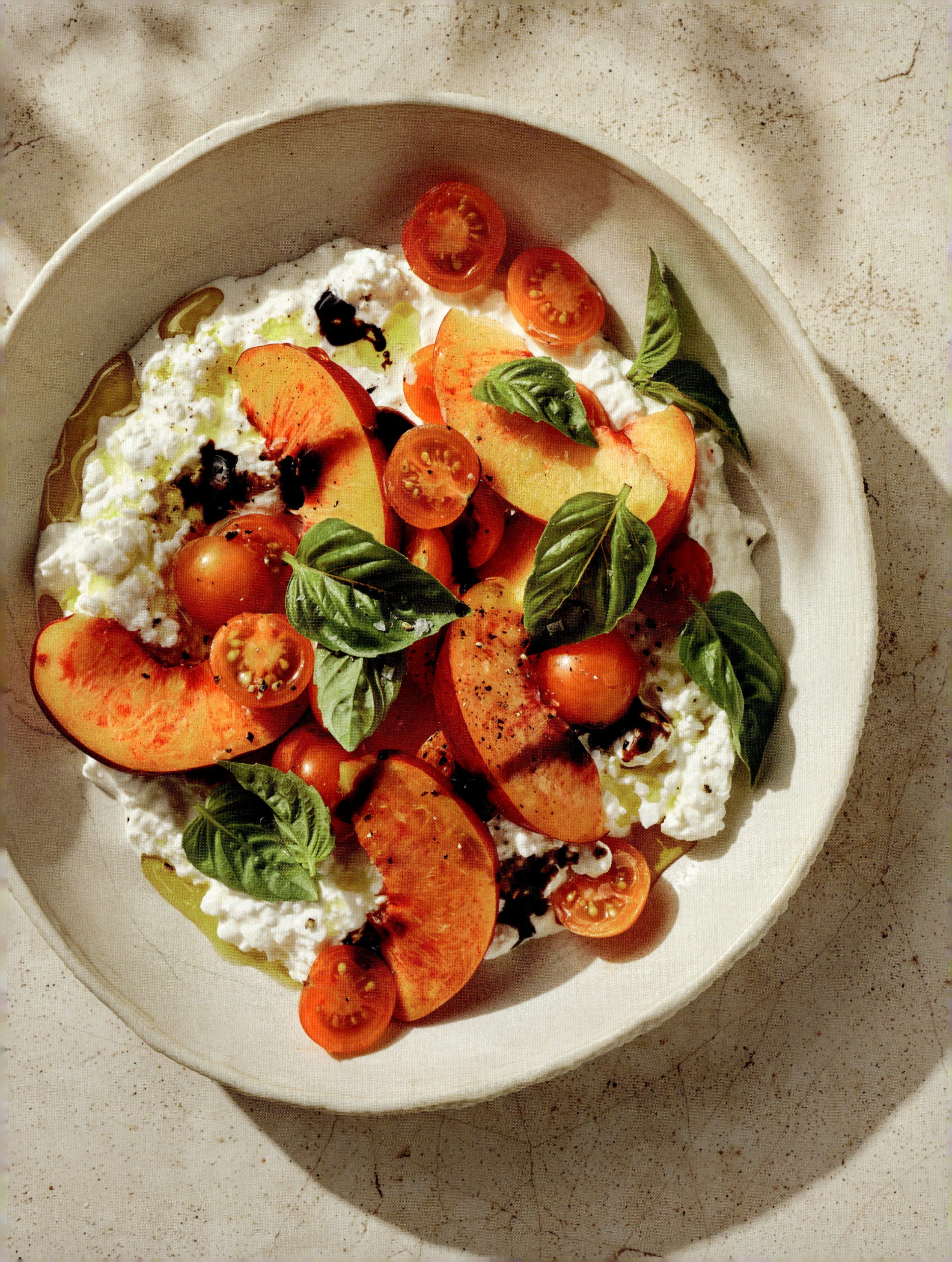

Cottage Cheese Caprese with Heirloom Tomatoes + Stone Fruit

PREP: 10 MINUTES (MORE IF MAKING BALSAMIC GLAZE) COOK: NONE SERVES 1

This life-saving recipe has prevented a blood sugar catastrophe for me countless times. It requires minimal effort, comes together in mere minutes, and is packed with protein and real, whole ingredients—making it far more satisfying (and delicious) than a protein bar or other packaged snack. I especially love it during my ovulatory phase as it spotlights seasonal produce rich in nutrients like vitamin C that support glowing skin, detoxification, and optimal egg quality—helping me feel my best inside and out.

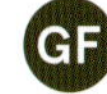

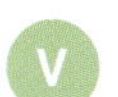

BF

- **1 cup organic full-fat cottage cheese**
- **½ cup orange Sungold cherry tomatoes (or other heirloom tomatoes of choice), halved**
- **1 ripe nectarine or apricot, pitted and chopped**
- **Drizzle of extra virgin olive oil**
- **Drizzle of Balsamic Glaze (page 180) or honey**
- **2 tablespoons chopped fresh basil leaves**
- **Sea salt and black pepper to taste**

Add the cottage cheese to a large, shallow bowl. Top with the tomatoes and nectarine or apricot and drizzle with olive oil and balsamic glaze. Sprinkle with basil and season with salt and pepper to taste.

OVULATORY PHASE BENEFITS

Supports vascular health • Supports liver function • Supports estrogen detoxification • Rich in probiotics • High in glutathione and antioxidants

Charred Cauliflower + Dates and Spiced Tahini Sauce

PREP: 10 MINUTES COOK: 30 MINUTES SERVES 4 (MAKES ⅔ CUP TAHINI)

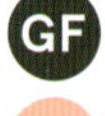

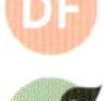

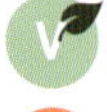

This side dish is so good it often accidentally ends up being the star of the show! The caramelized, crispy cauliflower bites are the most delicious way to up your cruciferous veggie intake. Cauliflower contains compounds to assist in excess estrogen elimination as it peaks, which is crucial for a symptom-free second half of your cycle. Sweet, plump dates make the ultimate fiber-rich topping and the spiced tahini sauce is *so* good you'll want to be sure to save the rest to reuse on bowls or salads.

Cauliflower

- **1 large cauliflower, chopped into small florets (about 4 cups)**
- **2 to 4 tablespoons avocado oil**
- **4 cloves garlic, minced**
- **Sea salt and black pepper to taste**

Spiced Tahini

- **¼ cup organic tahini**
- **3 tablespoons water**
- **1 tablespoon pure maple syrup**
- **Juice of 1 lemon (about 2 tablespoons)**
- **1 teaspoon coriander**
- **1 teaspoon cumin**
- **½ teaspoon paprika**
- **½ teaspoon chili powder**
- **½ teaspoon sea salt**

To Serve

- **¼ cup medjool dates, pitted and chopped, for topping**
- **¼ cup chopped pistachios, for topping**
- **2 tablespoons fresh mint leaves, for topping**
- **2 tablespoons fresh dill leaves, minced, for topping**

1. Preheat the oven to 425°F and line a large baking sheet with parchment paper.

2. *For the cauliflower:* Arrange the cauliflower florets on the baking sheet in an even layer and drizzle with enough avocado oil to evenly coat the florets. Add the garlic, salt, and pepper. Use your hands to mix everything together, making sure the cauliflower is evenly coated. Roast, flipping halfway through, for 25 to 30 minutes, until crispy and golden brown.

3. *For the spiced tahini:* While the cauliflower is roasting, combine all the ingredients in a blender and pulse until creamy and smooth. Set aside.

4. Sprinkle the cauliflower with the dates, pistachios, mint, and dill. Serve with a light drizzle of the tahini sauce.

NOTES: Make sure the cauliflower is chopped into very small pieces. This ensures they get extra charred and crispy!

OVULATORY PHASE BENEFITS

Supports liver function • Supports estrogen detoxification • Rich in fiber

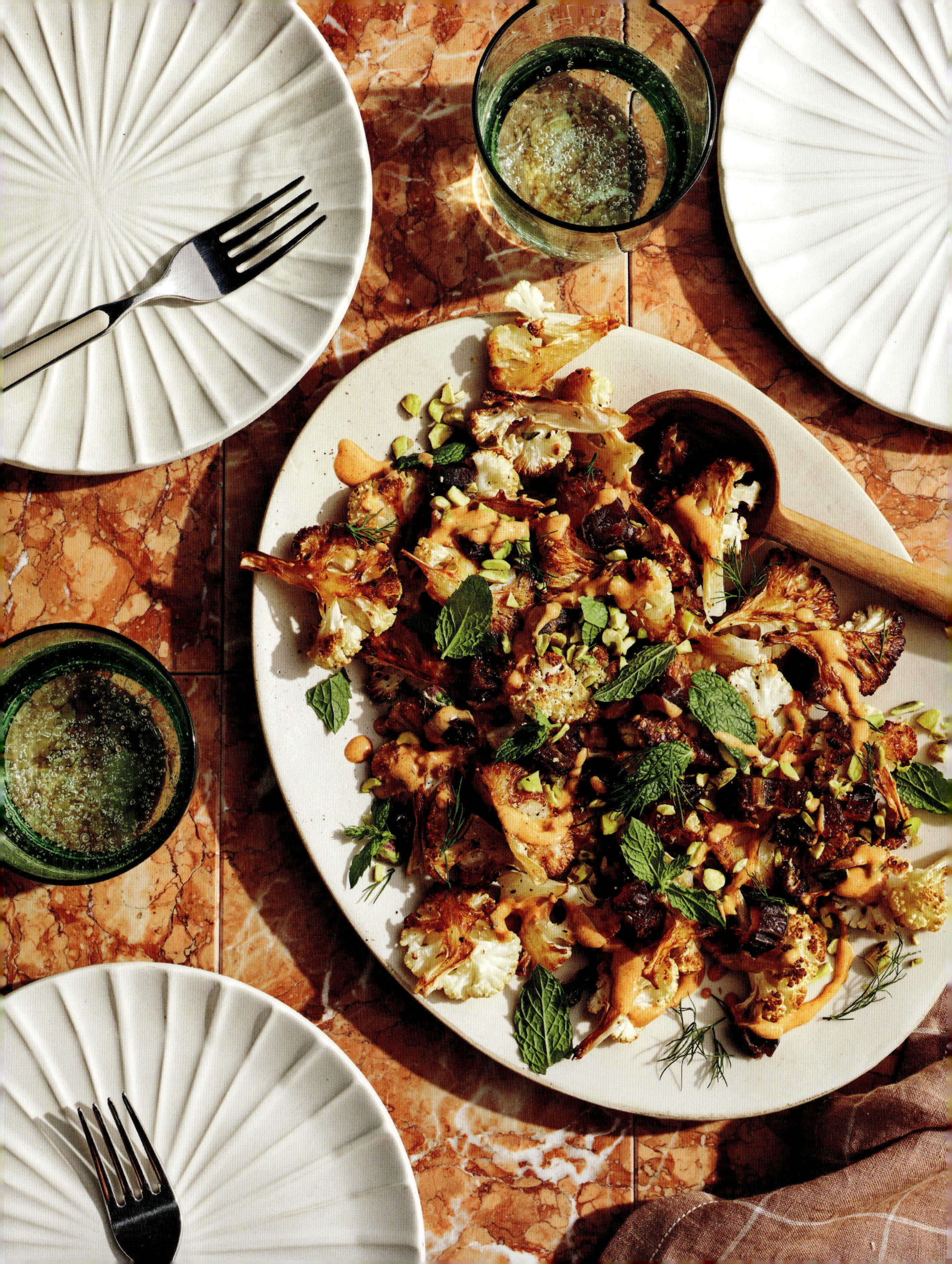

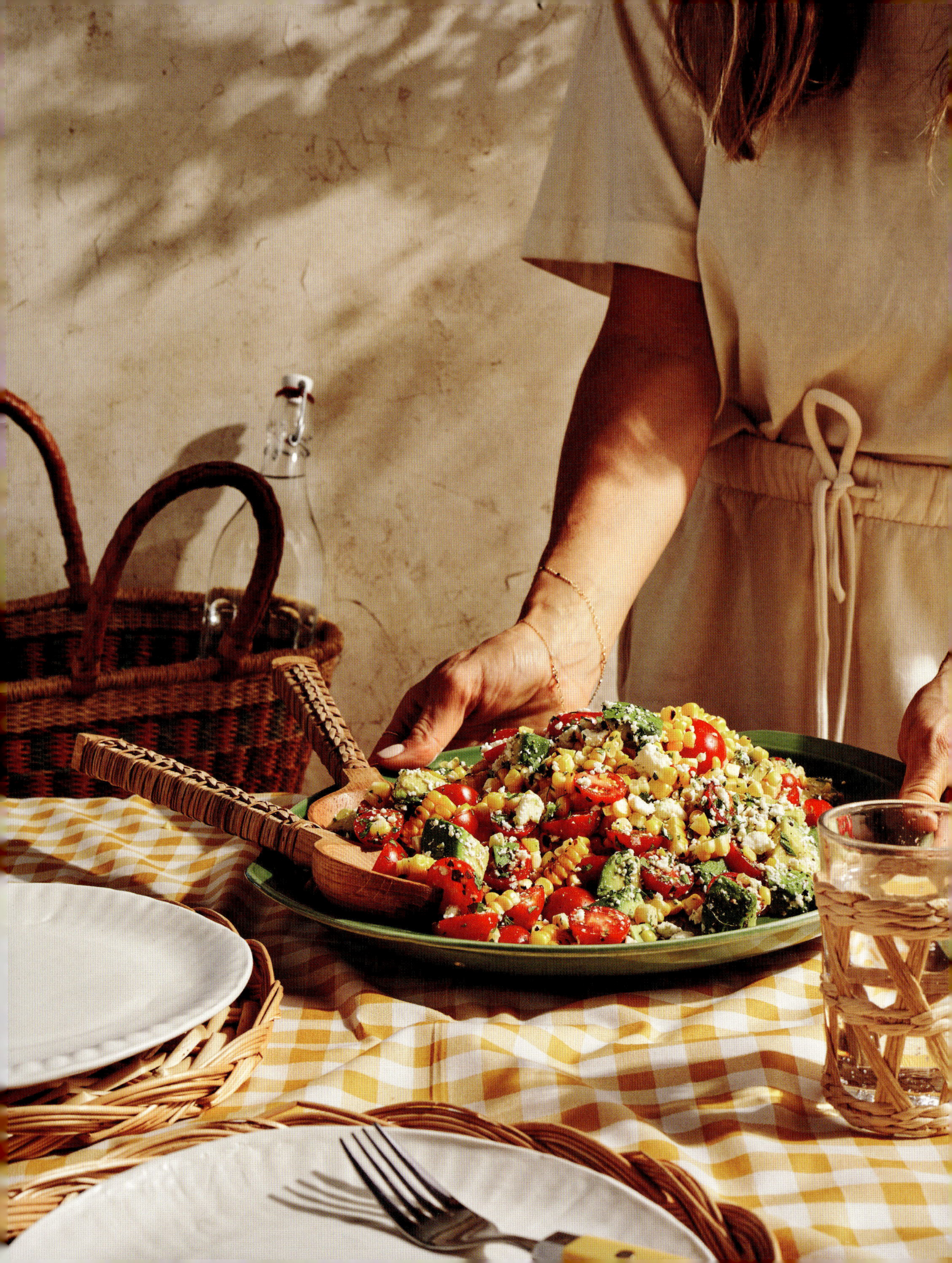

The GOAT Summer Corn Salad

PREP: 10 MINUTES COOK: 10 MINUTES SERVES 4

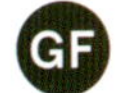
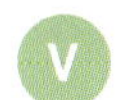

I've been making this salad every summer for over a decade and it's one of my most requested recipes to date. It's so easy to make, and it uses seasonal ingredients that stand out on their own (i.e., you really don't need to do much to enhance the flavor). It's also loaded with fiber to assist in excess estrogen elimination, along with antioxidant- and glutathione-rich produce, which further supports detoxification. I love serving it as a side dish with any grilled protein for a light and nourishing summer meal.

- 4 ears fresh sweet corn, shucked
- Avocado oil for brushing
- 1 pint organic cherry tomatoes, halved
- 2 ripe avocados, pitted, peeled, and chopped into large chunks
- Juice of 3 limes (about 6 tablespoons)
- 2 to 4 tablespoons extra virgin olive oil
- ¼ cup chopped cilantro leaves
- ¼ cup crumbled cotija cheese
- ½ teaspoon sea salt
- Black pepper to taste
- Flaky sea salt to serve

1. Preheat a grill to medium-high heat.
2. Brush the corn with avocado oil and grill for 2 to 3 minutes per side, until the corn is charred and the kernels have deepened in color. Set aside to cool.
3. Use a sharp knife to shave the grilled corn kernels off the cobs. Transfer to a large bowl and toss in all the remaining ingredients. Taste and add more seasoning accordingly. Sprinkle with flaky sea salt before serving.

NOTE: This salad dish tastes best when the corn is grilled, but you can also shave the corn kernels off the cob or use 2 drained (15-ounce) cans of sweet corn; sauté either one in a dry skillet over medium-high heat until toasted and slightly charred.

OVULATORY PHASE BENEFITS

Supports vascular health • Supports estrogen detoxification • Rich in fiber • High in glutathione and antioxidants

Beet and Citrus Salad + Goat Cheese and Avocado

PREP: 10 MINUTES COOK: 30 MINUTES SERVES 4

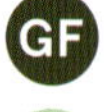

V

These flavors are a match made in heaven, and I've even converted some former beet skeptics after offering up this dish! Beets are often cited for their fertility-boosting properties, enhancing vascular and ovarian function and egg quality, as well as assisting the transition from ruptured follicle to a corpus luteum post-ovulation. The corpus luteum is what produces progesterone in the second half of your cycle, and is necessary for building a healthy uterine lining and for keeping PMS at bay.

Beets

- 2 large beets, peeled and cubed (about 3 cups)
- 2 tablespoons avocado oil
- 4 cloves garlic, minced
- Sea salt and black pepper to taste

Almonds

- ½ cup slivered almonds
- 1 to 2 tablespoons pure maple syrup
- Sea salt

Dressing

- ¼ cup fresh orange juice
- 2 tablespoons fresh lemon juice
- 2 tablespoons champagne vinegar
- 2 tablespoons raw honey
- 1 tablespoon Dijon mustard
- 1 teaspoon sea salt
- Black pepper to taste
- ½ cup extra virgin olive oil

Salad

- 4 cups arugula
- 2 avocados, pitted, peeled, and chopped into chunks
- 2 oranges, peeled and cut into segments
- ½ cup goat cheese, crumbled into large chunks
- Microgreens for topping

1. Preheat the oven to 425°F and line a large baking sheet with parchment paper.
2. *For the beets:* Arrange the beets on the baking sheet and coat with the avocado oil, garlic, and salt and pepper to taste. Roast for 30 minutes, flipping halfway through, until the beets are tender and pierce easily with a fork. Let cool for 5 minutes.
3. *For the almonds:* While the beets are roasting, heat a small skillet over medium heat and add the slivered almonds. Toast for 5 or so minutes, stirring frequently, until the almonds begin to turn golden brown. Drizzle in the maple syrup and stir vigorously until absorbed, about 1 minute. Sprinkle with salt, immediately remove from the heat, and place on parchment paper to cool. Use your hands to break the almonds apart into small clusters.
4. *For the dressing:* Whisk together all the dressing ingredients in a small mixing bowl and set aside.
5. *To assemble the salad:* In a large bowl, layer the arugula, roasted beets, avocados, oranges, goat cheese, almond clusters, and microgreens. Drizzle the dressing on top and enjoy.

NOTE: You can easily turn this salad into a full meal by adding a protein source such as cooked quinoa, lentils, or rotisserie chicken.

OVULATORY PHASE BENEFITS

Supports vascular health • Supports liver function • Supports estrogen detoxification • Rich in fiber • High in glutathione and antioxidants

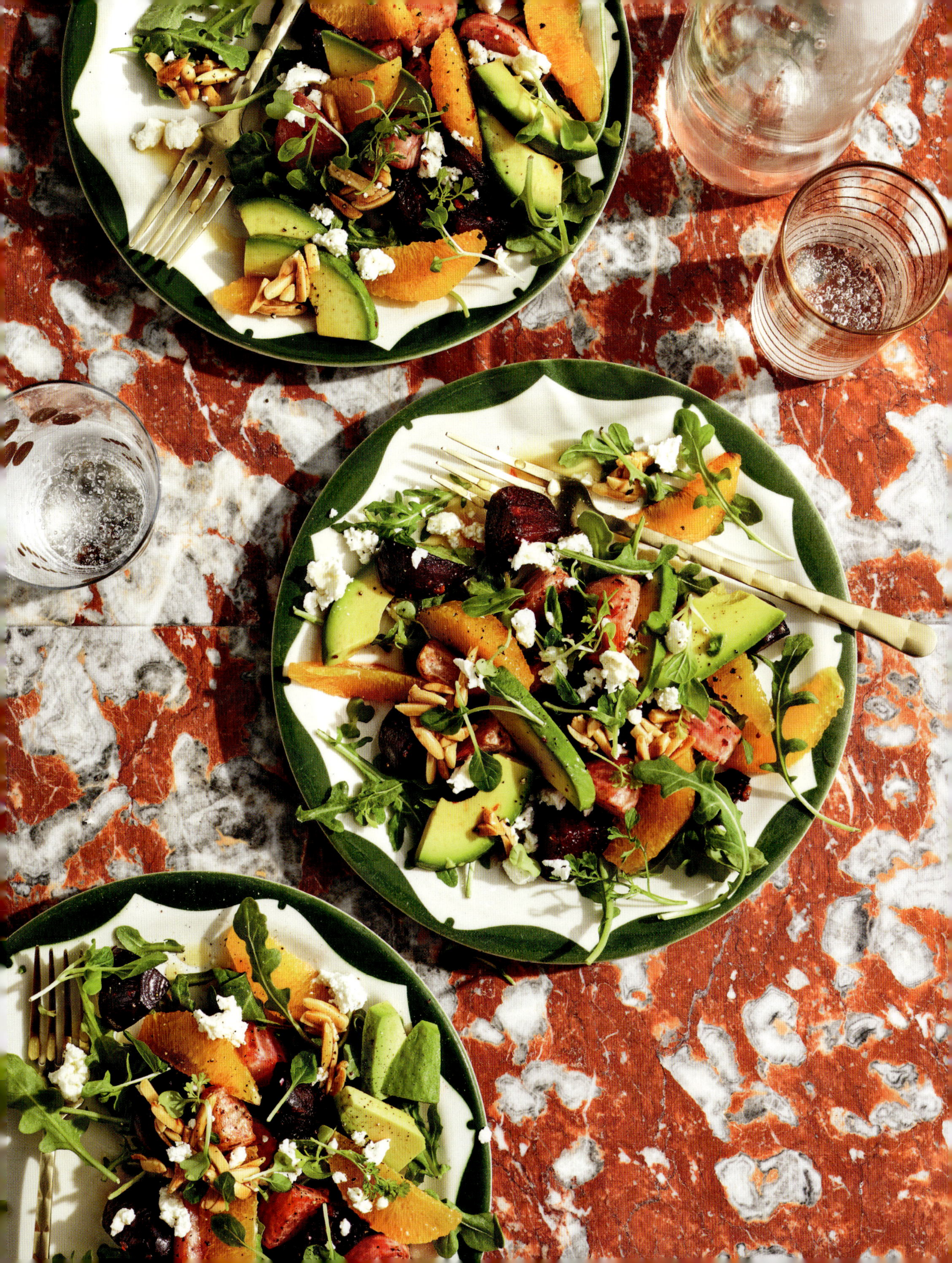

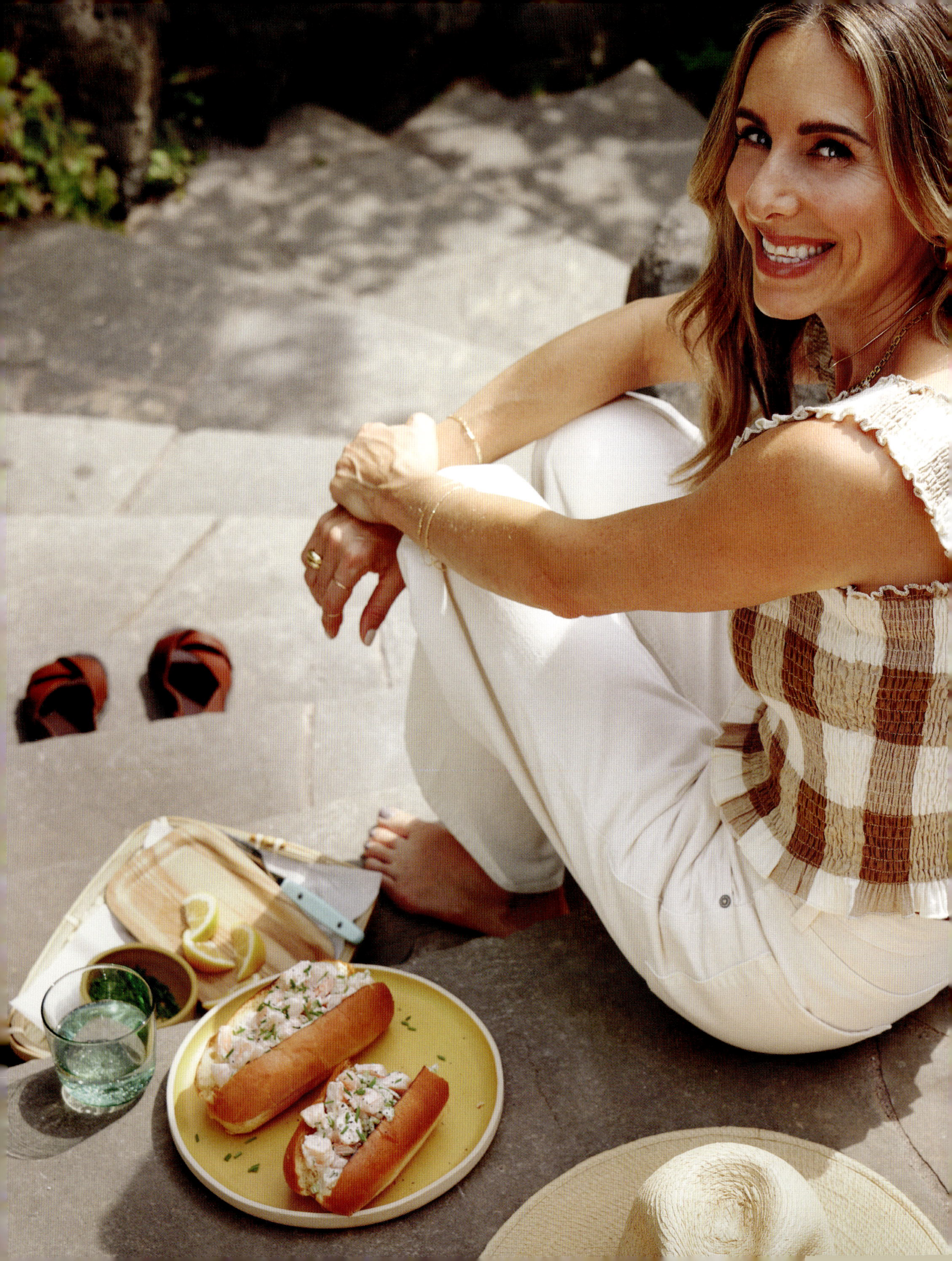

New England–Style Shrimp Rolls

PREP: 5 MINUTES COOK: 5 MINUTES SERVES 4

It doesn't get much more summery than this: Plump juicy shrimp are quickly cooked and cooled, then tossed in a simple lemon sauce and layered into buttery buns. Think lobster rolls, only easier and less expensive—but still delicious! We make this one on repeat every summer, and I especially love it when I'm ovulating as it is rich in minerals and antioxidants that support healthy ovarian function and fight off oxidative stress, which tends to peak during this phase.

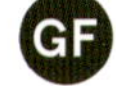

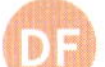

- ¼ cup avocado oil mayonnaise
- Juice of ½ lemon, plus wedges for serving
- ¼ cup minced celery
- 2 tablespoons minced fresh chives, plus more for garnish
- ½ teaspoon sea salt, plus more for serving
- Black pepper to taste
- 2 tablespoons grass-fed ghee, butter, or vegan butter substitute, plus more for the buns
- 1 pound wild-caught Patagonian Pink or Argentinian shrimp, peeled and deveined
- 4 gluten-free hot dog buns

1. Preheat the broiler.
2. In a large bowl, mix the mayo, lemon juice, celery, chives, salt, and pepper. Refrigerate until the shrimp are ready.
3. Melt the ghee or butter in a large sauté pan over medium-high heat. Add the shrimp and cook for 1 to 2 minutes on each side, until cooked through. Let the shrimp cool slightly on a cutting board, then cut into 1-inch chunks. Add the shrimp to the bowl with the mayonnaise sauce and mix well.
4. Place the hot dog buns open faced under the broiler and toast until golden brown. Coat each half with additional ghee or butter. Spoon the shrimp mixture generously in the middle of each bun. Option to top with more chives, salt, and pepper and serve with lemon wedges.

OVULATORY PHASE BENEFITS

Supports liver function • High in glutathione and antioxidants

Tropical Salmon Bites + Mango Avocado Salsa and Coconut Lime Rice

PREP: 15 MINUTES COOK: 20 MINUTES SERVES 4

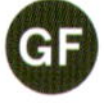

DF

Bright, refreshing, and loaded with flavor, this bowl gives major tropical paradise vibes. The salmon is rich in anti-inflammatory omega-3 fatty acids that promote a healthy vascular system, which is key for ovarian function and egg quality, while the salsa packs in plenty of antioxidants that boost glutathione production and support detoxification. This is *exactly* the kind of meal I crave during my inner summer phase, and I have a feeling you're going to love it as much as I do. And I'm offering both a stovetop and air-fryer option, to fit your preferences and needs!

Coconut Lime Rice

1 cup jasmine rice, rinsed three times in cold water and drained

1 cup full-fat coconut milk

¾ cup water

⅓ cup unsweetened coconut shreds or flakes

½ teaspoon sea salt

Grated zest and juice of 1 lime

½ cup cilantro leaves, chopped

Mango Avocado Salsa

1 large mango, pitted, peeled, and diced

1 large avocado, pitted, peeled, and diced

1 red bell pepper, seeded and diced

1 Persian cucumber (or ½ English cucumber), diced

½ jalapeño, seeded and diced

¼ cup cilantro leaves, chopped

Juice of 1 lime

½ teaspoon sea salt

Salmon

1 heaping tablespoon coconut sugar

2 teaspoons dried thyme

1 teaspoon smoked paprika

½ teaspoon sea salt

½ teaspoon black pepper

2 pounds wild-caught center-cut salmon fillets (such as Atlantic or king), skin removed, cut into 1-inch cubes

About 2 tablespoons Dijon mustard (enough to coat the salmon)

2 tablespoons avocado oil (for pan-searing, skip if air-frying)

Cilantro leaves and sesame seeds, for topping

1. *For the rice:* In a medium pot, combine the rinsed rice, coconut milk, water, coconut shreds or flakes, and salt. Whisk until well combined, cover the pot, and bring to a boil. Reduce the heat and simmer for 15 minutes. Remove from the heat and let steam for 5 more minutes. Gently fold in the lime zest and juice and the cilantro.

2. *For the salsa:* While the rice is cooking, combine all the salsa ingredients in a medium bowl and set aside.

3. *For the salmon:* Stir together the coconut sugar, thyme, paprika, salt, and pepper in a small bowl. Coat the cubed salmon with mustard and evenly rub on the seasoning mix.

4. *To air-fry the salmon:* Cook the salmon bites in a 400°F air fryer for 5 to 7 minutes, until the salmon flakes easily.

5. *To pan-sear the salmon:* Heat the avocado oil over medium-high heat and tilt the pan until evenly coated with oil. Add the salmon cubes and sear all over, 1 to 2 minutes per side or 4 minutes total, until the salmon flakes easily or registers an internal temperature of 125° to 130°F. Immediately remove from the heat.

6. *To serve:* Spoon the coconut lime rice into four bowls, then layer with generous portions of salmon bites. Top with the mango salsa and garnish with cilantro leaves and sesame seeds.

NOTE: Try to get center-cut fillets of wild-caught salmon (such as Atlantic or king), as the thicker cuts will keep the bites from drying out. You can also substitute wild-caught prawns for the salmon.

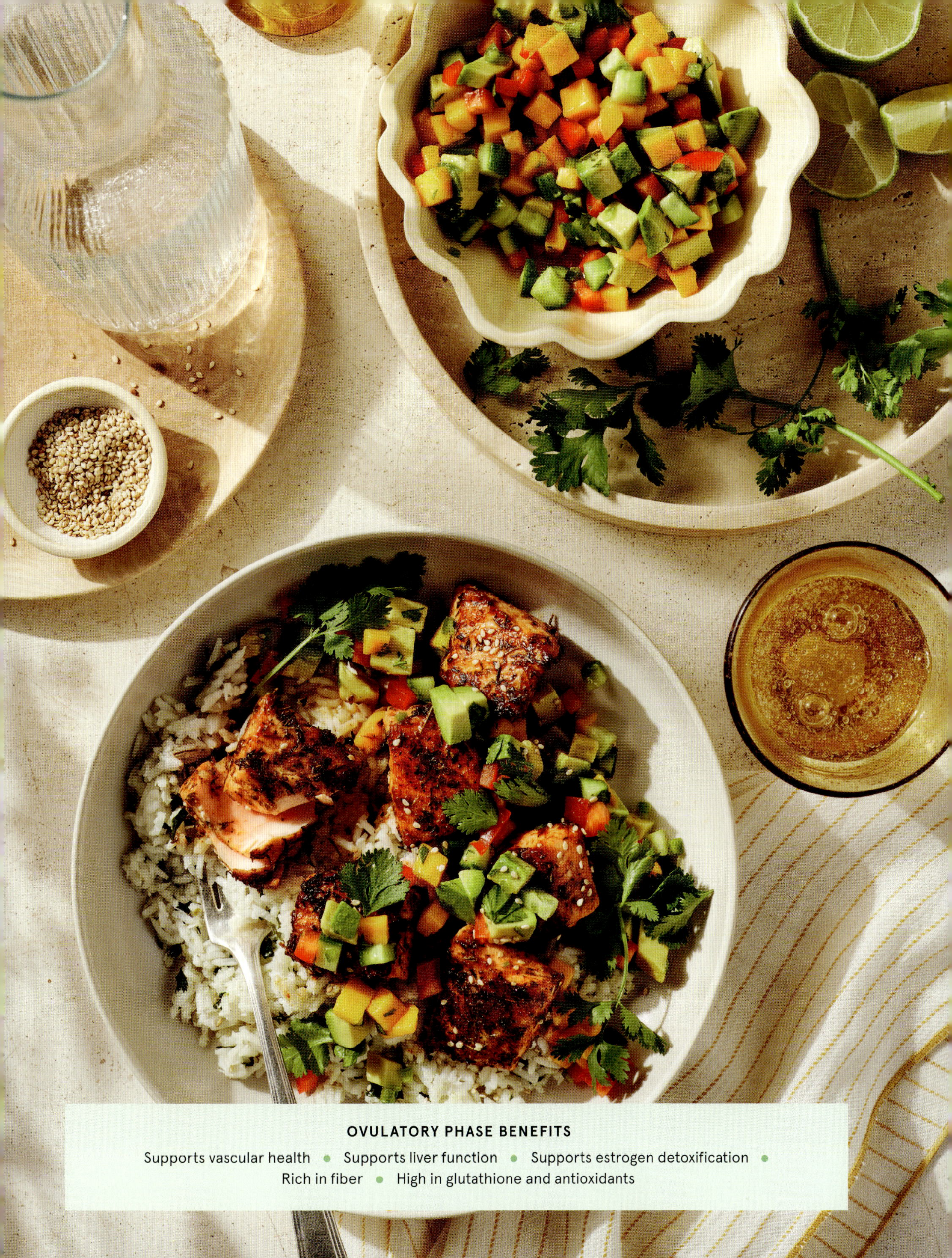

OVULATORY PHASE BENEFITS

Supports vascular health • Supports liver function • Supports estrogen detoxification • Rich in fiber • High in glutathione and antioxidants

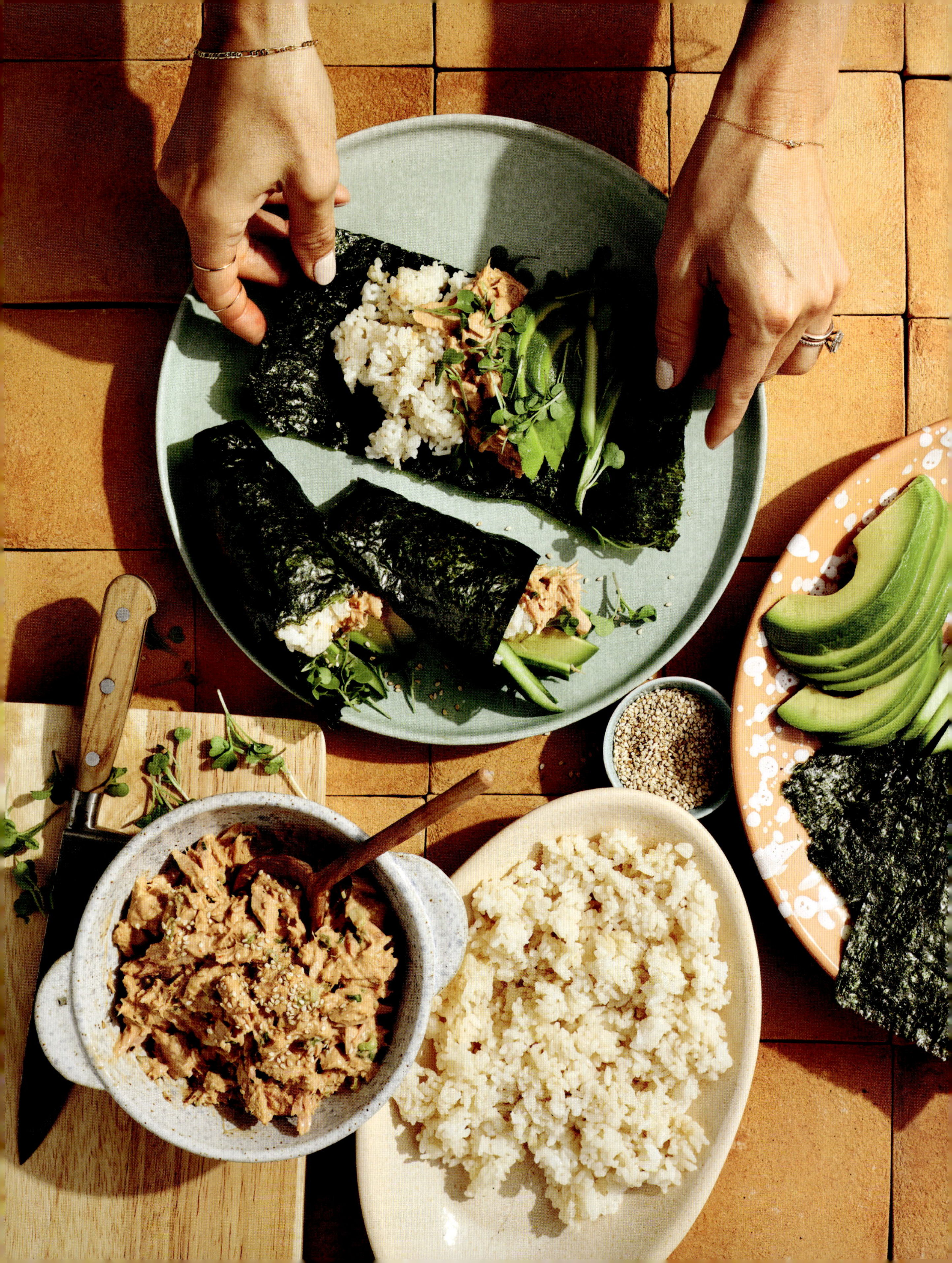

Quick and Spicy Tuna Hand Rolls

PREP: 25 MINUTES, PLUS 1 HOUR CHILLING   COOK: 25 MINUTES   SERVES 2 (MAKES 8 ROLLS)

These rolls are the next best thing to sushi, only less expensive and easier to make! They feature all those hallmark textures and flavors but swap out the raw fish for canned wild-caught tuna, which is much more accessible and budget-friendly. Using nori, the traditional seaweed wrap, packs in vitamins and iodine, a mineral crucial for optimal thyroid function that plays an intricate role in fertility, ovulation, and overall menstrual cycle health. You also have the option of cooking and cooling the rice a day before to create resistant starch, which boosts digestion and gut health, as well as enables this meal to come together quickly.

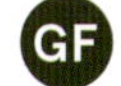

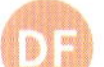

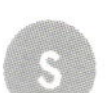

- **1 cup Japanese short-grain white rice (also known as sushi rice), rinsed three times and drained**
- **1 cup filtered water**
- **2 tablespoons unseasoned rice vinegar**
- **2 teaspoons coconut sugar**
- **½ teaspoon sea salt**
- **2 (5-ounce) cans wild-caught albacore tuna (or canned salmon), drained**
- **¼ cup avocado oil mayonnaise**
- **2 tablespoons coconut aminos or gluten-free soy sauce, plus more for dipping**
- **2 green onions, thinly sliced**
- **1 tablespoon white sesame seeds, plus more for sprinkling**
- **4 teaspoons sriracha**
- **½ teaspoon sea salt**
- **4 sheets nori**
- **1 avocado, pitted, peeled, and thinly sliced**
- **1 cup broccoli sprouts or other microgreens**
- **1 Persian cucumber (or small English cucumber), sliced into long thin strips**

1. *If you can, cook the sushi rice the day before:* Place the rinsed rice in a medium pot, add the water, and bring to a boil. Reduce to a simmer, cover, and cook for 20 minutes, or until the rice is cooked al dente.

2. Heat the rice vinegar, coconut sugar, and salt in a small pan over medium-high heat until barely simmering (it should be steaming but not boiling). Immediately remove from the heat and whisk until the sugar has dissolved.

3. Transfer the rice to a large glass container or bowl and pour the vinegar mixture over it, folding it in evenly with a spatula. Let cool to room temperature, then cover with an airtight lid and store in the refrigerator until cooled, about 1 hour.

4. In a small mixing bowl, combine the tuna, mayonnaise, coconut aminos, green onions, sesame seeds, sriracha, and salt until well mixed.

5. Fold the nori sheets in half lengthwise and use sharp scissors to cut along the fold. Place the nori shiny side down and place a spoonful of sushi rice on the left end, pressing flat with the back of a spoon. Top with a spoonful of the tuna filling, then two or three slices of avocado, a pinch of sprouts, and four thin slices of cucumber. Take the bottom left corner of the nori and fold it over the fillings, connecting it to the top center of the nori. Tuck in the sides of the nori as you continue rolling to form a cone. Once rolled, use a wet finger to seal the hand roll closed. Repeat until all nori sheets are filled. Sprinkle the tops with more sesame seeds and serve with a shallow bowl of coconut aminos for dipping.

NOTE: If you don't make the vinegar mixture when cooking the sushi rice, use this quick hack: Pour a little bit of rice vinegar over the cooked rice just before making the hand rolls.

OVULATORY PHASE BENEFITS

Supports vascular health • Rich in fiber • High in glutathione and antioxidants

Super Easy Chopped Chicken Salad Lettuce Wraps

PREP: 20 MINUTES   COOK: NONE   SERVES 2

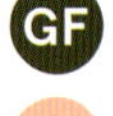

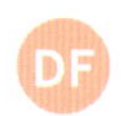

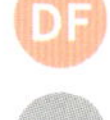

I make these wraps most weekdays for lunch during my follicular and ovulatory phases as they're easy, tasty, and packed with protein. They're also loaded with fresh raw fruits and veggies, which are rich in antioxidants that support vascular health and help create the healthiest egg possible. While I mostly opt for the lettuce wrap route, the salad also works well as a spread for gluten-free crackers or a sandwich filling with toasted gluten-free bread.

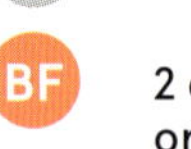
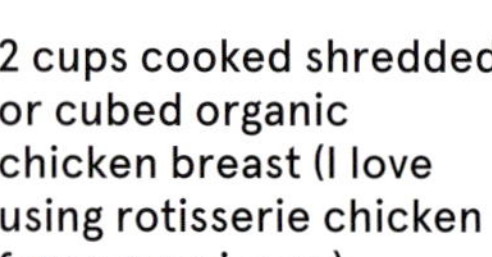

- 2 cups cooked shredded or cubed organic chicken breast (I love using rotisserie chicken for convenience)
- 2 small celery ribs, diced
- ½ cup purple grapes, rinsed and quartered
- ¼ cup pecans, chopped
- 1 green onion, diced
- 2 tablespoons finely chopped fresh parsley
- 1 tablespoon finely chopped fresh chives
- 1 tablespoon finely chopped fresh dill or tarragon (optional)
- ½ cup avocado oil mayonnaise or full-fat unsweetened Greek yogurt
- Juice of 1 small lemon (1 to 2 tablespoons)
- 1 teaspoon Dijon mustard
- ½ teaspoon sea salt
- Black pepper to taste
- 6 large romaine lettuce leaves, rinsed and patted dry

In a medium bowl, combine the chicken, celery, grapes, pecans, green onion, parsley, chives, and dill or tarragon (if using). Add the mayo, lemon juice, mustard, salt, and pepper to the bowl and stir until well mixed. Spoon the mixture onto the center of the romaine leaves and enjoy.

OVULATORY PHASE BENEFITS

Supports vascular health • Rich in fiber • High in glutathione and antioxidants

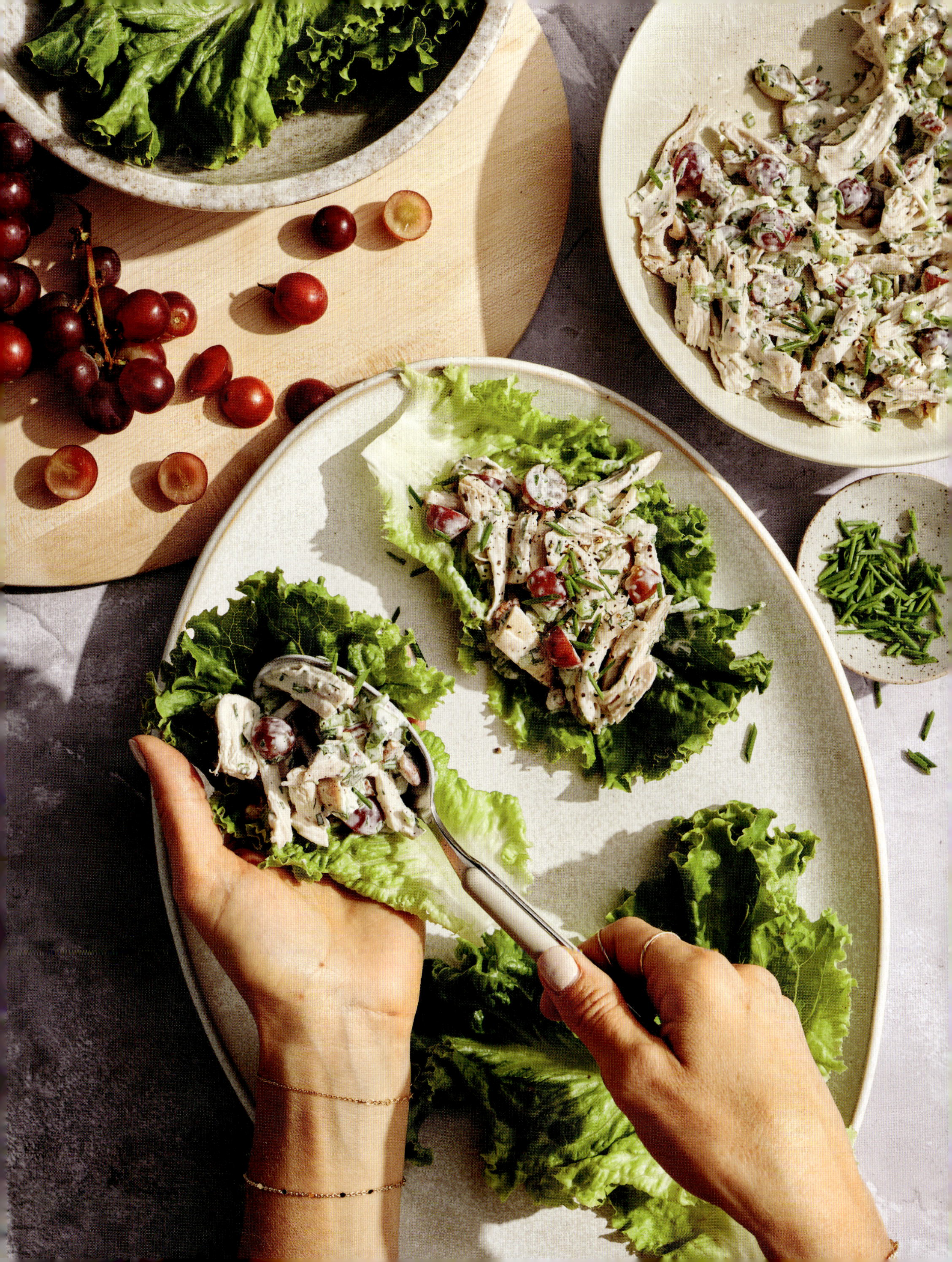

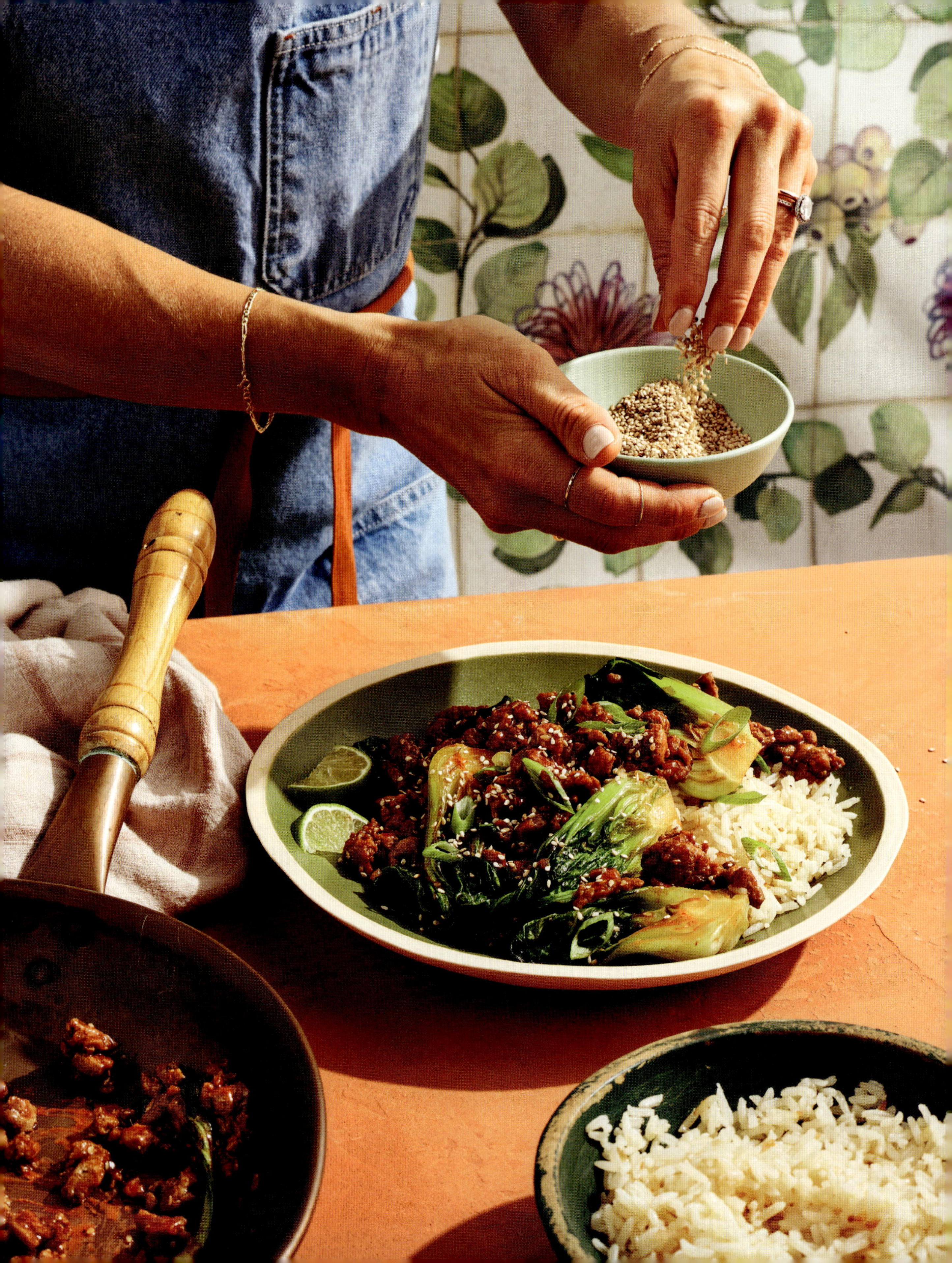

Ground Turkey Protein Bowls + Sriracha Honey Sauce

PREP: 10 MINUTES   COOK: 20 MINUTES   SERVES 2–4

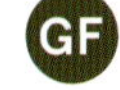

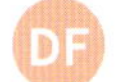

This is *the* weeknight meal I turn to time and again when I need something easy, delicious, and filling. It's packed with protein (hence the name) and healthy fats that support ovarian function and egg quality, as well as cruciferous vegetables and alliums that contain compounds that help your liver break down excess estrogen. It's also super versatile as you can easily swap out the ground turkey and bok choy for another protein or cruciferous vegetable of choice. Just don't skip the sriracha honey sauce, which adds loads of flavor, and feel free to add more sriracha if you like it extra spicy!

Rice

- **1 cup basmati rice, rinsed three times in cold water and drained**
- **1½ cups bone broth (try using the Super Simple Homemade Bone Broth on page 109)**
- **1 tablespoon grass-fed ghee**

Sriracha Honey Sauce

- **⅓ cup coconut aminos (or gluten-free soy sauce)**
- **¼ cup raw honey**
- **2 to 3 tablespoons sriracha**
- **Juice of 1 large lime (about 2 tablespoons)**
- **1 tablespoon minced fresh ginger**
- **1 teaspoon paprika**
- **1 teaspoon sea salt**
- **1 teaspoon sesame seeds**
- **Black pepper to taste**
- **1 tablespoon arrowroot starch**

Bowls

- **1 to 2 tablespoons grass-fed ghee**
- **1 shallot, minced**
- **4 cloves garlic, minced**
- **1 pound organic ground turkey (or ground chicken or beef)**
- **Sea salt and black pepper to taste**
- **1 pound (about 2 cups) baby bok choy, rinsed and ends trimmed**
- **Thai basil, cilantro, green onions (white and light green parts, thinly sliced), sliced avocado, lime, or more sesame seeds, for topping (optional)**

1. *For the rice:* Place the rice in a pot with the bone broth and top with the ghee. Cover the pot and bring to a boil. Reduce the heat and simmer for 15 minutes. Remove from the heat and let steam for 5 minutes.

2. *For the sauce:* Whisk together all the sauce ingredients in a small bowl and set aside.

3. *For the bowls:* Heat 1 to 2 tablespoons ghee (enough to evenly coat the pan) in a large skillet over medium-high heat. Add the shallot and garlic and cook for 1 to 2 minutes, until fragrant. Add the ground turkey and use a spatula or wooden spoon to separate any large chunks. Generously season with salt and pepper. Cook for about 5 minutes, until the meat is mostly cooked through. Add the bok choy and cook, stirring frequently, for 2 to 3 minutes, until the bok choy is bright green and tender. Pour the sauce evenly over the mixture and let cook for 2 to 3 more minutes, until thickened.

4. *To serve:* Divide the rice among two to four bowls, then layer in the turkey and bok choy mixture. Option to top with fresh herbs, green onions, avocado, and additional sesame seeds and serve with lime wedges.

OVULATORY PHASE BENEFITS

Supports liver function • Supports estrogen detoxification • Rich in fiber • High in glutathione and antioxidants

Sheet-Pan Miso-Glazed Black Cod + Veggies

PREP: 10 MINUTES   COOK: 25 MINUTES   SERVES 4

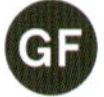
DF

This restaurant-worthy recipe is easier to make than it seems and comes together in less than 30 minutes. The buttery black cod is rich in anti-inflammatory omega-3 fatty acids that support circulation and vascular health, while the miso glaze packs in delicious umami flavor and probiotics that help you maintain a healthy gut flora (important for optimal estrogen elimination).

- 2 tablespoons organic white miso
- 2 tablespoons pure maple syrup
- 2 tablespoons coconut aminos
- 3 tablespoons avocado oil, divided
- 4 (6-ounce) fillets center-cut wild-caught black cod (sablefish)
- 1 bunch baby turnips, trimmed and quartered
- 1 cup shiitake mushrooms, halved
- 2 cloves garlic, minced
- Sea salt and black pepper to taste
- 1 tablespoon grated orange zest
- 2 tablespoons freshly squeezed orange juice
- 1 tablespoon grass-fed ghee
- Cooked jasmine rice, diced green onion, and sesame seeds, for serving (optional)

1. Preheat the oven to 425°F.

2. In a small bowl, whisk together the miso, maple syrup, coconut aminos, and 1 tablespoon of the avocado oil. Reserve half of the mixture and set aside to use later as a glaze.

3. Pour the remaining mixture evenly over the fillets in a shallow baking pan. Let marinate at room temperature while you roast the vegetables.

4. Combine the turnips and shiitake mushrooms on a large baking sheet and toss with the remaining 2 tablespoons avocado oil, the garlic, and salt and pepper. Roast for about 15 minutes, until the veggies have softened and begun to take on color. Transfer the vegetables to a plate with a spatula. Turn the oven to broil and place your oven rack on the top shelf.

5. Whisk the orange zest and juice into the reserved maple miso glaze. Drizzle the vegetables with about half of the reserved miso glaze and coat evenly with the ghee. Cover to keep warm.

6. Place the marinated black cod on the baking sheet and broil for about 8 minutes. Return the vegetables to the baking sheet and broil an additional 2 to 4 minutes, until the veggies have charred and the black cod is cooked through, opaque, and flaky, or registers an internal temperature of 145°F.

7. If you like, serve the cod and vegetables on a bed of rice. Pour the rest of the glaze evenly over the cod and vegetables. Further option to garnish with green onion cut on a bias and sesame seeds.

NOTE: If you can't find black cod, wild-caught salmon and true cod make for tasty swaps.

OVULATORY PHASE BENEFITS

Supports vascular health • Supports estrogen detoxification • Rich in probiotics

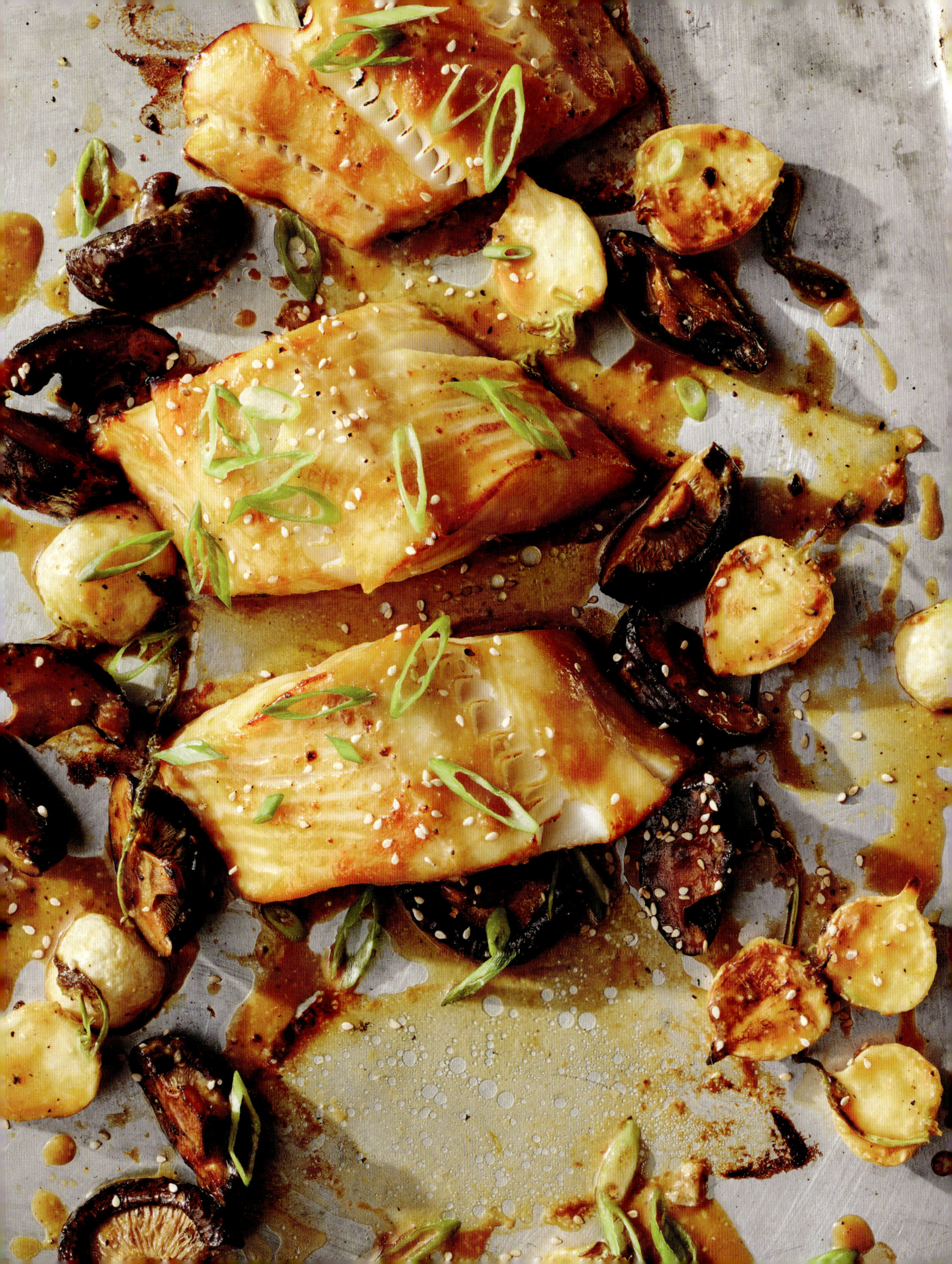

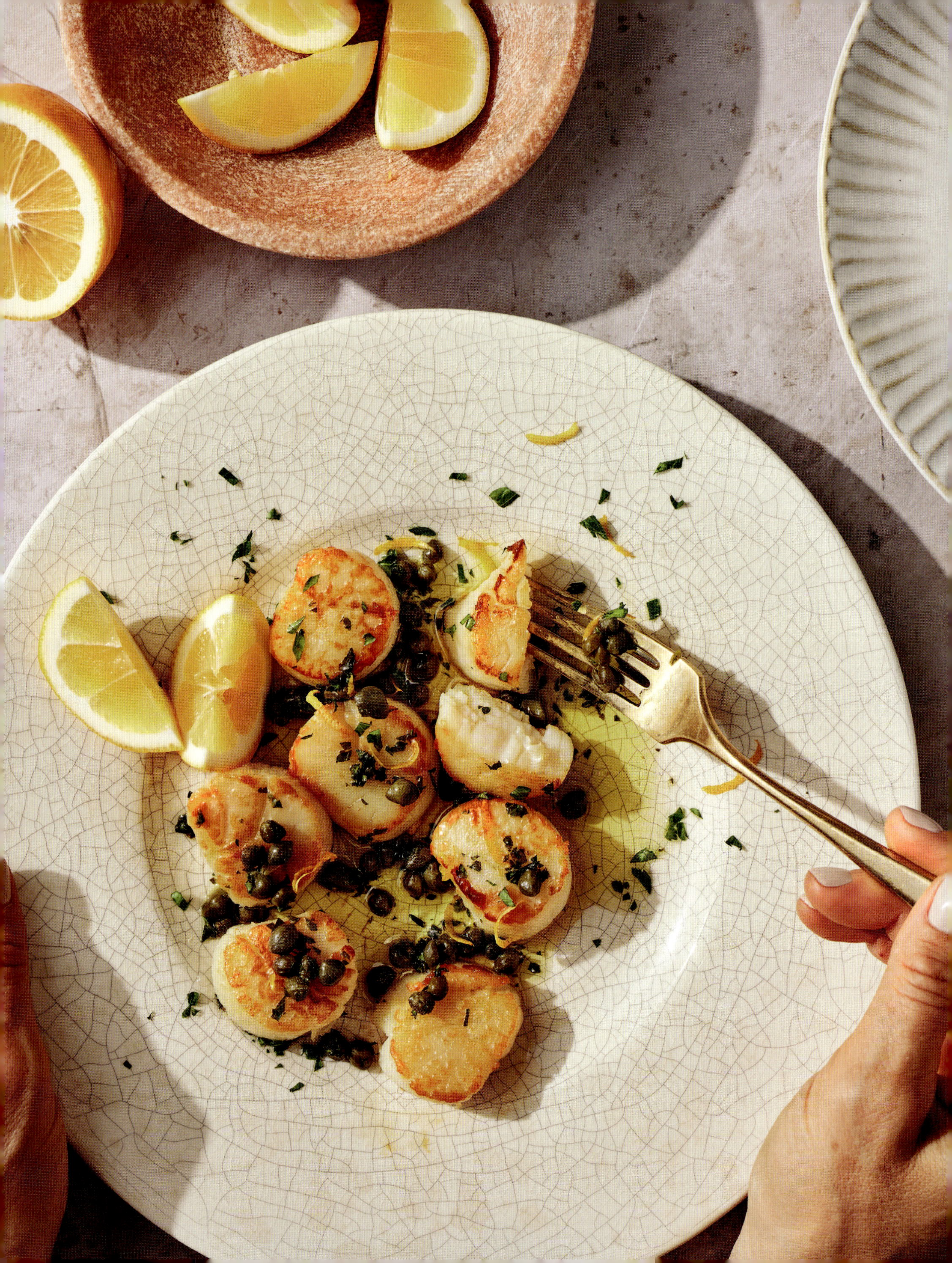

Buttery Seared-Scallop Piccata

PREP: 5 MINUTES　COOK: 10 MINUTES　SERVES 4

GF

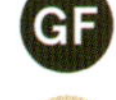

Scallops are not something I typically cook at home, but when I'm able to get my hands on high-quality ones you can rest assured I'm making this recipe. I love to serve this when I'm ovulating for two reasons: 1) Scallops are rich in trace minerals vital for healthy ovulatory function; and 2) I'm usually feeling social during this phase and this dish is a surefire way to impress guests. Try serving them with the Whole Roasted Lemony Artichokes (page 149) and thank me later.

- **1½ pounds U15 dry sea scallops (harvested from Atlantic waters; see Note)**
- **Sea salt and black pepper to taste**
- **2 tablespoons avocado oil**
- **¼ cup grass-fed ghee or butter**
- **½ cup capers, drained**
- **2 tablespoons chopped fresh flat-leaf parsley**
- **Grated zest and juice of 1 small lemon**
- **Lemon wedges, flaky sea salt, and black pepper, for serving**

1. Season each side of the scallops generously with salt and pepper.

2. Heat the avocado oil in a large stovetop or cast-iron skillet over medium-high heat. When the pan is piping hot, add the scallops, spacing them evenly apart (work in batches if needed to avoid crowding the pan). Let them cook without disturbing for 2 to 4 minutes, until a golden-brown crust forms on the bottom of each scallop. Flip each scallop over carefully, then immediately add the ghee or butter, capers, and parsley to the pan, swirling to coat the pan evenly. Cook, using a spoon to baste the scallops, for 2 to 3 more minutes, until the scallops are opaque and cooked through (or until they reach an internal temperature of 165°F). Remove the skillet from the heat and transfer the scallops to a plate. Add the lemon zest and juice to the sauce in the pan, stirring to mix. Season the sauce with salt and pepper, then pour over the scallops.

3. Garnish the scallops with more chopped parsley, sea salt, and pepper and serve with lemon wedges.

NOTE: The quality of the scallops really matters here. Look for U15 dry sea scallops when purchasing. "U15" indicates there are fewer than 15 scallops per pound (the U stands for "under"), while "dry" ensures the scallops have not been treated with preservatives. U15 dry sea scallops are hand-harvested from Atlantic waters and have a tender, sweet, and briny texture similar to crab or lobster meat. If you're unable to find scallops, large wild-caught Argentinian or Patagonian Pink shrimp would be ideal swaps.

OVULATORY PHASE BENEFITS

Supports liver function • High in glutathione and antioxidants

BBQ Chicken Ranch Quinoa Bowls

PREP: 10 MINUTES COOK: 30 MINUTES SERVES 4–6

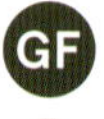

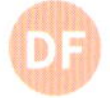

S

BF

These bowls are a virtual rainbow loaded with colorful fiber- and antioxidant-rich foods that support liver detoxification and estrogen elimination, not to mention deliver the quintessential flavors of a summer potluck. The shredded BBQ chicken is also high in protein and super tender, and the leftovers are great in tacos or wraps. While purchasing premade sauces (see Note) will save you time, the homemade Jalapeño Ranch adds *so* much delicious, zingy flavor that it truly takes this bowl to the next level.

BBQ Shredded Chicken

- 1 cup bone broth (try using the Super Simple Homemade Bone Broth on page 109)
- 2 pounds (6 to 8) organic boneless skinless chicken thighs
- 1 tablespoon coconut sugar
- 1 teaspoon paprika
- ½ teaspoon onion powder
- ½ teaspoon garlic powder
- ½ teaspoon sea salt
- Black pepper to taste
- 2 teaspoons gluten-free Worcestershire sauce
- 2 to 3 cups barbecue sauce of choice, to taste

Jalapeño Ranch

- ½ cup Greek-style coconut yogurt or Greek yogurt
- ⅓ cup avocado oil mayonnaise
- Grated zest and juice of 1 lime (about 1 teaspoon zest and 2 tablespoons juice)
- 1 cup fresh cilantro leaves
- ½ jalapeño, seeded and diced
- 2 tablespoons chopped fresh chives
- 1 teaspoon garlic powder
- 1 teaspoon onion powder
- ½ teaspoon sea salt

Quinoa Bowls

- 1 cup quinoa, cooked according to package instructions (typically with 1½ cups water or bone broth for 15 minutes)
- 2 cups organic baby spinach (or shredded romaine)
- ½ small red cabbage, shredded
- 2 Roma or plum tomatoes or 1 cup cherry tomatoes, chopped
- 1 (15-ounce) can organic black beans, drained
- 1 (15-ounce) can organic sweet corn, drained (or kernels from 2 ears fresh corn, if in season)
- 1 to 2 avocados, pitted, peeled, and chopped
- Fresh cilantro, limes, and optional cotija cheese for topping

1. *For the chicken:* Add the bone broth to a large pot and evenly arrange the chicken thighs on the bottom of the pot. Sprinkle with the coconut sugar, paprika, onion powder, garlic powder, salt, and pepper and pour the Worcestershire over all. Pour in 1 cup of the barbecue sauce. Bring everything to a boil, cover, and reduce the heat. Simmer for 30 minutes, until the chicken is tender. You can also cook the chicken, seasonings, and sauce in a pressure cooker: Cook on high pressure for 15 minutes, then let the pressure naturally release for 10 minutes.

2. Transfer the chicken to a medium mixing bowl and drizzle about ½ cup of liquid on top. Use two forks to shred. Stir in 1 to 2 cups barbecue sauce (to taste) and set aside.

3. *For the jalapeño ranch:* Combine all the ingredients in a blender or food processor and mix until creamy and well combined.

4. *To assemble the bowls:* Divide the quinoa among four to six bowls. Arrange the spinach, cabbage, tomatoes, black beans, corn, avocados, and shredded chicken on top. Drizzle with the jalapeño ranch. Top with cilantro and cotija cheese and serve with lime wedges if you like.

NOTE: If you're looking to save time, you can purchase a ranch dressing; just make sure to select a brand with minimal, real ingredients!

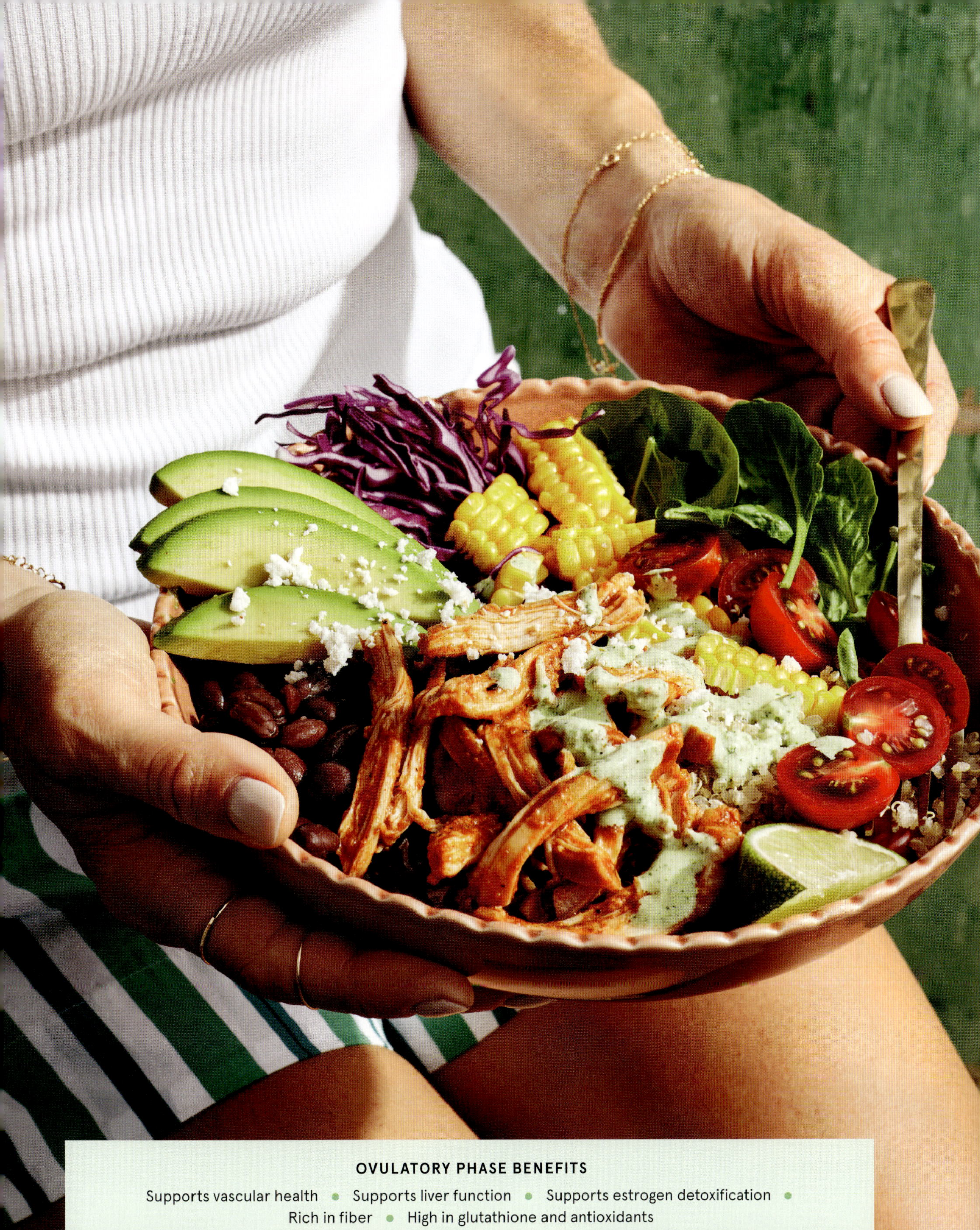

OVULATORY PHASE BENEFITS

Supports vascular health • Supports liver function • Supports estrogen detoxification • Rich in fiber • High in glutathione and antioxidants

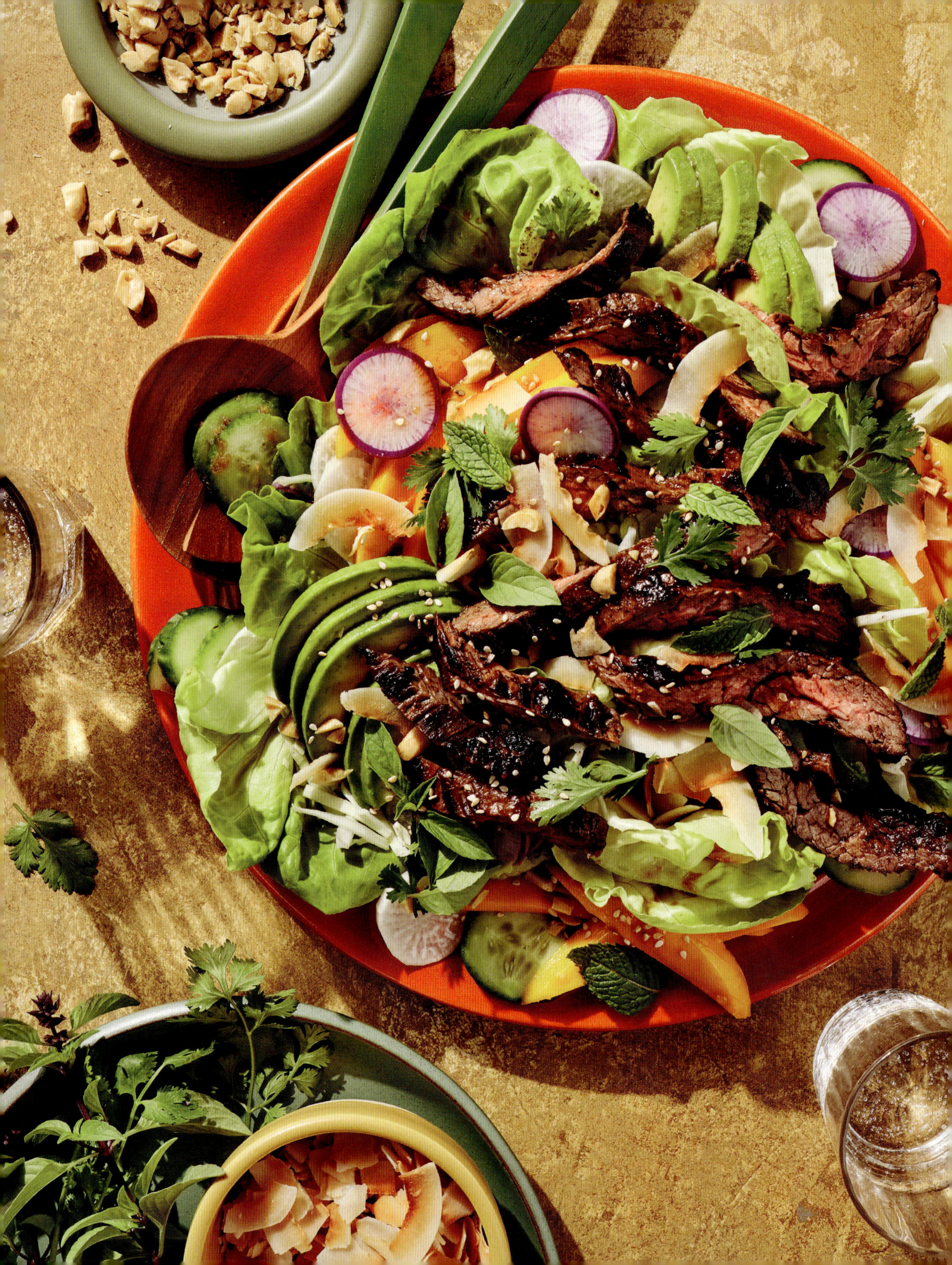

Seriously Refreshing Thai Steak Salad

PREP: 15 MINUTES, PLUS 2 HOURS MARINATING COOK: 10 MINUTES SERVES 4

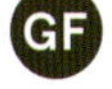
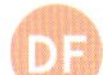
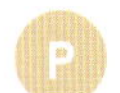

A few summers ago my family and I were vacationing in Bend, Oregon, and ate at an Asian fusion restaurant after a long day in the sun on the river. I was hot and hungry and craving something filling but also refreshing. The waiter suggested the Thai steak salad and I will forever be grateful! It was insanely flavorful, filled with cooling herbs, crunchy veggies, and juicy, seared strips of steak, and I knew I had to attempt to re-create it at home. It's become an ovulatory phase staple ever since, not only for its serious freshness, but for its excellent source of amino acids, which are essential cofactors during phase-two liver detoxification. The salad is especially beneficial during this time of increased uterine energy demand by supplying energy to reproductive tissues and boosting egg quality.

Marinade/Dressing and Steak

- **½ cup coconut sugar**
- **¼ cup chicken bone broth (try using the Super Simple Homemade Bone Broth on page 109)**
- **¼ cup coconut aminos or gluten-free soy sauce**
- **¼ cup toasted sesame oil**
- **2 tablespoons fish sauce**
- **Grated zest and juice of 2 limes**
- **1 tablespoon minced fresh ginger**
- **2 cloves garlic, minced**
- **½ to 1 red chili pepper (optional, and to taste according to spice tolerance), thinly sliced**
- **2 pounds grass-fed and grass-finished skirt steak**
- **2 tablespoons avocado oil**

Salad

- **1 (5-ounce) package butter lettuce**
- **1 small green cabbage, cored and thinly sliced (or another package of butter lettuce)**
- **1 mango, pitted, peeled, and sliced**
- **1 large or 2 small avocados, pitted, peeled, and sliced**
- **1 daikon radish, thinly sliced**
- **1 cucumber, thinly sliced into rounds**
- **1 cup fresh Thai basil leaves, torn**
- **1 cup fresh mint leaves, torn**
- **1 cup fresh cilantro leaves, chopped**
- **2 green onions, thinly sliced on the bias**

- **Flaky sea salt and black pepper**
- **Sesame seeds, toasted coconut flakes, and crushed peanuts**

1. *For the marinade/dressing:* Whisk together the coconut sugar, bone both, coconut aminos, sesame oil, fish sauce, lime zest and juice, ginger, garlic, and optional chili in a small mixing bowl until well combined.

2. *For the steak:* Place the steak in a large glass dish and pour half to three-fourths of the marinade over the top, making sure the steak is fully submerged in the marinade (if not, you may need to flip the steak halfway through). Marinate in the fridge for 2 to 4 hours. Store the remaining marinade in a glass jar in the fridge until ready to use as the salad dressing.

3. Heat the avocado oil in a large cast-iron skillet over medium-high heat. Remove the steak from the marinade using tongs and shake to remove any excess liquid; discard any remaining marinade. Add the steak to the hot skillet and sear for 4 minutes. Flip the steak and cook for another 4 minutes for medium-rare. Let the steak rest for 5 to 10 minutes, then slice thinly against the grain.

4. *To assemble the salad:* Arrange all of the salad ingredients on a large platter or in individual bowls. Top with the sliced steak and pour the reserved dressing evenly over. Sprinkle with flaky sea salt and black pepper, top with garnishes of choice, toss, and serve.

OVULATORY PHASE BENEFITS

Supports liver function • Supports estrogen detoxification • High in glutathione and antioxidants

Pineapple-Turmeric Gut Gummies

PREP: 20 MINUTES, PLUS 2–4 HOURS CHILLING   COOK: 10 MINUTES   SERVES 16

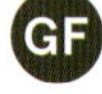

DF

These gummies evoke the nostalgia and sweet flavor of a beloved childhood treat, but that's about where the similarities end. You won't find refined sugar or preservatives in this recipe, but rather beef gelatin, which is a crucial thickening agent. It provides a chewy, elastic texture as well as an abundance of amino acids that improve GI health and assist in phase-two liver detoxification (necessary to eliminate excess estrogen). The pineapple juice adds a dose of fun flavor, vitamin C, and an enzyme called bromelain that reduces bloating, while the turmeric fights inflammation and oxidative stress. The process might seem intimidating at first, but these gummies are actually pretty simple to make and have become a favored little sweet bite to cap off a meal.

1 (32-ounce) jar (4 cups) unsweetened pure pineapple juice, divided

6 tablespoons grass-fed beef gelatin

¼ cup raw honey (or pure maple syrup)

1 teaspoon ground turmeric

¼ teaspoon black pepper

1 to 2 tablespoons coconut oil, for greasing the dish (and a piña colada flavor!), optional

1. Add 1 cup of the pineapple juice to a small bowl and slowly sprinkle in the beef gelatin 1 tablespoon at a time, stirring vigorously with a whisk. This is known as "blooming," which will help even out the texture and get rid of any clumps. Let sit for 5 minutes, until set.

2. Add the remaining 3 cups juice to a small pot and stir in the honey, turmeric, and black pepper. Bring to a simmer over medium heat, making sure the juice only comes to a bare simmer (steaming) and is not boiling, as this will denature the gelatin. Slowly add the bloomed gelatin mixture, whisking until well combined, completely even, and with no visible clumps. Remove from the heat.

3. Grease a 9 by 13-inch Pyrex dish with the coconut oil. (You can also use four ungreased 2 ml silicone molds with at least 16 indentations each.) Pour the gelatin mixture into the greased dish or molds. Refrigerate for a minimum of 2 hours to set (I like at least 4 hours to firm up). Make sure to refrigerate uncovered so the gummy mixture doesn't "sweat."

4. Once completely firm, remove from the fridge and cut into 16 squares (or remove the gummies from the molds). Store in an airtight container in the fridge for up to 1 week.

NOTE: For a more Jell-O-like consistency, use less gelatin (5 tablespoons). If you prefer your gummies firmer, add more gelatin (7 to 8 tablespoons).

OVULATORY PHASE BENEFITS

Supports liver function • Supports estrogen detoxification • High in glutathione and antioxidants

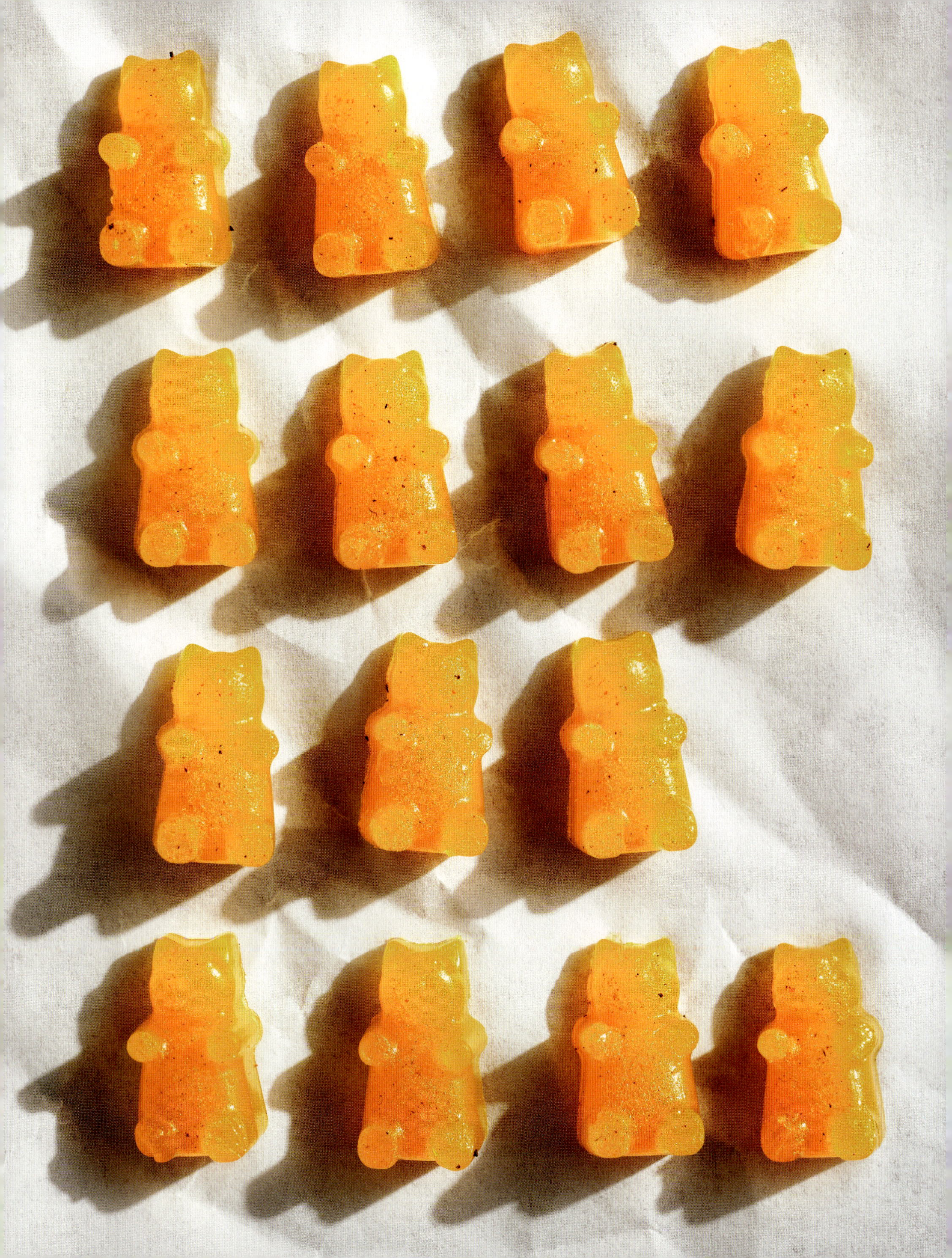

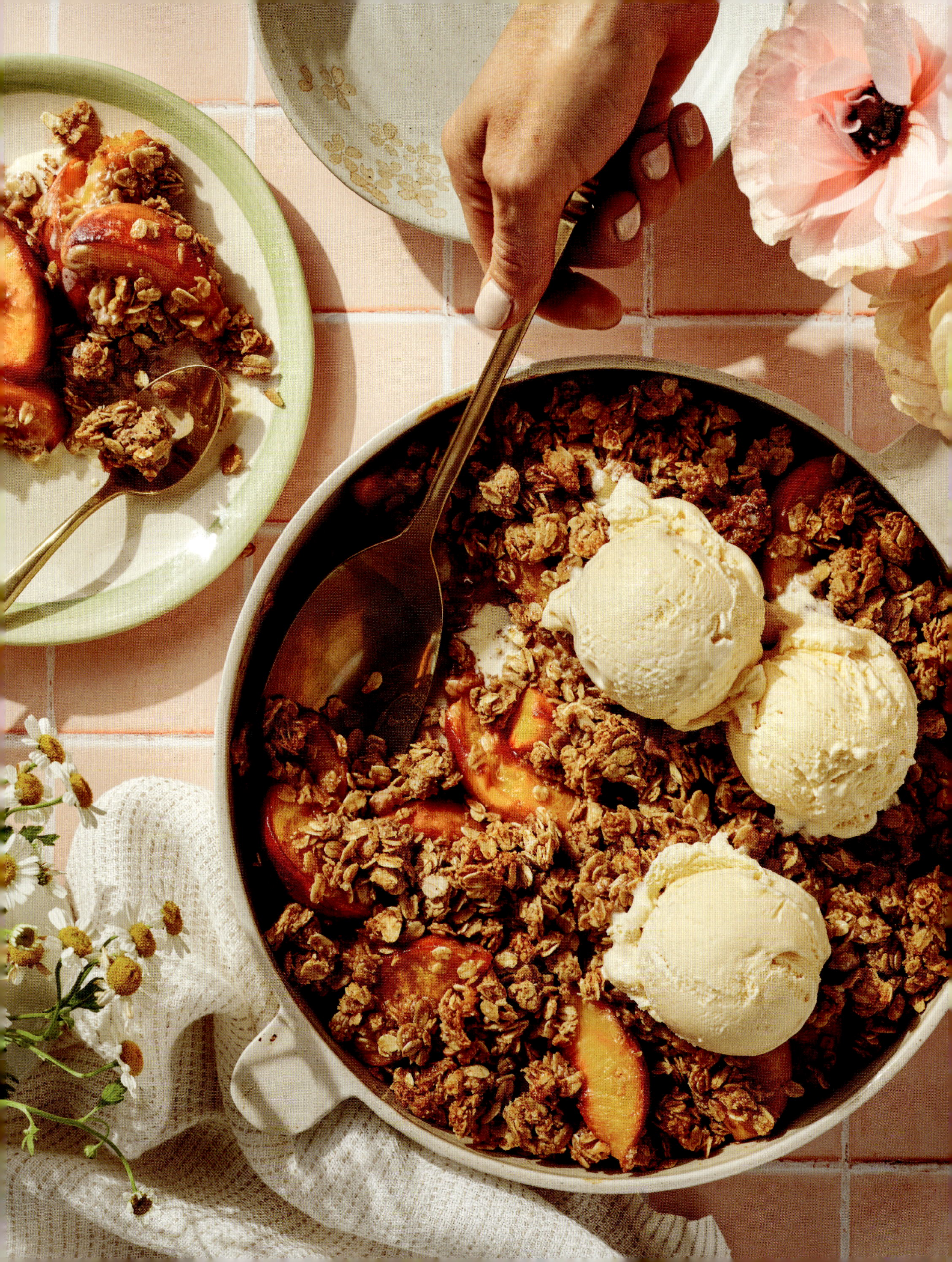

Perfect Peach–Almond Butter Oat Crisp

PREP: 10 MINUTES COOK: 30–40 MINUTES SERVES 4–6

This dessert is a must when peaches are in season and at their peak—juicy, fresh, sweet, and packed with antioxidants that combat oxidative stress. (**PRO TIP:** Fresh peaches have higher levels of antioxidants than canned.) The nutty oat clusters are still my favorite part of the dessert, and they happen to sneak in some fiber and protein to boot. Try serving the crisp with dollops of Coconut Whipped Cream (see page 110) or vanilla bean ice cream for the perfect dessert that aligns with your inner summer phase.

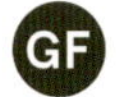

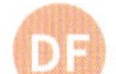

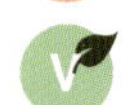

S

- Avocado oil spray, for greasing the pan
- 6 ripe organic peaches, pitted and sliced (about 4 cups)
- 1 tablespoon plus ¼ cup pure maple syrup, divided
- 1 tablespoon fresh lemon juice
- 1 tablespoon arrowroot starch
- 1½ teaspoons cinnamon, divided
- 1½ cups gluten-free protein oats (or sprouted gluten-free oats)
- ¼ cup almond flour
- ¼ cup creamy almond butter
- ¼ cup coconut sugar
- 1 teaspoon pure vanilla extract
- ½ teaspoon sea salt

1. Preheat the oven to 350°F and lightly grease a 9-inch pie pan or oven-safe skillet with avocado oil. Set aside.

2. Mix the peaches, the 1 tablespoon maple syrup, lemon juice, arrowroot, and ½ teaspoon of the cinnamon in a medium bowl until well combined. Transfer to the prepared pan or skillet.

3. Rinse out and dry the mixing bowl. Add the remaining ¼ cup maple syrup, remaining 1 teaspoon cinnamon, the oats, almond flour, almond butter, coconut sugar, vanilla, and salt and stir until well combined. The texture should be chunky and stick together thanks to the almond butter acting as a binder.

4. Spread the mixture evenly over the peaches. Bake for 30 to 40 minutes, until the peaches are bubbling and the crisp is golden brown. (If using ripe peaches, they will cook more quickly, whereas underripe peaches may need more baking time to allow them to release juices.) Let cool for 5 to 10 minutes and serve.

NOTE: I absolutely love this dessert with fresh peaches, but any other stone fruit or berry would taste delicious, as well as a combination (such as peaches and blueberries or raspberries). Just make sure to use a total of 4 cups chopped fruit!

OVULATORY PHASE BENEFITS

Supports vascular health • Rich in fiber • High in glutathione and antioxidants

Raspberry Cheesecake Froyo + Dark Chocolate Magic Shell

PREP: 10 MINUTES, PLUS 30 MINUTES FREEZING   COOK: NONE   SERVES 4 (8 OUNCES EACH)

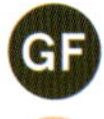
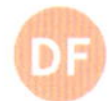
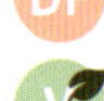

I'm a girl who likes a little bit of dessert every night after dinner, so I'm constantly trying to come up with recipes that satisfy my sweet tooth without negatively impacting my hormonal health, and this treat gets the job done. It's packed with vitamin C, probiotics, protein, and healthy fats and tastes legit like raspberry swirled cheesecake with a graham cracker crust and dark chocolate topping. Every bite is magic and everyone who tries it is obsessed. I recommend always keeping a batch in your freezer, but especially during your inner summer phase, when froyo just hits differently.

- 1 (16-ounce) container full-fat unsweetened Greek or coconut yogurt
- ⅓ cup full-fat vegan cream cheese (or regular cream cheese)
- ¼ cup coconut sugar
- 2 servings vanilla protein powder
- 1 teaspoon pure vanilla extract
- ½ teaspoon sea salt, plus more for topping
- 1 cup organic raspberries, rinsed and lightly mashed
- 1 cup crushed gluten-free graham-style crackers, plus more for topping
- ½ cup dark chocolate chips
- 1 teaspoon unrefined organic coconut oil

1. Combine the yogurt, cream cheese, coconut sugar, protein powder, vanilla, and salt in a medium mixing bowl. Beat with a hand or stand mixer on high for 1 to 2 minutes, scraping the sides with a spatula to evenly mix, until fluffy. Stir in the mashed raspberries and crushed graham crackers until well combined. Set aside.

2. Combine the chocolate chips and coconut oil in a small microwave-safe bowl. Melt in the microwave in 30-second increments, stirring each time, until the chocolate chips have melted.

3. Use a spatula to spoon the froyo base into four 8-ounce glass jars (or serving jars or bowls of choice). Pour the chocolate mixture evenly on top of each. This is what will create a "magic shell." Sprinkle more salt and crushed graham crackers on top. Place in the freezer for 30 minutes, until the base has chilled through.

4. To enjoy, use a spoon and tap with force through the top of the magic shell, then scoop some into each bite.

NOTE: I love to always have a batch of these in the freezer; they'll keep for up to 2 months. Just make sure to use airtight glass jars or containers with lids and defrost at room temperature for at least an hour before serving.

OVULATORY PHASE BENEFITS

Supports vascular health • Supports estrogen elimination • Rich in probiotics • Rich in glutathione and antioxidants

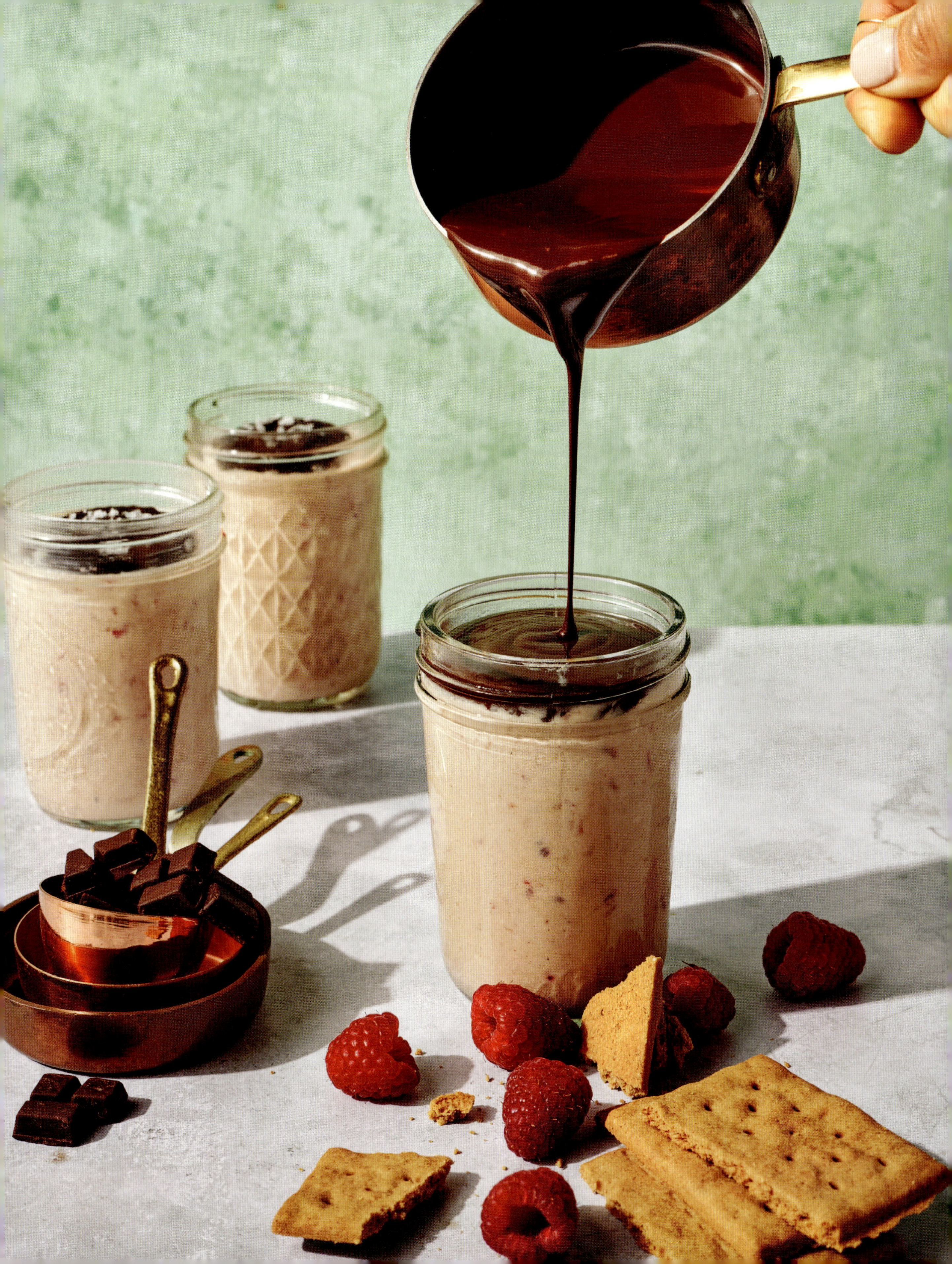

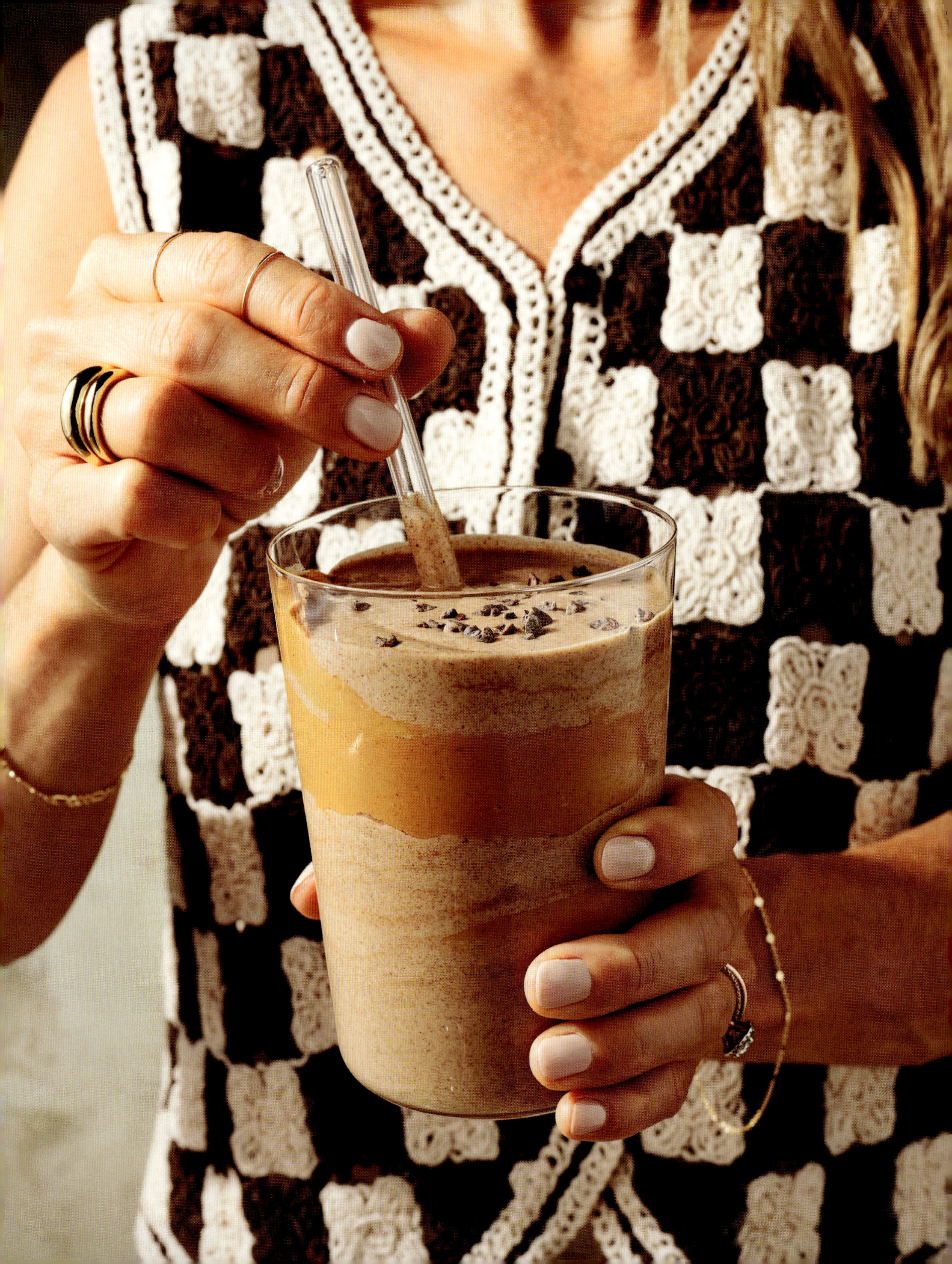

Tastes-Like-Dessert Snickers Smoothie

PREP: 10 MINUTES COOK: NONE SERVES 1 (24 OUNCES)

This smoothie may taste like a candy bar, but it packs a serious nutrient punch that leaves me feeling energized and satiated until lunch. Maca root (see Note) adds a caramel note and optimizes ovulation in a myriad of ways, from reducing the negative effects of chronic stress to naturally boosting testosterone levels (and libido) and stimulating luteinizing hormone (which triggers ovulation).

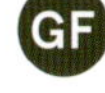

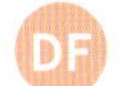

- 1 cup almond milk (or homemade Brazil Nut Milk, page 163)
- 1½ servings caramel protein powder (or chocolate or vanilla flavor)
- 2 dates, pitted
- 2 tablespoons ground flaxseeds
- 2 tablespoons cacao nibs
- 2 tablespoons unsweetened organic peanut butter
- 1 teaspoon cinnamon
- 1 teaspoon gelatinized red maca root powder
- ¼ to ½ teaspoon sea salt
- 1 cup frozen cauliflower (this adds nutrients, fiber, and bulk to thicken the smoothie without impacting the taste!)
- ½ frozen banana

Pour the almond milk into a high-speed blender, then add all the remaining ingredients. Blend at the lowest setting, slowly increasing in speed until all the ingredients are completely blended and the smoothie is rich and creamy.

NOTE: Women should take the red phenotype of maca for ovulation support, while men can take black to help with sperm production and motility. I always encourage checking with your medical practitioner before incorporating herbs or adaptogens like maca root into your routine, especially if taking medications. Additionally, maca should be avoided if you have Hashimoto's or thyroid issues, as it contains a significant amount of iodine.

OVULATORY PHASE BENEFITS

Supports liver function • Supports estrogen detoxification • Rich in fiber

Tart Cherry Pie Smoothie

PREP: 10 MINUTES COOK: NONE SERVES 1 (24 OUNCES)

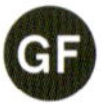

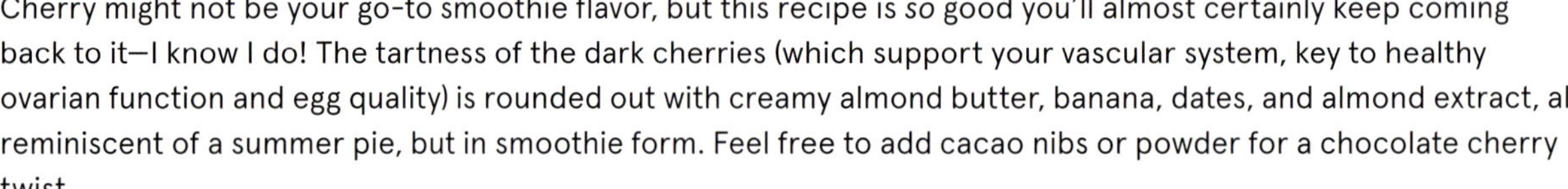
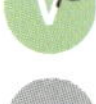
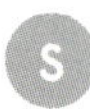

Cherry might not be your go-to smoothie flavor, but this recipe is *so* good you'll almost certainly keep coming back to it—I know I do! The tartness of the dark cherries (which support your vascular system, key to healthy ovarian function and egg quality) is rounded out with creamy almond butter, banana, dates, and almond extract, all reminiscent of a summer pie, but in smoothie form. Feel free to add cacao nibs or powder for a chocolate cherry twist.

- **1½ cups almond milk (or other nondairy milk)**
- **1 serving vanilla protein powder (or enough to provide 20 to 30 grams protein)**
- **2 tablespoons almond butter**
- **2 tablespoons flaxseeds**
- **2 dates, pitted**
- **1 teaspoon pure vanilla extract**
- **¼ teaspoon almond extract**
- **¼ teaspoon sea salt**
- **1 cup frozen cauliflower**
- **⅔ cup frozen organic tart cherries (or dark sweet cherries)**
- **½ frozen banana**
- **1 to 2 tablespoons cacao powder or nibs (for a chocolate twist, optional)**

Pour the almond milk into a high-speed blender, then add all the remaining ingredients. Blend at the lowest setting, slowly increasing in speed until all the ingredients are completely blended and the smoothie is rich and creamy.

OVULATORY PHASE BENEFITS

Supports vascular health • Supports liver function • Supports estrogen detoxification • Rich in fiber • High in glutathione and antioxidants

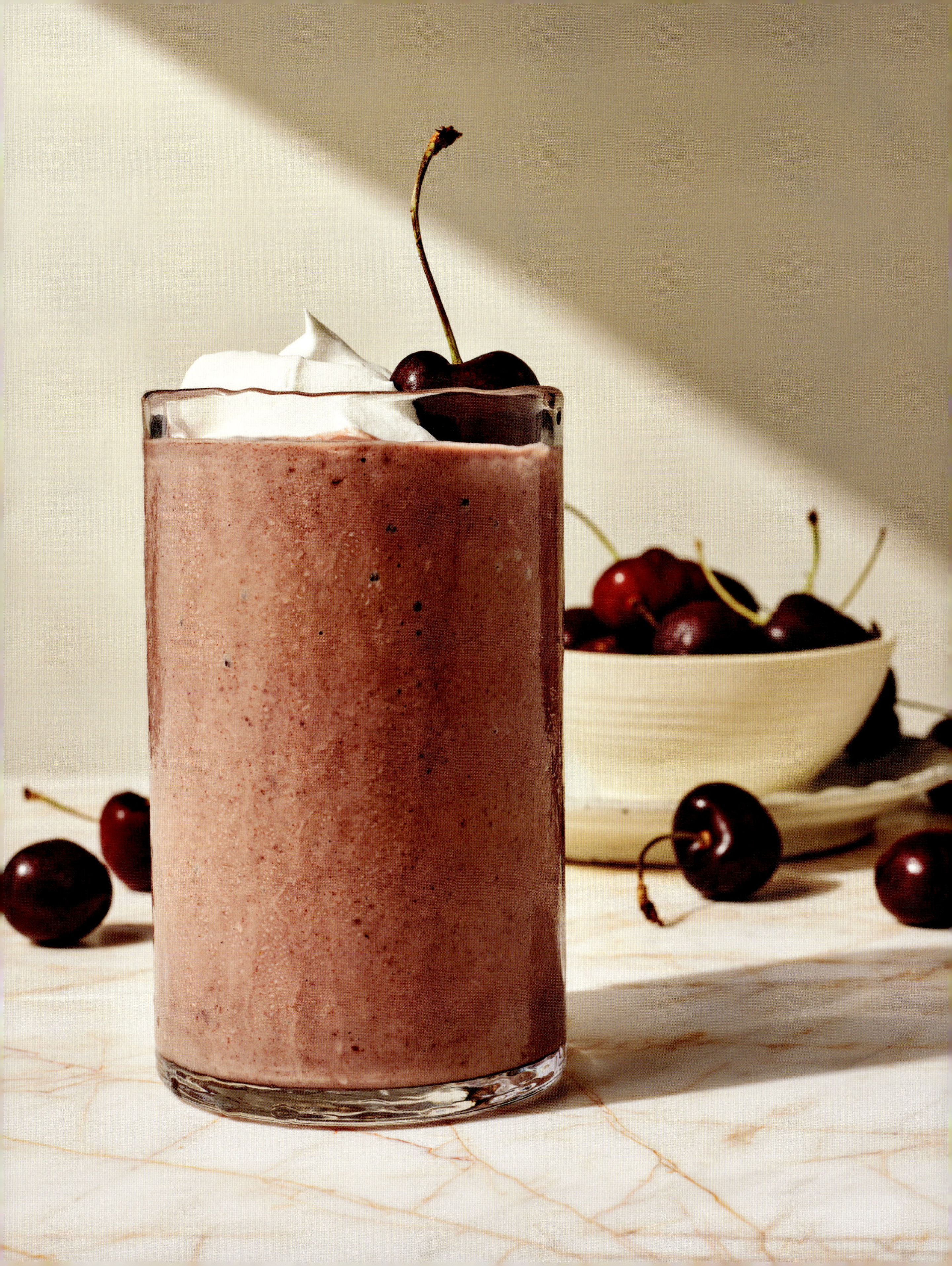

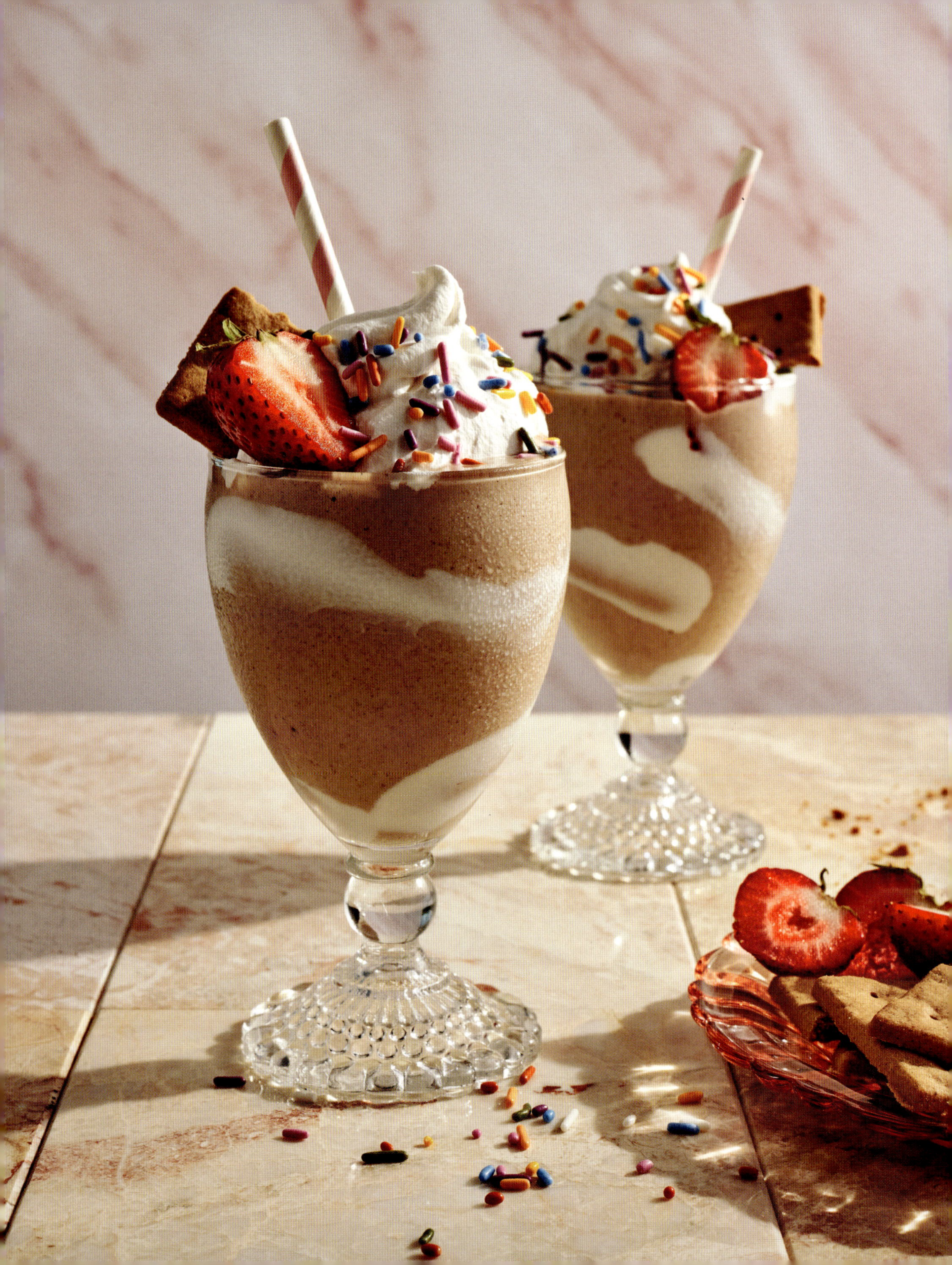

Strawberries 'n' Cream Dream Smoothie

PREP: 10 MINUTES   COOK: NONE   SERVES 1 (24 OUNCES)

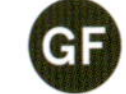
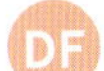

This smoothie is reminiscent of the milkshakes I enjoyed during childhood, minus the blood sugar spike and subsequent crash. It's also packed with fiber and antioxidants that help fight off oxidative stress and metabolize excess estrogen. While incredibly delicious as is, if you desire an even creamier texture, reduce the coconut milk to 1 cup and add ½ cup full-fat unsweetened cottage cheese, Greek yogurt, or whole-milk kefir, which also ups the protein and gut-friendly probiotic factor.

- 1½ cups full-fat canned coconut milk
- 1½ servings vanilla protein powder (or enough to provide 30 grams protein)
- 2 tablespoons hemp seeds
- 2 dates, pitted and chopped (or 1 to 2 tablespoons raw honey)
- 2 tablespoons cashew butter
- 1 teaspoon pure vanilla extract
- ¼ teaspoon Himalayan pink salt
- 1 cup frozen strawberries
- ½ cup frozen cauliflower
- ½ frozen banana

- Coconut Whipped Cream (page 110), sprinkles, or crushed gluten-free graham crackers for topping (optional)

1. Pour the coconut milk into a high-speed blender, then add all remaining ingredients. Blend at the lowest setting, slowly increasing in speed until all the ingredients are completely blended and the smoothie is rich and creamy.

2. If you like, add some optional toppings for a fun milkshake factor.

NOTE: This smoothie is super thick (just the way I like it!), but feel free to add more milk based on your texture preference.

OVULATORY PHASE BENEFITS

Supports vascular health • Supports liver function • Supports estrogen detoxification • Rich in fiber • High in glutathione and antioxidants

Slightly Spicy Blood Orange Adrenal Cocktail

PREP: 10 MINUTES COOK: NONE SERVES 2 (8 OUNCES EACH)

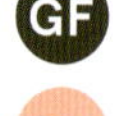
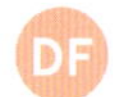
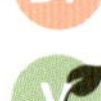

If you love margaritas or any sort of citrus-y beverage with loads of color, flavor, and a hint of spice, then you are going to *love* this (non-alcoholic) adrenal cocktail. It's got all the aforementioned components, plus packs a powerhouse combo of vitamin C, potassium, and sodium that nourishes your adrenal glands and combats oxidative stress, which tends to increase right before ovulation. This is such a great one to whip up when you're entertaining guests on warm sunny days, or if you're craving a fun, thirst-quenching mocktail. It pairs especially well with the Fish Tacos (page 134), and you can't go wrong serving it alongside chips and guac.

- Fresh or dried blood orange slices, plus sea salt or Tajin spice, for the glass rims (optional)
- Ice cubes (try using a pebble ice cube tray if you're feeling fancy)
- ⅓ cup freshly squeezed blood orange juice (or regular orange juice)
- ¼ cup fresh lime juice
- ¼ cup organic coconut water
- 2 slices jalapeño (optional)
- 1 tablespoon coconut cream
- Orange slices, for garnish

1. If you like, slide an orange slice around the rims of two 8-ounce glasses, then dip the rims into a shallow bowl of sea salt or Tajin spice. Add ice cubes to the glasses and set aside.

2. Combine the orange juice, lime juice, coconut water, jalapeño slices (if using), and coconut cream in a cocktail shaker with ice and shake vigorously for 12 to 15 seconds, until the concoction is chilled and well mixed.

3. Strain into the rimmed glasses with the ice cubes, then garnish with a fresh orange slice and enjoy.

OVULATORY PHASE BENEFITS

Supports vascular health • Supports liver function • Rich in glutathione and antioxidants

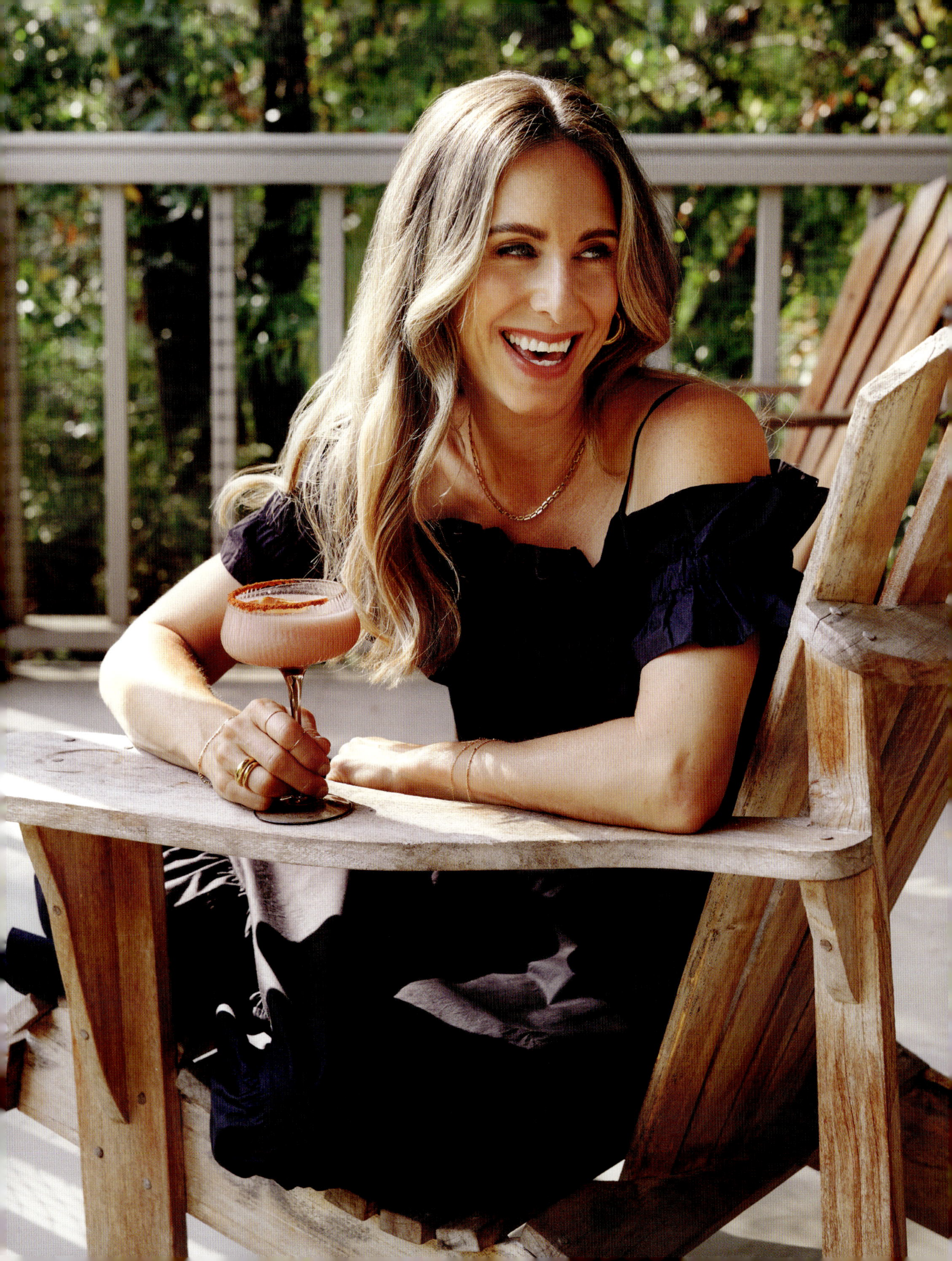

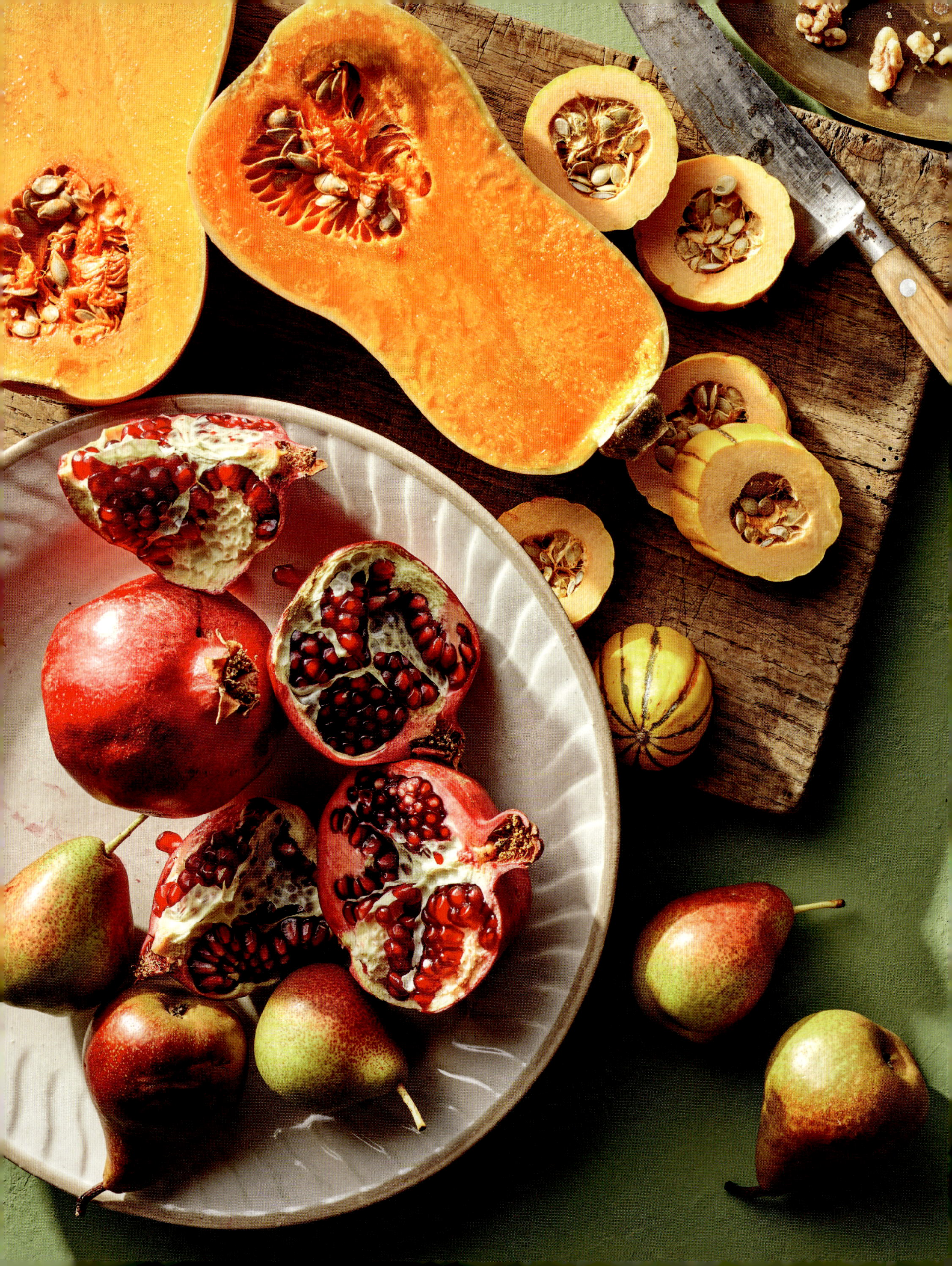

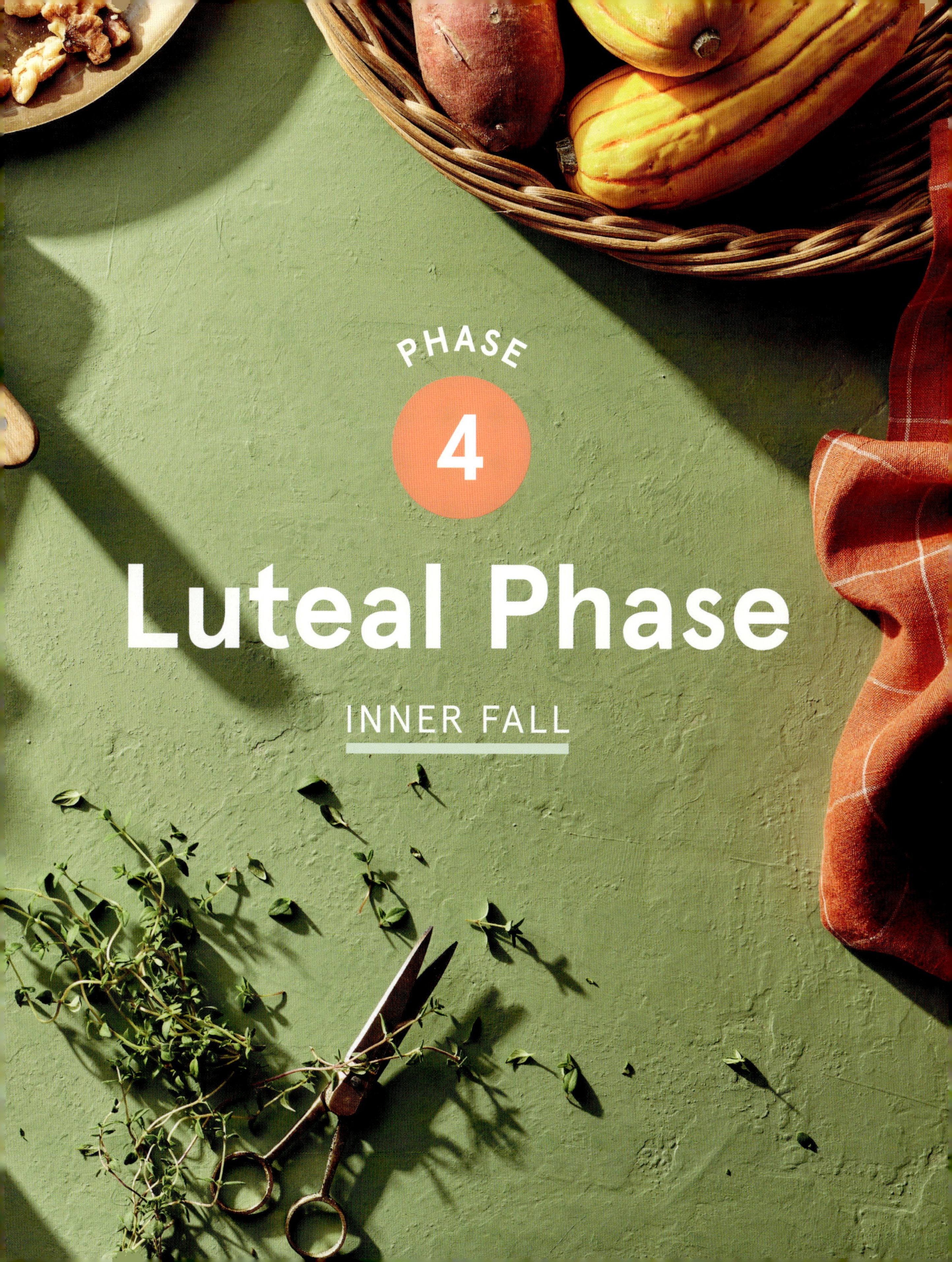

PHASE 4

Luteal Phase

INNER FALL

RECIPES

WHAT'S HAPPENING

Immediately after ovulation, your dominant follicle transforms into the corpus luteum and begins producing progesterone. Progesterone takes over for estrogen, which, up until ovulation, was building a cushy endometrium lining in anticipation of a potential pregnancy. Progesterone completes the maturation process and renders the lining receptive for egg implantation. If an egg was fertilized, the corpus luteum will continue producing progesterone throughout pregnancy. If not, it breaks down 12 to 14 days post-ovulation, beginning your period and a new menstrual cycle.

This shift often feels gradual, just like that slow transition from late summer to early fall, and we're often still riding high off the feel-good effects of ovulation for about the first half of the phase. But, as progesterone production increases, it naturally inclines us to turn our attention inward and focus on routines, organization, self-care regimens, and completing important tasks and goals.

While a dwindle in energy and a more introspective mood are normal during this time, many women experience symptoms of PMS that are common but not normal—insomnia, bloat, cravings, fatigue, headaches, cramping, anxiety, acne, or depression—making this phase often the most dreaded of the entire cycle. However, as someone who struggled with PMS for many, many years, I can assure you that when your hormones are operating in harmony this can actually be a really beautiful and enjoyable time in your cycle, and the autumnal-themed foods and recipes happen to be some of my favorites.

Speaking of food, the increase in progesterone during the luteal phase also stimulates appetite and increases body temperature and resting metabolic rate, which may require women to consume anywhere between 100 and 300 more calories per day. This is *especially* not the time to count calories, restrict foods, or skip meals, as doing so can destabilize blood sugar, dysregulate feel-good hormones like serotonin and dopamine, and increase cortisol production (which also turns on fat storage). I also want to point out if you *do* feel hungrier during this phase, it is completely normal, and I encourage you to listen to your body. (I say this as someone who ignored hunger signals for years to adhere to the same calorie intake day after day, with major PMS to show for it.)

By the same token, you'll most likely find a reduction in PMS-related symptoms when you're consistently consuming a variety of nutrient-dense foods throughout your cycle, including fewer cravings and the ability to satisfy your increased energy needs easily and sufficiently. In fact, women with PMS report more cravings and show a 30 percent higher energy intake during this phase, while women without PMS experienced mild cravings and a 6.5 percent increase in energy intake.[1]

My hope is that you can find a way to be kinder and more compassionate to your body all of the time—but especially during this phase. For women who struggle with dieting or disordered eating, it can be extremely difficult to let go of the less-is-more mentality. I used to push myself so hard through this phase, dealing with extreme guilt if I consumed more calories than usual or caved to cravings. Please know it's not a matter of willpower, it's simply a matter of increased energy needs, and you'll find an abundance of comforting, cozy, and nourishing recipes in this chapter to help you support your female physiology in a very delicious way.

PILLARS OF EATING FOR YOUR LUTEAL PHASE

Due to the hormonal fluctuations that take place during this phase, it's important to consume plenty of nutrients that support progesterone production, stable blood sugar levels, and healthy mood and brain function. Note that while adequate progesterone levels are critical, they can naturally slow digestion (hi, bloat and constipation), so it's helpful to eat plenty of warm, well-cooked, fiber-rich foods, which support large intestine functionality and increase transit time, leading to regular bowel movements.

Optimal Foods to Support Your Luteal Phase

B VITAMIN-RICH FOODS

B vitamins (especially B_6 and B_9) support optimal progesterone production (crucial to reducing PMS-related symptoms) as well as help stabilize blood sugar levels, helping you avoid energy dips, mood swings, and cravings. **Optimal B vitamin–rich foods for your luteal phase include:**

- Liver and other organ meats
- Poultry
- Tuna
- Wild-caught salmon and other fatty fish
- Full-fat ricotta or cottage cheese
- Gluten-free oats
- Potatoes
- Bananas
- Citrus

FIBER-RICH FOODS

The increase in progesterone naturally slows digestion, which can lead to bloat and constipation during this phase. Eating a variety of fiber-rich foods supports large intestine functionality and increases transit time, leading to regular bowel movements. **Optimal fiber-rich foods for your luteal phase include:**

- Walnuts
- Starchy root vegetables
- Chickpeas and other legumes
- Gluten-free whole grains (quinoa, millets, oats, buckwheat, etc.)
- Leafy greens
- Pears
- Apples

COMPLEX CARBOHYDRATES

Consuming adequate complex carbohydrates (i.e., slow-burning carbs) helps to regulate serotonin and dopamine levels, preventing mood swings, providing your cells with energy, and blunting cravings. As always, you'll want to make sure you pair these with quality sources of protein and fat to prevent a blood sugar spike or crash. **Optimal complex carbs for this phase include:**

- Potatoes
- Sweet potatoes
- Squash
- Pumpkin
- Carrots
- Buckwheat
- Millet
- Oats
- Brown rice

MAGNESIUM-RICH FOODS

Magnesium is an essential mineral involved in over 300 biochemical reactions in the body, including muscle and nerve function (helping to lower prostaglandin levels tied to menstrual cramps), regulating blood sugar and improving insulin sensitivity, and supporting a healthy immune system. Magnesium deficiency is extremely common among women, especially those with PCOS, and has been

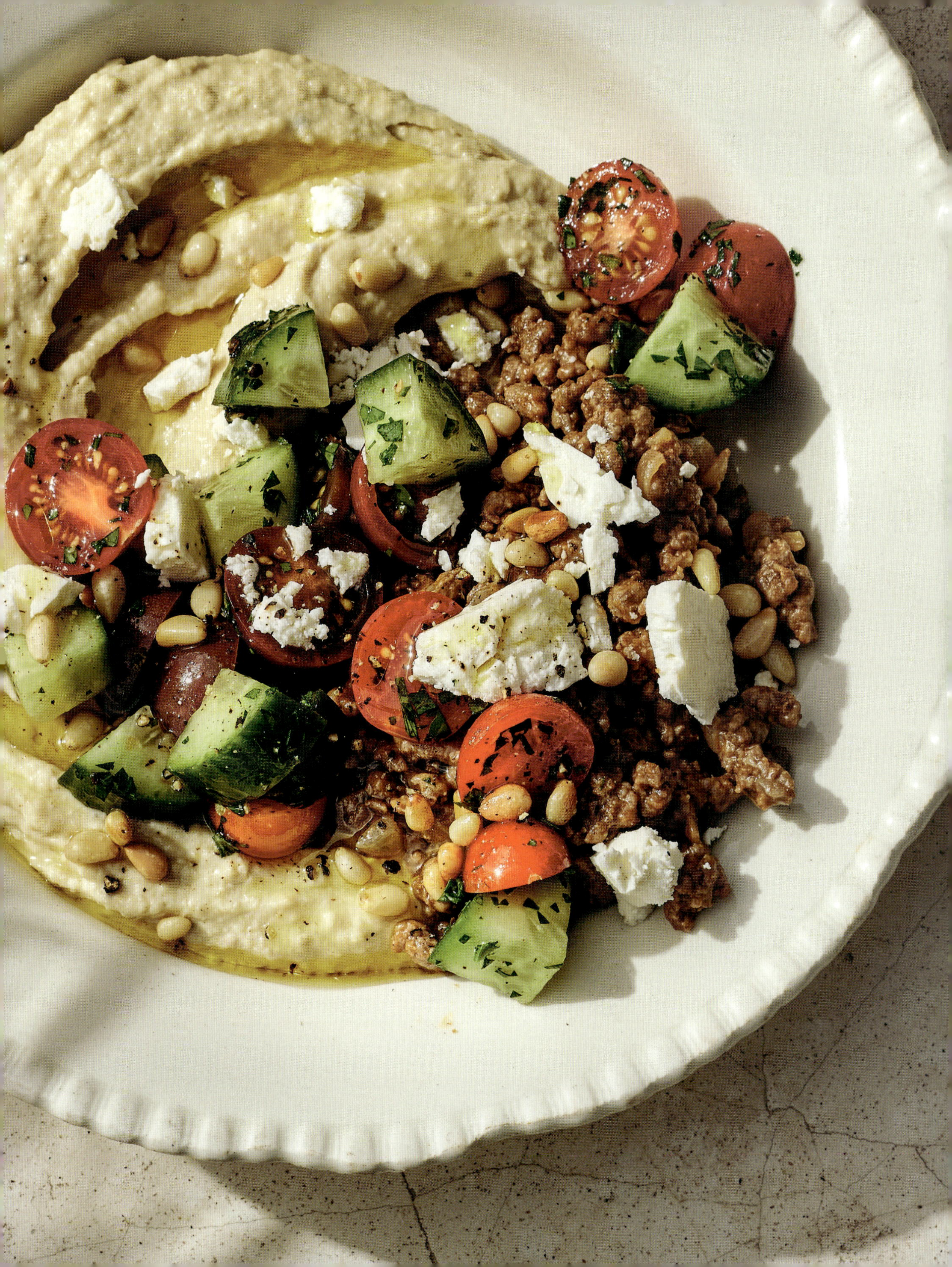

associated with a variety of metabolic problems including insulin resistance, high blood pressure, and inflammation. You'll want to ensure you're consuming plenty of magnesium-rich foods regularly, with an emphasis during this phase to keep PMS-related symptoms at bay. **Optimal food sources include:**

- Fish (salmon, cod, halibut, etc.)
- Nuts and seeds
- Legumes (chickpeas, navy beans, black beans, cannellini beans, etc.)
- Gluten-free whole grains (quinoa, brown rice, etc.)
- Avocado
- Spinach, kale, and other dark leafy greens
- Dark chocolate

FOODS HIGH IN OMEGA-3 FATTY ACIDS

As you learned earlier, omega-3 fatty acids are highly anti-inflammatory and have been shown to lower prostaglandins that if elevated can lead to cramping and period pain. **Optimal sources include:**

- Fatty fish (wild-caught salmon, sardines, tuna, mackerel, herring)
- Oysters
- Pasture-raised egg yolks
- Walnuts
- Hemp seeds
- Chia seeds
- Spirulina

ANTI-INFLAMMATORY HERBS AND SPICES

Herbs and spices have been used in traditional Chinese medicine for over 2,000 years and have been clinically proven to help reduce cramping, nausea, bloating, fatigue, and headaches, as well as boost immunity and digestion and promote cycle regularity. **Optimal herbs and spices to incorporate in your luteal phase include:**

- Garlic
- Ginger
- Burdock root
- Dandelion root
- Red raspberry leaf
- Peppermint
- Cinnamon
- Oat straw

Luteal Phase Cooking and Eating Tips

INCREASE DAILY CALORIC INTAKE, IF NEEDED

As mentioned earlier, your resting metabolic rate increases during this phase, naturally burning 10 to 20 percent more calories, which is often accompanied by an increase in appetite. If you feel hungrier during this phase, I highly encourage you to meet this increased energy expenditure with more food (which also supports metabolism and blood sugar levels, key for a decrease in fat storage and for stable weight).

Try adding a protein-rich snack or two if needed or increasing the caloric density of your meals with a drizzle of olive oil or a few avocado slices, extra-large servings of protein, chopped nuts and seeds, or an egg.

OPT FOR WARM, WELL-COOKED FOODS

Progesterone, your calming and relaxing hormone, tends to *slooow* things down, especially your digestion, by relaxing the muscles in your digestive tract, which can lead to uncomfortable symptoms like constipation and bloat. Cooking most of the foods featured in this chapter (especially starches and grains, vegetables and fruits, and meat and poultry) helps optimize digestion and nutrient extraction. This all works to support large intestine functionality and increase transit time, leading to more regular bowel movements.

DON'T CUT OUT CARBS

Slow-burning complex carbohydrates help to stabilize blood sugar levels and boost your feel-good neurotransmitter serotonin, which acts as a natural appetite suppressant and mood stabilizer. Opt for the fiber- and nutrient-rich carbs listed in this section, paired with a source of high-quality protein and fat to prevent a blood sugar spike.

NOTE: If grains don't work well for you, as can be the case for those with an autoimmune condition, starchy root vegetables and fruits are great fiber-rich sources.

EAT REGULARLY AND OFTEN

Because blood sugar is less stable and resting cortisol levels are higher during your luteal phase, skipping meals or eating irregularly signals to your adrenals to pump out cortisol to compensate for fluctuating blood sugar levels. This means you have more stress hormones circulating in your bloodstream, which can lead to an increase in mood swings, cravings, sleep issues, anxiety, and fat storage, to name a few issues. Focus on eating three consistent, nourishing meals per day, adding a snack or two if needed.

BOOST HYDRATION WITH ELECTROLYTES AND SALT

You know how important it is to drink water regularly, but to maintain proper fluid levels you'll also want to prioritize electrolytes and salt. These contain essential minerals—sodium, potassium, chloride, calcium, and magnesium—that provide a myriad of benefits, from supporting energy levels, adrenal health, and fluid balance to maintaining the correct plasma volume in your bloodstream to supplying adequate stomach acid necessary for the absorption of vitamins and minerals and facilitating protein digestion.

Low salt intake has been associated with a higher risk for PMS, most likely because it triggers the adrenal glands to release a hormone called aldosterone, which leads to fluid and sodium retention. If you experience fluid retention during this phase, it's likely you need to consume more salt, not less. Additionally, an insufficient intake of electrolytes like magnesium and calcium has been shown to contribute to cycle issues including cramping, breast tenderness, fluid retention (i.e., bloat), headaches or migraines, and mood changes. Drinking plenty of fluids—like the beverage recipes at the end of the chapter—along with consuming these recipes (naturally rich in hydrating minerals!) will work to naturally combat these symptoms.

> “
>
> FOCUS ON EATING THREE CONSISTENT, NOURISHING MEALS PER DAY, ADDING A SNACK OR TWO IF NEEDED.

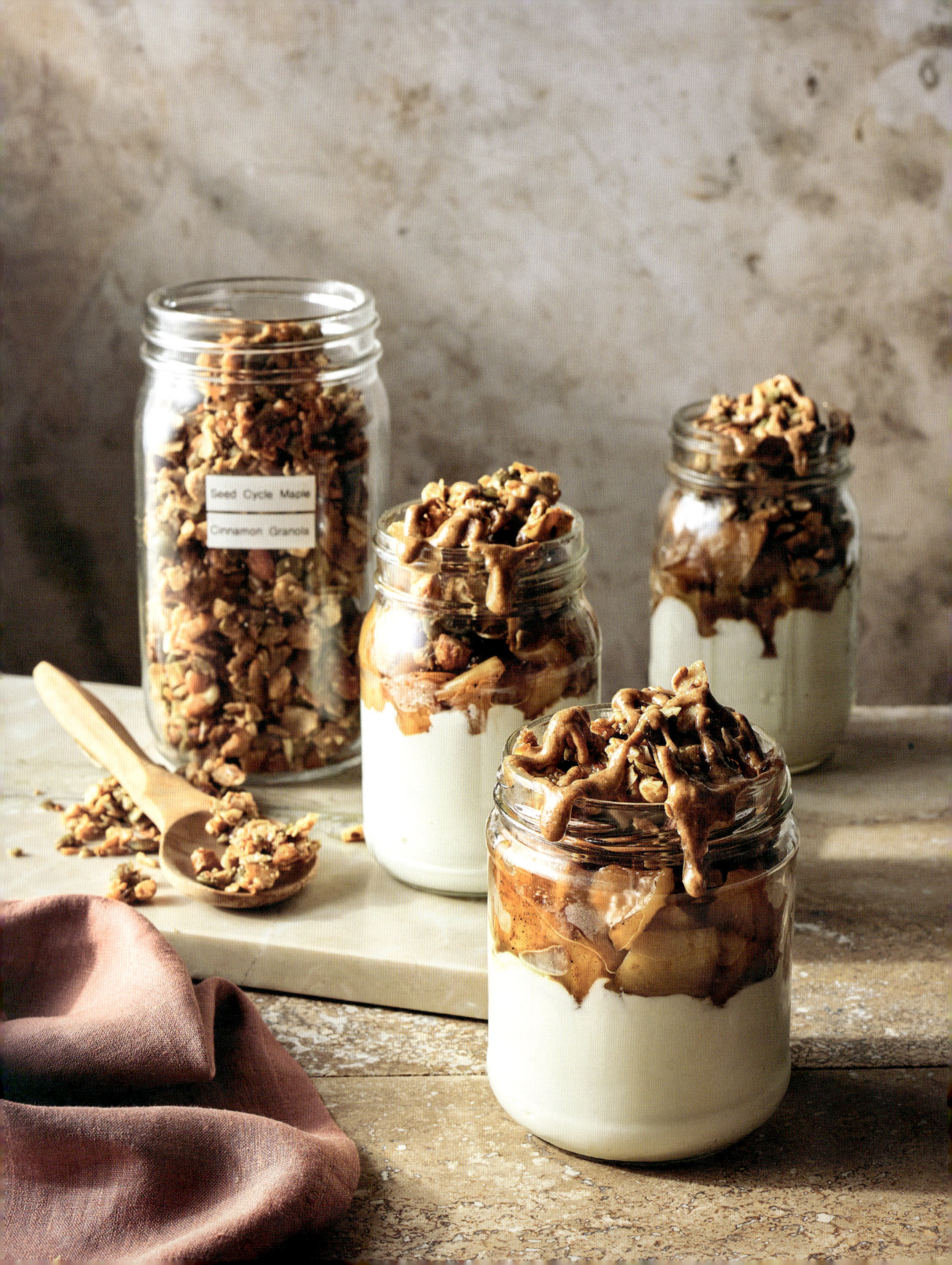
Seed Cycle Maple
Cinnamon Granola

Stovetop Apple-Cinnamon Breakfast Parfaits

PREP: 5 MINUTES COOK: 15 MINUTES SERVES 4

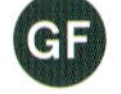

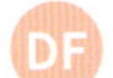

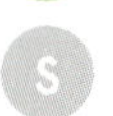

BF

I could (and often do) make this breakfast on repeat during the latter half of my cycle. It reminds me of eating warm apple pie filling, but with way less sugar, plus a healthy dose of protein and fats to keep energy and mood stable. The apples are also rich in fiber and an antioxidant called quercetin, which has been shown to lower inflammation and keep blood sugar levels in check (critical for managing PMS). Eating a nutrient-dense, protein-rich breakfast during the luteal phase is one of the most impactful ways to balance blood sugar and lower stress in the body, and this recipe is a quick meal prep option to ensure you're doing just that!

Stovetop Cinnamon Apples

4 small Fuji or Honeycrisp apples, cored and chopped into bite-size chunks (3 to 4 cups)

2 tablespoons water

1 heaping tablespoon unrefined organic coconut oil or grass-fed ghee

1 tablespoon pure maple syrup

1 teaspoon pure vanilla extract

1 teaspoon cinnamon

½ teaspoon cardamom

¼ teaspoon sea salt

Parfaits

2 to 3 cups full-fat unsweetened Greek yogurt, coconut yogurt, or skyr

1 cup Seed-Cycle Maple Cinnamon Granola (page 65)

Raw honey, creamy nut butter, and flaky sea salt, for topping (optional)

1. *For the apples:* In a large skillet over medium-high heat, combine the chopped apples and water. Cover and cook for 5 minutes, stirring frequently, until most of the water has been absorbed. Reduce the heat to medium, stir in the coconut oil or ghee, and cook for 5 more minutes, stirring frequently, until the apples have softened. Add the maple syrup, vanilla, cinnamon, cardamom, and salt and cook for 3 to 5 minutes more, stirring frequently until the apples are caramelized and fragrant. Remove from the heat and let cool for 3 to 5 minutes.

2. *To assemble the parfaits:* Layer the yogurt of choice into four glass jars or serving dishes and top each with a generous portion of the cinnamon apples. Sprinkle each with some granola and drizzle with optional honey, nut butter, and flaky sea salt.

NOTE: If making for one, store the remaining apple topping in an airtight glass container in the fridge for up to 5 days. Reheat throughout the week for a quick and delicious breakfast! If meal prepping in advance, I prefer storing each element in a separate container, then combining before serving.

LUTEAL PHASE BENEFITS

Rich in fiber • Anti-inflammatory • Slow cooked for maximum nutrient absorption

Sweet Potato Toast 4 Ways

PREP: 5 MINUTES COOK: 30 MINUTES SERVES 2

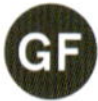

BF

Sweet potato toast might not be novel, but it is a delicious and easy way to get yourself out of a breakfast or lunch rut, especially during your luteal phase, when you need more of those slow-burning, complex carbs to regulate feel-good hormones like serotonin and dopamine (critical to preventing mood swings and PMS). Swapping out bread for thinly sliced sweet potatoes also provides a budget-friendly option for my gluten-free girlies, as sourcing high-quality gluten-free bread can sometimes be difficult and spendy! Below I offer up four topping options for the delicious, fiber-filled vehicle: two savory and two sweet. You can't go wrong, whichever you choose—or mix and match to your heart's desire.

2 medium orange-fleshed or Japanese sweet potatoes, scrubbed and patted dry

Avocado oil spray

With Jammy Eggs and Avocado

Whipped Ricotta Cheese (see page 175)

1 large avocado, pitted, peeled, and thinly sliced

½ cup microgreens

4 pasture-raised organic eggs, soft-boiled (see Notes)

Minced fresh chives, extra virgin olive oil, flaky sea salt, and red chile flakes, for garnish

With Lox and Cucumber

Hummus or cream cheese

1 Persian cucumber, thinly sliced

½ cup lox-style smoked salmon

Chopped fresh dill, extra virgin olive oil, flaky sea salt, and red chile flakes, for garnish

With Ricotta and Pears

Whipped Ricotta Cheese (see page 175)

1 small pear, cored and thinly sliced

Chopped walnuts, honey, and cinnamon, for garnish

With Nut Butter and Banana

¼ cup creamy almond butter or peanut butter

1 small banana, thinly sliced

¼ cup organic blueberries

Honey, cacao nibs, hemp seeds, and flaky sea salt, for garnish

1. Preheat the oven to 400°F and line a baking sheet with parchment paper.

2. Using a sharp knife or mandoline, slice the sweet potatoes lengthwise into ½-inch-thick slices. Lightly coat them with avocado oil spray and arrange on the lined baking sheet. Bake for 25 to 30 minutes, flipping halfway through, until the slices are soft, tender, and slightly crispy on the outside. Let cool for a few minutes.

3. Top the toasts with your choice from the following combinations (or mix and match your own favorites):

For savory jammy eggs and avocado: Top with whipped ricotta, avocado, microgreens, and soft-boiled eggs, then garnish with chives, a drizzle of olive oil, flaky sea salt, and red chile flakes.

For savory lox and cucumber: Top with hummus or cream cheese, sliced cucumber, and lox-style salmon, then garnish with dill, a drizzle of olive oil, flaky sea salt, and red chile flakes.

For sweet ricotta and pear: Top with whipped ricotta and sliced pear, then garnish with walnuts, a drizzle of honey, and cinnamon.

For sweet nut butter and banana: Top with almond or peanut butter, sliced banana, and blueberries, then garnish with a drizzle of honey, cacao nibs, hemp seeds, and flaky sea salt.

NOTES: If you want to make the sweet potato toast in a standard toaster, you will need to place the oiled sweet potato slices in the slots and toast 5 to 8 times, until the sweet potato is cooked all the way through. You can also cook in an air fryer at 400°F for about 20 minutes.

To soft-boil eggs, place in a small pot of water, cover, and bring to a boil. Immediately remove from the heat and let sit covered for 4 minutes. Make an ice water bath with 1 tablespoon apple cider vinegar (to help remove the shell). With a slotted spoon, transfer the eggs to the water bath and let cool for 5 minutes, then peel.

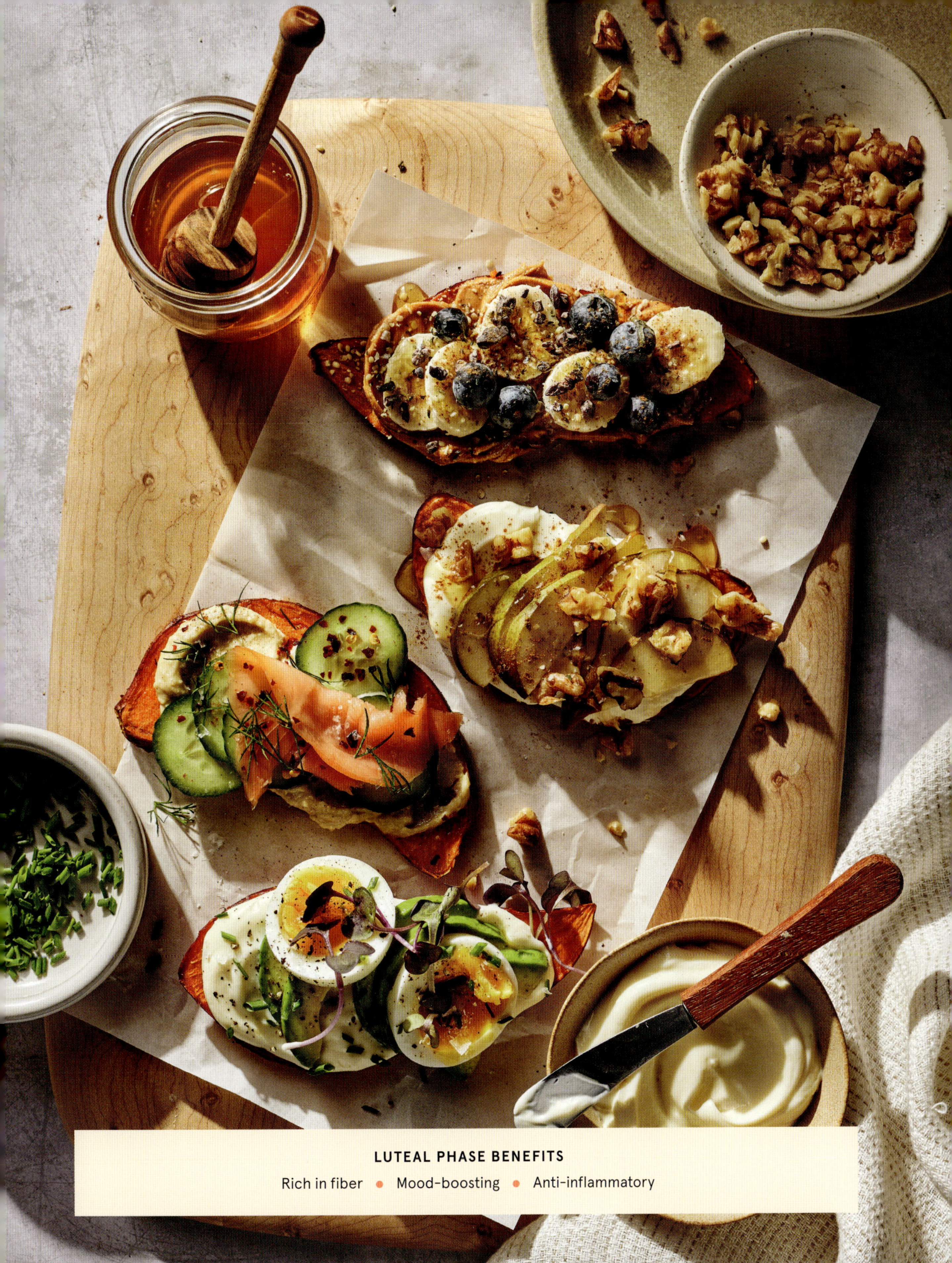

LUTEAL PHASE BENEFITS

Rich in fiber • Mood-boosting • Anti-inflammatory

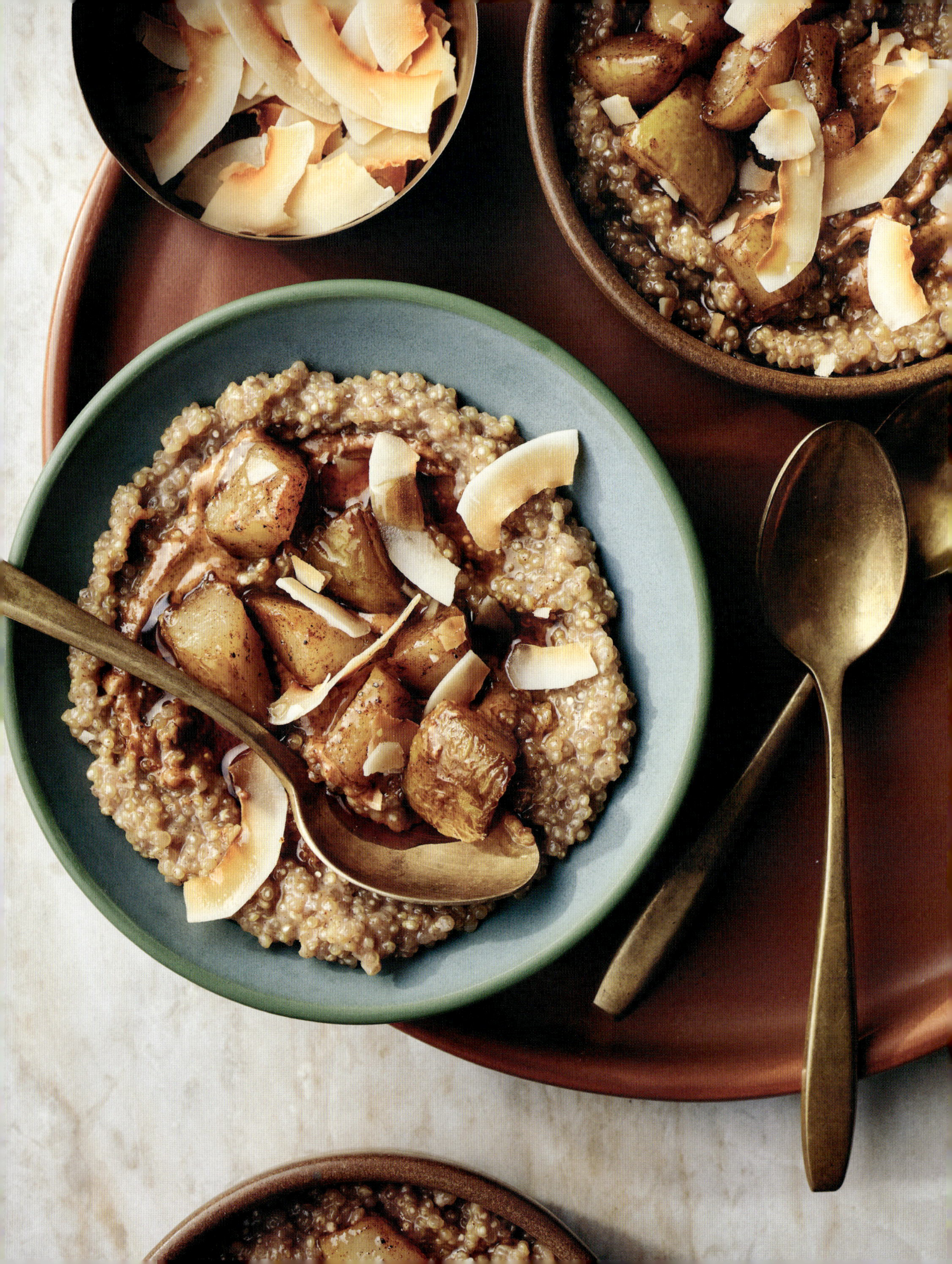

Creamy Quinoa Porridge + Cardamom-Spiced Pears

PREP: 10 MINUTES COOK: 15 MINUTES SERVES 2

A friend of mine once described this recipe as a warm hug in a bowl, and I couldn't agree more. It's truly such a cozy, nourishing breakfast and one I crave often during my luteal phase. I love that it satisfies my sweet and carb cravings without wrecking my blood sugar, thanks to hefty doses of quality protein, fat, and dietary fiber. The cardamom spice adds loads of flavor and has been used medicinally for years to help relieve excess gas and bloating.

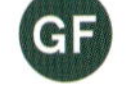

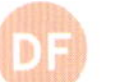

Creamy Quinoa Porridge

- **1 (13.5-ounce) can full-fat unsweetened coconut milk (or 1½ cups other nondairy milk of choice)**
- **2 tablespoons pure maple syrup, plus more for topping**
- **1 teaspoon pure vanilla extract**
- **1 teaspoon cinnamon**
- **¼ teaspoon sea salt**
- **1 cup sprouted quinoa**
- **1 to 2 servings protein powder or collagen peptides (optional)**

Cardamom-Spiced Pears

- **2 large pears, cored and chopped into chunks**
- **1 tablespoon water**
- **1 tablespoon unrefined organic coconut oil, grass-fed ghee, or vegan butter**
- **1 tablespoon pure maple syrup**
- **½ teaspoon cardamom**
- **½ teaspoon cinnamon**
- **¼ teaspoon sea salt**

- **Grass-fed ghee or vegan butter (optional)**
- **Creamy nut butter, maple syrup, coconut flakes, or other chopped nuts and seeds, for topping (optional)**

1. *For the porridge:* Combine the coconut milk, maple syrup, vanilla, cinnamon, and salt in a small pot and bring to a boil. Stir in the sprouted quinoa, then reduce to a simmer, cover, and cook for 12 to 15 minutes, until the liquid is mostly absorbed. (**Note:** Cooking instructions may differ based on the type of quinoa, so be sure to check the label first.) Remove from the heat. If you like, stir in the protein powder or collagen peptides.

2. *For the pears:* While the porridge is cooking, heat a medium pot over medium-high heat and add the pears and water. Cover and cook for 5 minutes to let the pears soften. Reduce the heat to medium, remove the lid, and stir in the coconut oil, ghee, or butter. Cook the pears for 3 to 5 minutes, then stir in the maple syrup, cardamom, cinnamon, and salt. Cook for 3 to 5 minutes, until the pears are soft, fragrant, and caramelized.

3. *To serve:* Scoop generous portions of quinoa porridge into two bowls and stir in ghee, if using. Top with the pears, then any toppings of choice: nut butter, maple syrup, coconut flakes, or chopped nuts and seeds.

NOTE: I like to save the leftovers, then add more coconut milk when I reheat the quinoa to replicate that creamy texture, since it will harden in the fridge. The pears also taste amazing in yogurt bowls, over cottage cheese, or with vanilla bean ice cream as a dessert.

LUTEAL PHASE BENEFITS

Rich in fiber • Mood-boosting • Slow cooked for maximum nutrient absorption and digestion

High-Protein Pumpkin-Spice Pancakes

PREP: 10 MINUTES COOK: 15 MINUTES SERVES 4 (MAKES 8–10 PANCAKES)

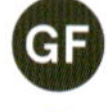
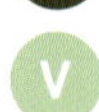
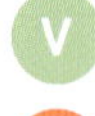

Packed with protein (20 to 30 grams per serving!), these pancakes are the MVPs of keeping blood sugar balanced. This is especially important during your luteal phase, as rising progesterone levels tend to destabilize blood sugar, resulting in many of those dreaded PMS symptoms. Additionally, the oats, egg yolks, and cottage cheese are all rich in B vitamins that support optimal mood and energy levels. If you tend to crave sweet breakfasts and struggle with PMS, I highly recommend giving this recipe a go. **PRO TIP:** Pair with the Maple Turkey Breakfast Sausage on page 129.

- 1½ cups gluten-free rolled oats (I like to use protein or sprouted oats)
- 1 cup full-fat unsweetened cottage cheese
- ½ cup organic pumpkin puree
- 3 pasture-raised eggs
- 2 tablespoons pure maple syrup
- 1½ teaspoons baking powder
- 1 teaspoon cinnamon
- ½ teaspoon pumpkin spice
- ¼ teaspoon sea salt
- 1 teaspoon pure vanilla extract
- 1 to 2 servings vanilla protein powder or collagen peptides (optional)
- Avocado oil spray, coconut oil, or grass-fed ghee, for the pan
- Dark chocolate chips, blueberries, nut butter, grass-fed ghee or butter, or maple syrup, for mixing in or topping (optional)

1. Add the oats to the blender and mix until they turn into a flour-like consistency. Add the cottage cheese, pumpkin puree, eggs, maple syrup, baking powder, cinnamon, pumpkin spice, salt, vanilla, and protein powder (if using) to the blender, making sure to scrape up any flour stuck to the bottom or sides so that it mixes well, then blend until the mixture is smooth.

2. Heat a large skillet over medium-low heat, then grease evenly with avocado oil spray, coconut oil, or ghee. When the skillet is hot, add batter in ¼-cup portions, leaving a bit of space between each pancake, until the pan is filled but not overcrowded, and sprinkle with any desired mix-ins. Cook until bubbles appear on top, 2 to 3 minutes, then flip with a spatula and cook until both sides are golden brown, 1 to 2 more minutes. Transfer the pancakes to a plate, then continue the process to cook all the batter. Serve with toppings of choice.

NOTE: You can store the batter in the fridge for 3 to 4 days to make a super quick and convenient fresh batch of pancakes every morning. Store leftover cooked pancakes in the freezer for up to 2 months and defrost as needed.

LUTEAL PHASE BENEFITS

Rich in fiber • Mood-boosting • High in B vitamins • Supports progesterone production

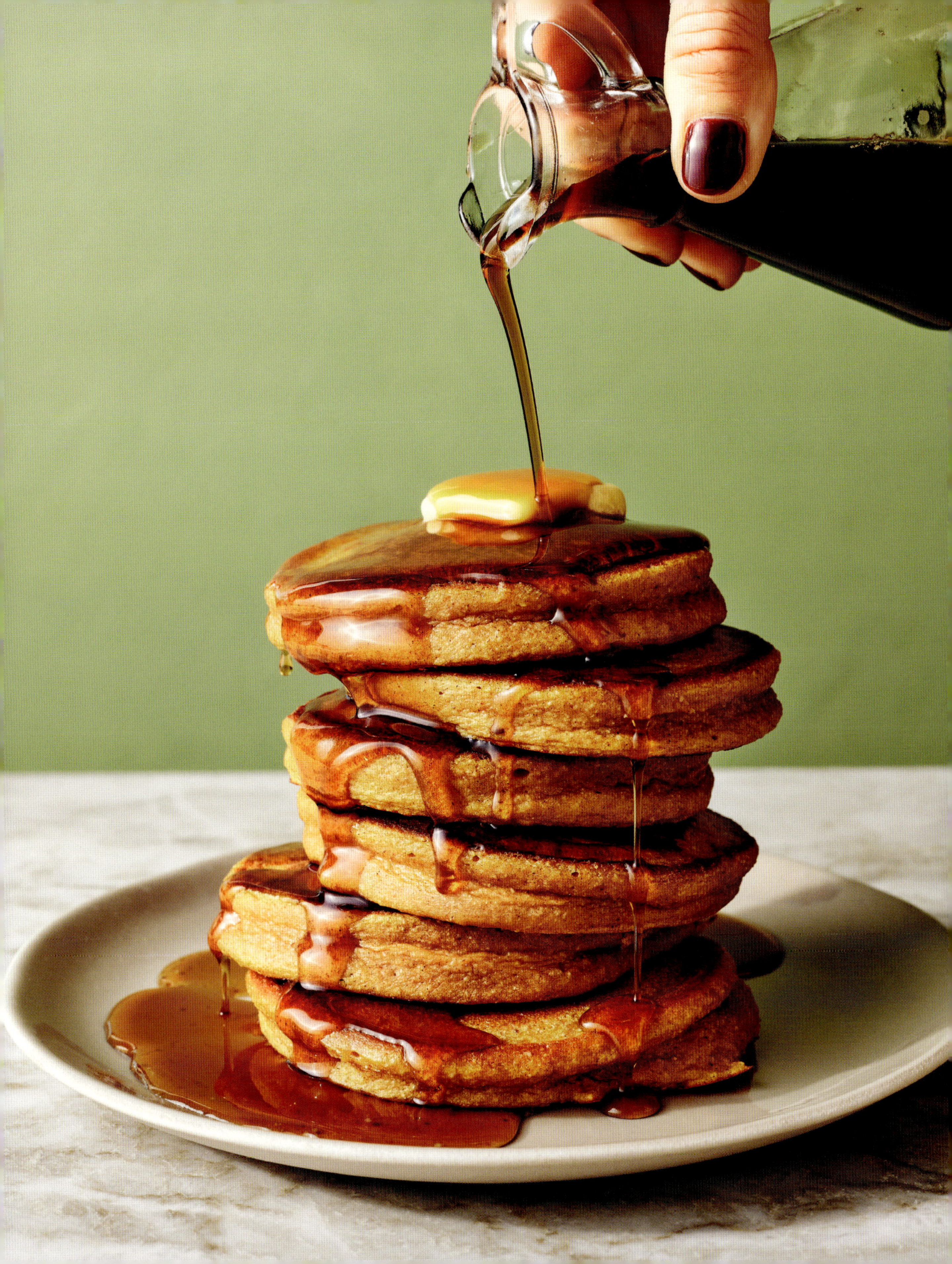

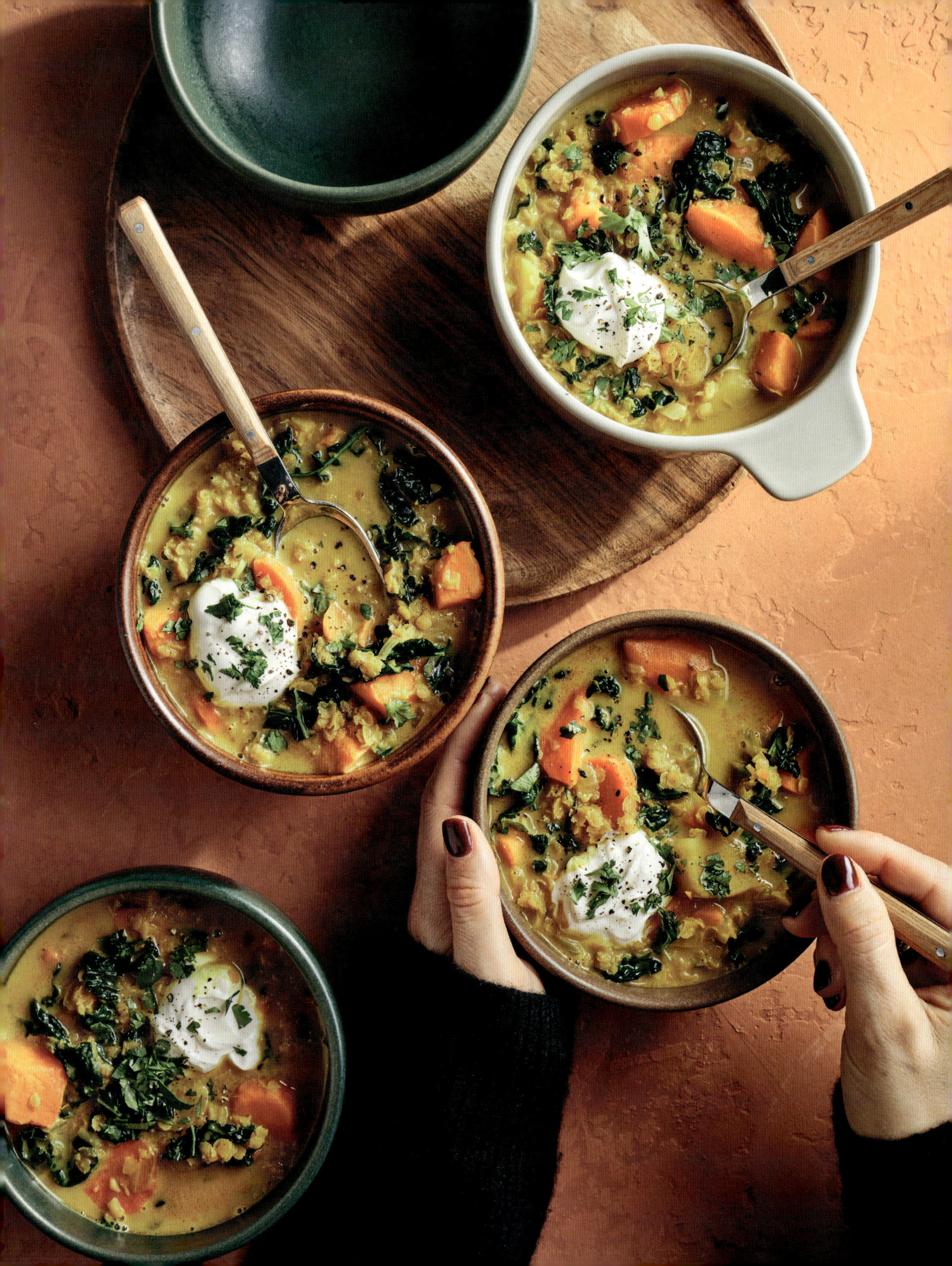

Curried Coconut Lentil and Sweet Potato Soup

PREP: 10 MINUTES COOK: 25 MINUTES SERVES 4–6

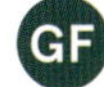

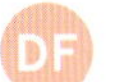

BF

This cozy bowl of soup is packed with plant protein and is incredibly filling. It's warm and well cooked, helping with digestion and nutrient extraction, as well as loaded with fiber that helps to speed up transit time. The spices are anti-inflammatory and add lots of earthy, complex flavors to an otherwise simple dish. I especially enjoy this as leftovers for a quick and satisfying weekday lunch.

- **2 tablespoons unrefined organic coconut oil**
- **1 medium yellow onion, diced**
- **2 medium sweet potatoes, peeled and cut into 1-inch chunks**
- **2 large carrots, peeled and sliced into rounds**
- **1 tablespoon minced fresh ginger**
- **4 cloves garlic, minced**
- **1 teaspoon coriander**
- **1 teaspoon cumin**
- **1 teaspoon ground turmeric**
- **1 teaspoon smoked paprika**
- **½ teaspoon cinnamon**
- **¼ teaspoon cardamom**
- **1 teaspoon sea salt, plus more for serving**
- **Black pepper to taste**
- **1 cup red lentils, rinsed and drained**
- **4 cups bone broth (try using the Super Simple Homemade Bone Broth recipe on page 109)**
- **1 (13.5-ounce) can full-fat unsweetened coconut milk**
- **1 small bunch lacinato kale, leaves torn from stems, then rinsed and chopped**
- **Coconut yogurt (or full-fat Greek yogurt) and cilantro leaves for topping (optional)**

1. Melt the coconut oil in a large pot over medium heat. Add the onion and cook until translucent, 3 to 5 minutes. Add the sweet potatoes and carrots and cook, stirring frequently, until softened, about 5 minutes. Add the ginger, garlic, coriander, cumin, turmeric, paprika, cinnamon, cardamom, salt, and pepper. Stir again, making sure to coat all the vegetables, and cook for 1 minute longer, until fragrant.

2. Stir in the lentils and bone broth and bring the mixture to a boil. Reduce to a simmer and cook until the lentils are fully cooked and the vegetables are tender, 15 to 20 minutes.

3. Stir in the coconut milk and kale and simmer for 5 more minutes, until the kale is just cooked through. Remove from the heat and season with more salt and pepper. Top with coconut yogurt or Greek yogurt and cilantro if you like.

LUTEAL PHASE BENEFITS

Rich in fiber • Mood-boosting • Anti-inflammatory • Rich in magnesium • Supports progesterone production

Rustic Split Pea Soup + Crispy Bacon

PREP: 10 MINUTES   COOK: 1 HOUR AND 20 MINUTES   SERVES 6–8

GF
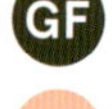
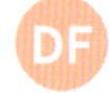

BF

This soup takes me back to childhood, as my mom would often make it for us. She convinced us to eat it by calling it "magic green goblin soup," and now I do the exact same thing for my daughters. The split peas provide that green hue, as well as packing in B vitamins and dietary fiber (16 grams per cup!), which helps speed up digestion and combat bloat. The fresh herbs and crispy bacon impart loads of flavor, and the root vegetables make it feel extra hearty. **PRO TIP:** Serve with buttery toasted GF bread or grilled cheese to make it feel extra special and nostalgic.

- 1 (8-ounce) package uncured organic bacon (look for a brand with no added sugar, nitrates, or MSG), diced
- 1 small yellow onion, diced
- 1 leek, white part only, sliced into thin rounds (or 1 sliced shallot)
- 3 large carrots, peeled and sliced into thin rounds
- 4 cloves garlic, minced
- 1 teaspoon sea salt
- Black pepper to taste
- 1 pound dried green split peas, rinsed and drained
- 6 to 8 cups chicken or beef bone broth (use 7 or 8 cups if you prefer a thinner texture) (try using the Super Simple Homemade Bone Broth on page 109)
- 2 bay leaves
- 1 tablespoon minced fresh thyme or 1 teaspoon dried thyme
- 1 large sweet potato, peeled and diced (about 2 cups)
- Red chile flakes to taste (optional)
- Grated Parmesan and more fresh thyme or flat-leaf parsley, for topping (optional)

1. Cook the bacon in a large pot or Dutch oven over medium heat, stirring occasionally, until crisped up, 7 to 10 minutes. Transfer the bacon with a slotted spoon to a paper towel–lined plate and pat off excess grease. Set aside.

2. Add the onion, leek, and carrots to the pot with the bacon grease and cook until softened, 8 to 10 minutes. Add the garlic, salt, and pepper and cook for another minute. Stir in the split peas, bone broth, bay leaves, and thyme and bring to a boil. Reduce the heat to low, cover, and simmer, stirring occasionally for 30 minutes. Add the sweet potatoes and simmer until they are tender and the split peas are fully cooked, another 20 to 30 minutes.

3. Stir in the bacon and simmer until heated through, 2 to 3 more minutes. Discard the bay leaves and season with additional salt and pepper, and chile flakes if needed.

4. Ladle into large bowls and top with optional Parmesan and thyme or parsley to serve.

NOTE: This soup is thick, and the split peas will continue to absorb some of the liquid overnight, so if you prefer a thinner texture, you may need to add more broth or some water, both when cooking and reheating leftovers.

LUTEAL PHASE BENEFITS

Rich in fiber • Mood-boosting • Rich in magnesium • Supports progesterone production

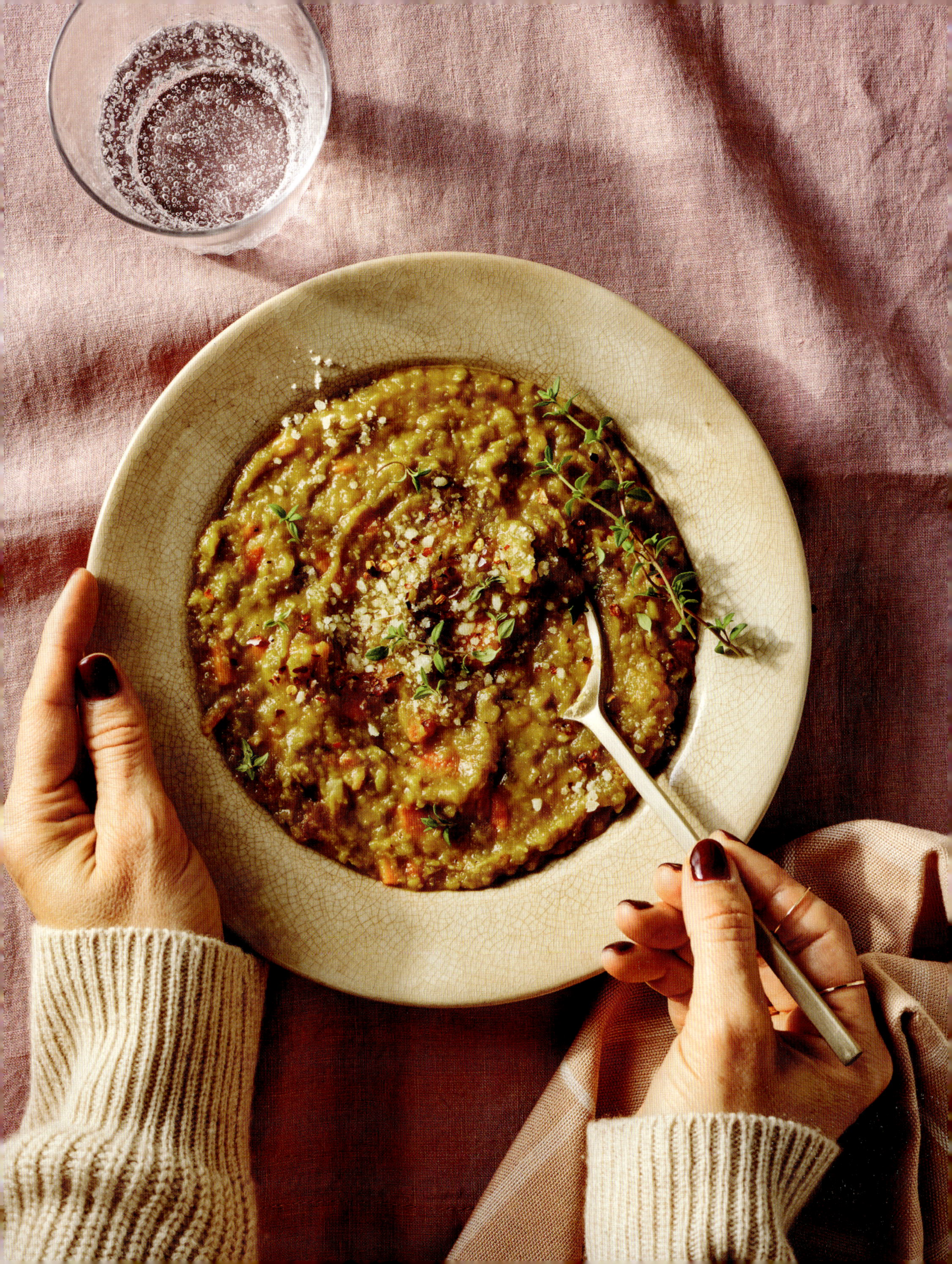

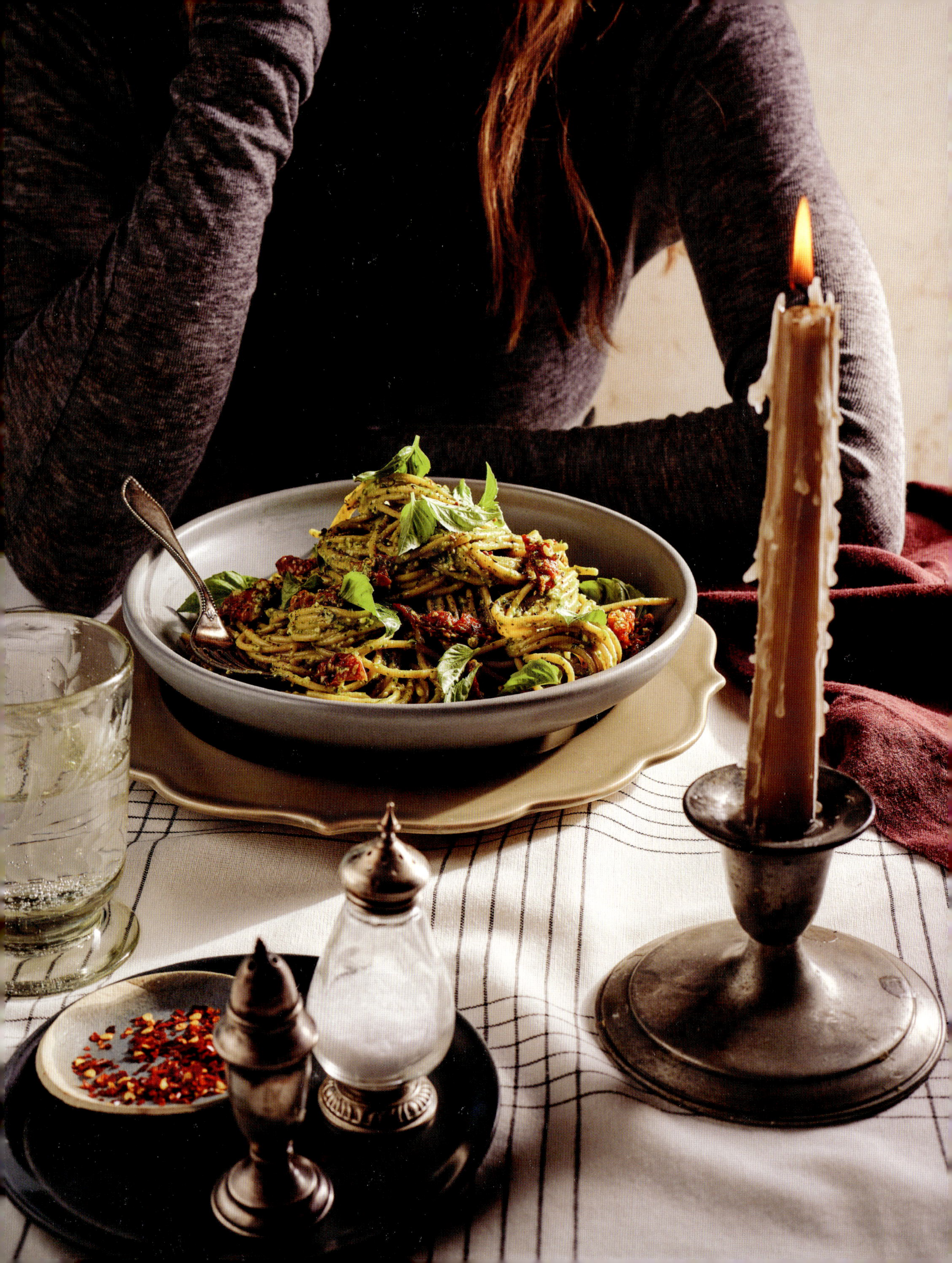

Creamy Cashew-Pesto Protein Pasta

PREP TIME: 10 MINUTES   COOK: 15 MINUTES   SERVES 4

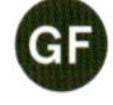

There's nothing quite as satisfying as pasta when the pre-period cravings hit, but it's also important to focus on complex, slow-carb options that are rich in vitamins and minerals—which is why I opt for legume pasta in this dish. It's rich not only in dietary fiber, but blood sugar–stabilizing protein (13 grams per serving) to boot, helping to prevent mood swings, crashes, and other symptoms related to PMS. The cashew pesto provides a dose of healthy, satiating fats and serious flavor. The optional rotisserie chicken or smoked salmon provides an additional protein boost.

Cashew Pesto

- **2 cups fresh basil leaves**
- **¼ cup arugula**
- **½ cup raw organic cashews**
- **Grated zest and juice of 1 lemon**
- **1 tablespoon nutritional yeast (or grated Parmesan)**
- **2 cloves garlic, minced**
- **1 teaspoon sea salt**
- **Black pepper to taste**
- **½ cup extra virgin olive oil**
- **½ teaspoon red pepper flakes (optional)**

Pasta

- **1 (8-ounce) package chickpea, lentil, or other high-protein legume pasta**
- **½ cup sun-dried tomatoes, oil drained**
- **2 tablespoons fresh basil leaves, torn**
- **2 tablespoons melted grass-fed ghee or butter**
- **Smoked salmon, shredded rotisserie chicken, grated Parmesan, or other protein of choice for topping (optional)**

1. Bring a large pot of salted water to a boil.
2. *For the pesto:* While water is heating, combine all the pesto ingredients in a food processor and mix until creamy and well combined; set aside.
3. Cook the pasta in the boiling water according to package instructions. Drain. Toss the drained pasta with the pesto, sun-dried tomatoes, basil, and ghee or butter. Add protein or toppings of choice.

NOTE: This recipe makes a large batch, but leftovers hold up well. Just store in an airtight container in the fridge for up to 3 days. I sometimes have extra pesto, which I'll keep in the fridge for up to a week and use on toast or with eggs, bowls, etc.

LUTEAL PHASE BENEFITS

Rich in fiber • Mood-boosting • Rich in magnesium • Supports progesterone production

Roasted Cauliflower Shawarma Bowls + Herby Green Tahini Sauce

PREP: 10 MINUTES COOK: 30 MINUTES SERVES 4

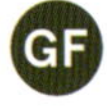
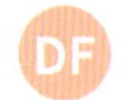

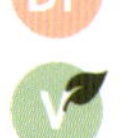

This bowl is packed with Middle Eastern flavors thanks to the earthy and smoky shawarma spice blend (rich in anti-inflammatory and digestive-boosting properties) and herby, creamy tahini sauce (high in gamma-linolenic acid, which naturally supports progesterone production). While this is a vegetarian dish, it contains plenty of plant protein thanks to the chickpeas and quinoa, making it quite filling. However, it also tastes amazing topped with grilled chicken or the spiced lamb from my Loaded Spiced-Lamb Hummus Bowls (page 264).

- 1 head cauliflower, florets chopped (roughly 3 cups)
- 1 (15-ounce) can organic chickpeas, rinsed and drained
- 2 to 4 tablespoons avocado oil
- Shawarma spice blend: ½ teaspoon each ground turmeric, coriander, cumin, paprika, garlic powder, and sea salt (or use a premixed brand)
- 2 cloves garlic, minced
- 1 cup quinoa
- 1¼ cups water or bone broth

Herby Green Tahini Sauce

- ¼ cup organic tahini
- ¼ cup extra virgin olive oil
- ¼ cup filtered water
- ½ cup fresh cilantro leaves
- ½ cup fresh flat-leaf parsley leaves
- Juice of 1 lime (about 2 tablespoons)
- 1 tablespoon raw honey
- 2 cloves garlic, minced
- ½ teaspoon sea salt
- Black pepper to taste

- 2 Persian cucumbers, chopped
- 1 cup cherry tomatoes, halved
- Chopped fresh parsley and cilantro, sesame seeds, and feta cheese, for topping (optional)

1. Preheat the oven to 425°F and line a large baking sheet with parchment paper.

2. Add the chopped cauliflower and chickpeas to the baking sheet and coat evenly with the avocado oil, spice mix, and minced garlic, using your hands to ensure they're evenly mixed. Roast for 25 to 30 minutes, flipping halfway through, until the cauliflower is crispy and golden brown with a slight char to the edges.

3. Cook the quinoa according to package instructions (typically simmered in 1¼ cups liquid for 15 minutes), with the option to use bone broth for the liquid (this adds flavor and nutrients!).

4. *For the tahini sauce:* Combine all the ingredients in a high-speed blender and mix until smooth and creamy.

5. Add the quinoa to the base of each bowl, followed by the roasted chickpeas and cauliflower. Drizzle the green tahini over the bowls and top with chopped cucumbers, tomatoes, and optional toppings.

NOTE: This dish also tastes delicious as a wrap, in which case you can skip the quinoa and add all the other components to a gluten-free wrap or pita.

LUTEAL PHASE BENEFITS

Rich in fiber • Mood-boosting • Anti-inflammatory • Rich in magnesium • Supports progesterone production

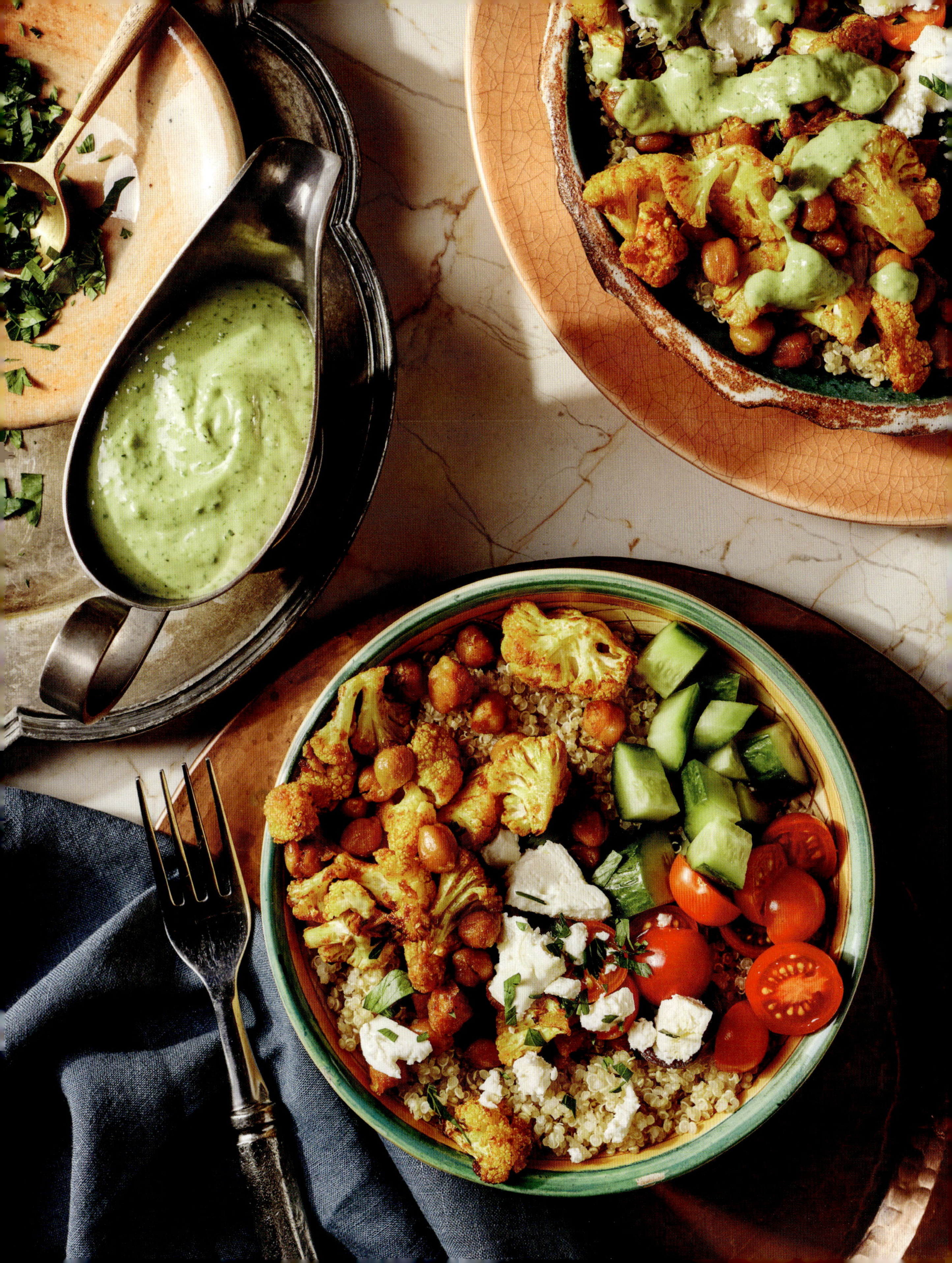

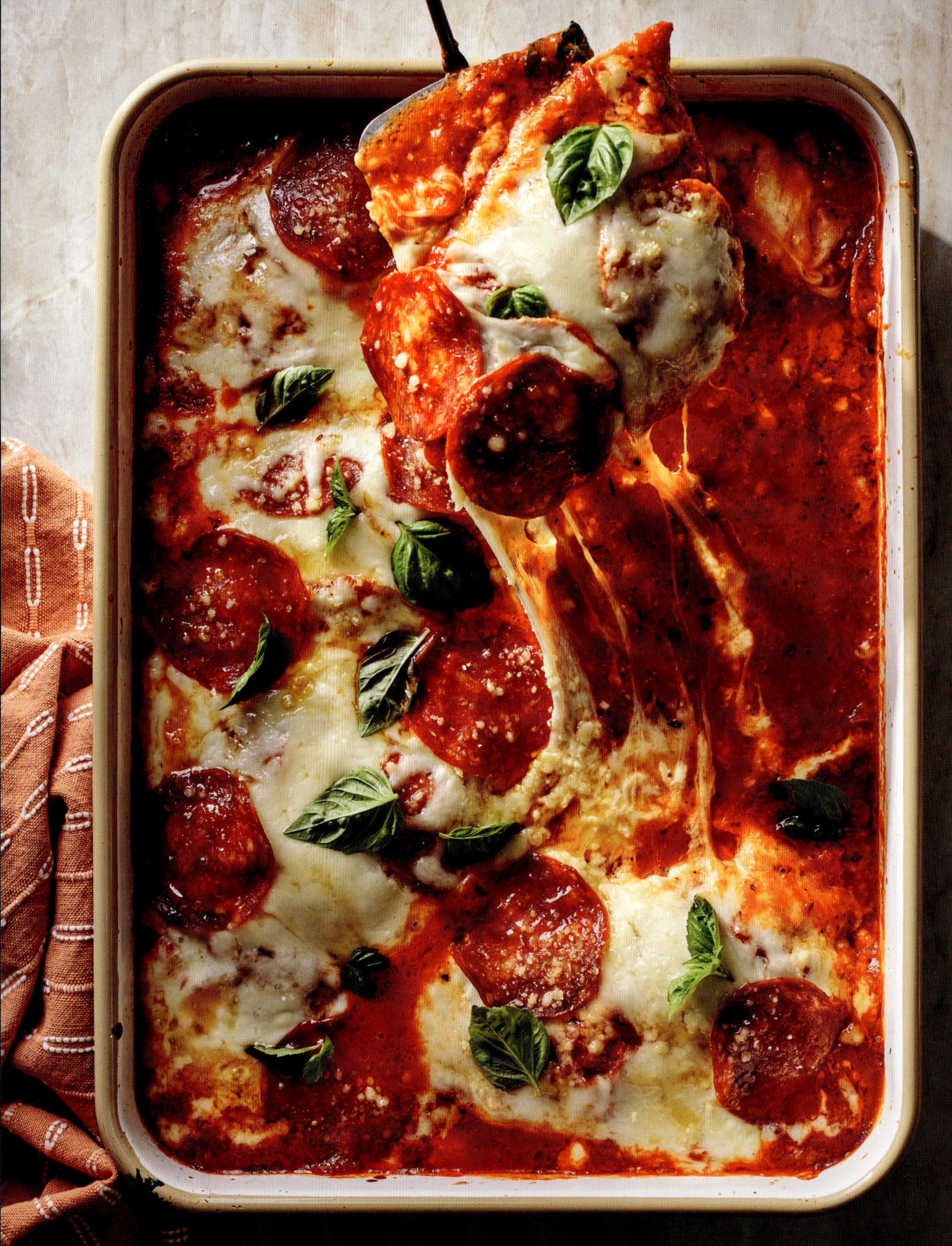

Crustless Chicken Pizza Bake + Hot Honey with Basil

PREP: 10 MINUTES COOK: 30 MINUTES SERVES 4–6

This is my go-to when I'm craving all the flavors of pizza (right before my period—always) but want something high in protein that leaves me feeling satisfied, not sluggish. It's easy to make, requires only one pan, and tastes cheesy and super delicious. While it's not traditional pizza, it's kind of the next best thing? The kiddos love it too, sans the hot honey.

GF
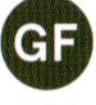
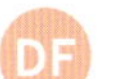

- Avocado oil spray
- 1 (32-ounce) jar marinara, divided
- 1 pound organic skinless boneless chicken breasts, sliced in half widthwise
- 2 tablespoons olive oil or avocado oil
- 1 tablespoon Italian seasoning
- 2 teaspoons garlic powder
- 1 teaspoon sea salt
- Black pepper to taste
- 8 ounces sliced rounds of whole-milk mozzarella (or a dairy-free version)
- ½ cup organic pepperoni slices, divided
- 1 (16-ounce) package (2 cups) shredded mozzarella or goat cheese (or a dairy-free version)
- 1 cup grated Parmesan (can omit, or use dairy-free version)
- 2 to 4 tablespoons hot honey (or regular honey) for drizzling
- Fresh basil leaves for topping

1. Preheat the oven to 400°F and coat an 11 by 13-inch baking pan with avocado oil spray.

2. Using a spatula, evenly spread half of the marinara on the bottom of the pan. Add the halved chicken breasts in an even layer and drizzle with the oil. Evenly sprinkle with the Italian seasoning, garlic powder, salt, and pepper. Pour the rest of the marinara evenly over the chicken, then add the mozzarella rounds in an even layer. Top with half of the pepperoni slices, then sprinkle the shredded mozzarella over everything. Top with the Parmesan, then the remainder of the pepperoni. Bake for 25 to 30 minutes, until the thickest parts of the chicken register 165°F. Let cool for 5 minutes.

3. Drizzle the chicken with the honey and top with fresh basil before serving.

NOTE: If dairy tends to cause digestive stress for you, try cashew or shredded goat mozzarella or another nondairy cheese made with minimal ingredients. There are plenty of options out there that taste delicious in this dish.

LUTEAL PHASE BENEFIT

High in B vitamins • Slow cooked for maximum nutrient absorption and digestion

Fish en Papillote (Cod in Parchment Paper)

PREP: 10 MINUTES COOK: 20 MINUTES SERVES 4

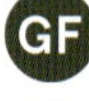

GF

P

Don't let this French cooking method intimidate you—it's honestly one of the easiest and *best* ways to cook white fish (which can dry out easily). Using homemade parchment packets creates a seal that keeps the steam in while the veggies and fish cook, infusing all of the delicious flavors of the herby sauce into the cod and fingerlings and resulting in tender potatoes and perfectly flaky and moist fillets. I love to make this recipe in the first few days of my luteal phase, as it's a bit on the lighter side but still super nourishing and loaded with B vitamins to support progesterone production and omega-3 fatty acids that combat inflammation, both of which are helpful in reducing PMS.

- **1 small bunch asparagus, ends trimmed**
- **1 pound (about 2 cups) fingerling potatoes, halved**
- **4 tablespoons extra virgin olive oil, divided**
- **2 tablespoons Dijon mustard**
- **3 tablespoons chopped fresh flat-leaf parsley**
- **2 tablespoons chopped fresh thyme leaves**
- **Grated zest and juice of 1 lemon**
- **½ teaspoon sea salt**
- **Black pepper to taste**
- **2 leeks, white and light green stems, sliced**
- **4 (6-ounce) fillets lingcod (or another white fish like halibut), patted dry**
- **½ cup kalamata olives, pitted (optional)**
- **Lemon wedges, chopped parsley or thyme, and flaky sea salt, for serving (optional)**

1. Preheat the oven to 425°F and set out a large baking sheet along with four large sheets of parchment paper. Bring a large pot of salted water to a boil. Prepare an ice bath by filling a medium bowl with cold water and ice.

2. When the water is boiling, drop in the asparagus and blanch for 30 seconds. With tongs, immediately transfer the spears to the ice bath to chill (this keeps it from overcooking).

3. In the same pot of boiling water, cook the halved fingerling potatoes for 10 minutes, until fork tender. Drain and set aside.

4. While the potatoes are cooking, in a small bowl, whisk together 3 tablespoons of the olive oil with the Dijon, parsley, thyme, lemon zest and juice, and salt and pepper and set the sauce aside.

5. Heat the remaining 1 tablespoon olive oil in a skillet over medium-high heat. Stir in the leeks and sauté until softened, 3 to 5 minutes. Remove from the heat.

6. Fold one sheet of parchment in half (like a book), then open up again. Place one-fourth of the potatoes in the center of the right-hand side of the sheet. Top with a piece of cod, then layer with one-fourth of the leeks. Chop the asparagus spears in half and place one-fourth on top. Top with the olives, if using. Drizzle evenly with one-fourth of the sauce, using your hands to rub it in evenly. Fold the left-hand, top side of the parchment paper over the right. To seal, tightly roll the edges of the parchment together around the fish and vegetables. If you want to create an extra tight seal you can brush oil along the border of the parchment paper on both sides before rolling. Repeat the process to make four parchment packets.

7. Place the packets on the large baking sheet and bake for 15 to 18 minutes, until the cod is opaque and easily flakes with a fork (or registers an internal temperature of 165°F).

8. Use a knife to pierce the center of each packet and open before serving, letting the steam release. Serve with optional lemon wedges, more chopped fresh herbs, and flaky sea salt.

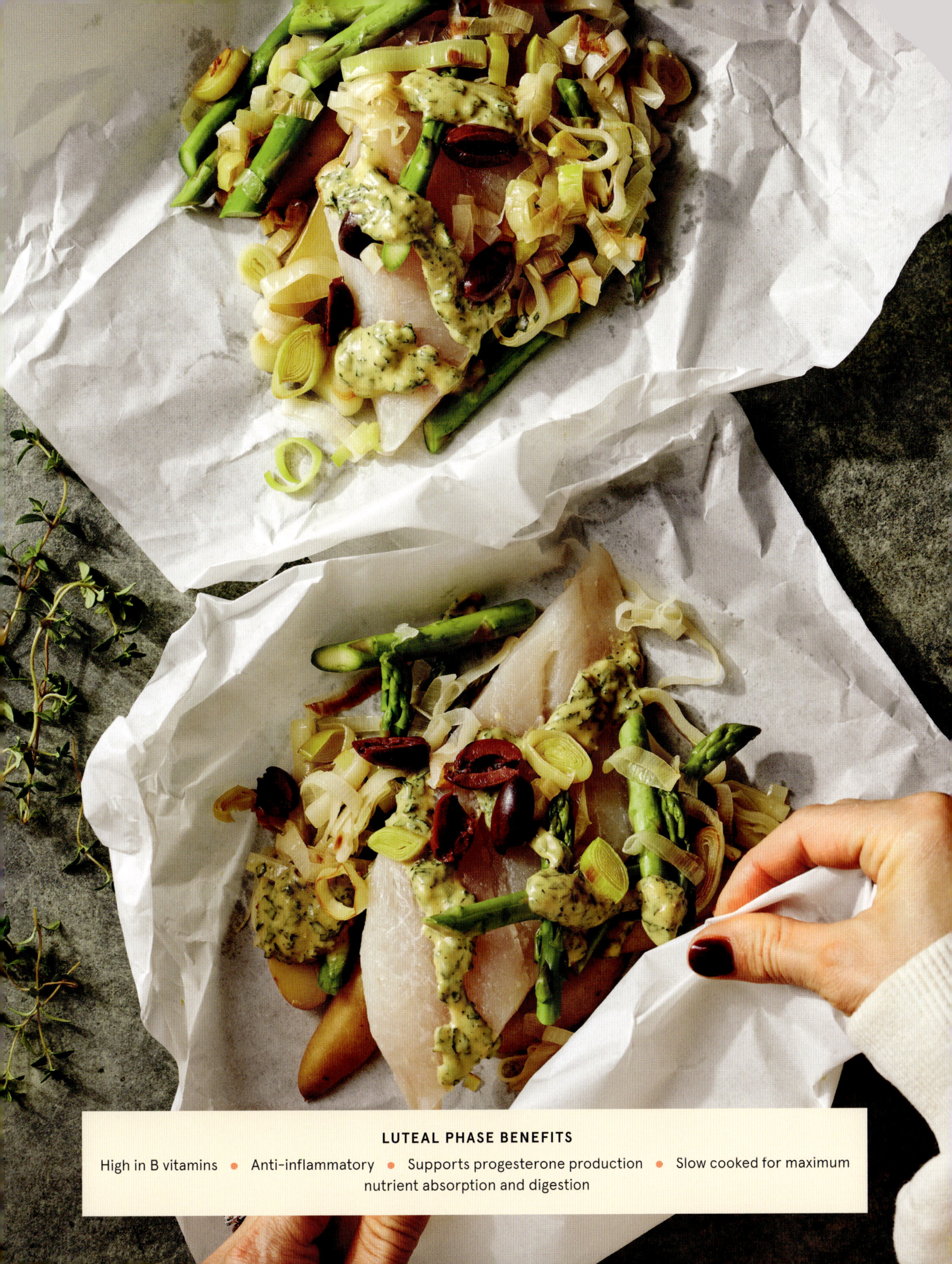

LUTEAL PHASE BENEFITS

High in B vitamins • Anti-inflammatory • Supports progesterone production • Slow cooked for maximum nutrient absorption and digestion

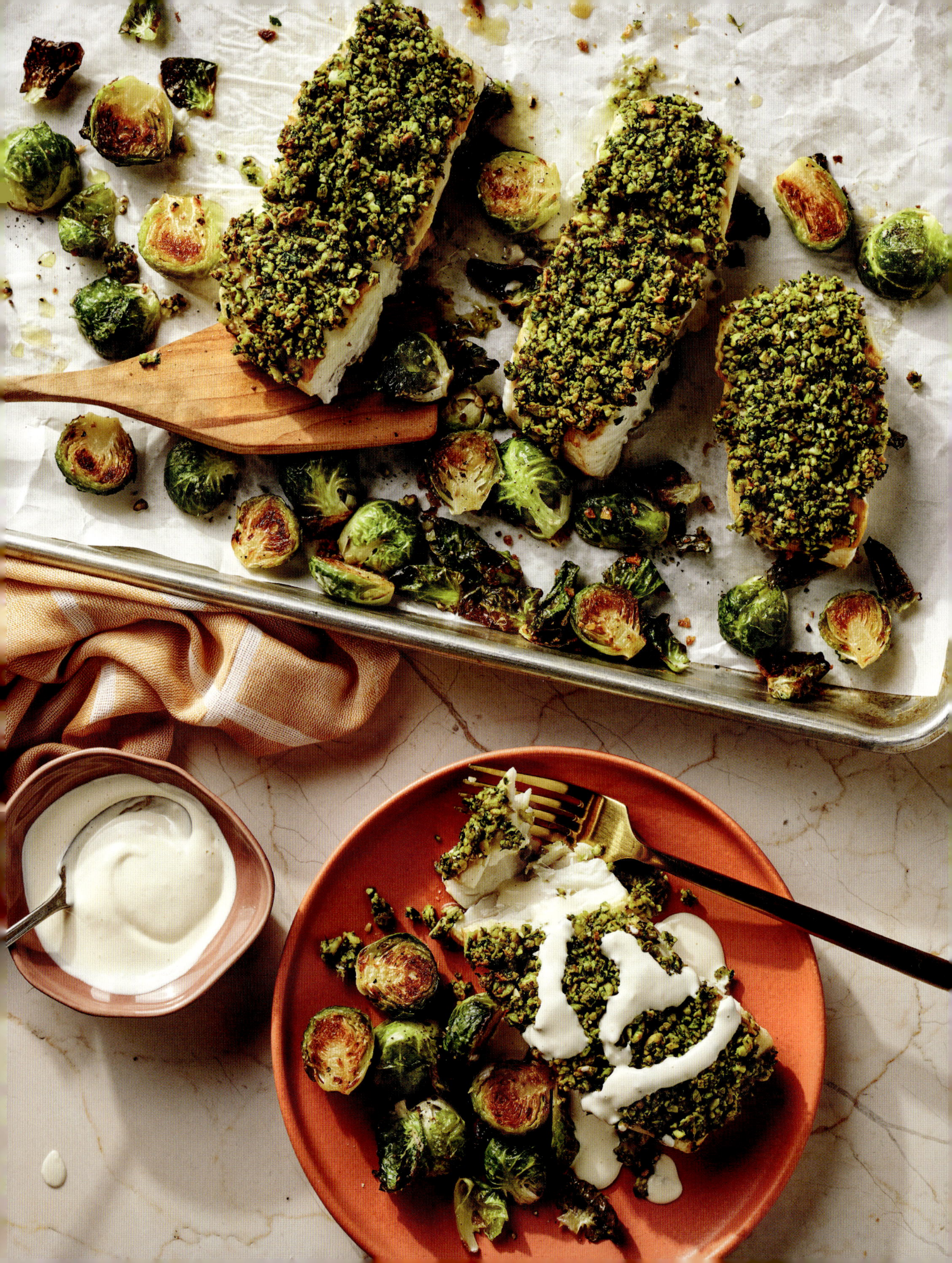

Roasted Pistachio-Crusted Halibut and Brussels Sprouts + Dijon Aioli

PREP: 10 MINUTES COOK: 25 MINUTES SERVES 4

Wild-caught Alaskan halibut is a great source of protein that is also rich in anti-inflammatory omega-3 fatty acids that help to lower prostaglandins, which if too high can lead to cramping and period pain—making halibut an awesome option to include during your luteal phase. The herby pistachio crust adds tons of flavor and crunch to the mild, fatty fillets, the roasted Brussels are the perfect fiber-rich side, and the creamy Dijon aioli is just... [chef's kiss].

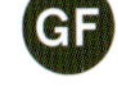

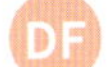

Dijon Aioli

- **¾ cup full-fat unsweetened Greek yogurt (or coconut yogurt)**
- **¼ cup avocado oil mayonnaise (or organic sour cream)**
- **1 tablespoon Dijon mustard**
- **Juice of 1 small lemon (1 to 2 tablespoons)**
- **2 cloves garlic, minced**
- **1 teaspoon sea salt**

Pistachio-Crusted Halibut and Brussels Sprouts

- **2 cups (about 1 pound) Brussels sprouts, ends trimmed and cut in half**
- **2 tablespoons avocado oil**
- **4 cloves garlic, minced**
- **Sea salt and black pepper to taste**
- **½ cup shelled pistachios**
- **½ cup chopped fresh flat-leaf parsley**
- **1 tablespoon grated lemon zest**
- **⅓ cup Dijon mustard**
- **4 (6-ounce) fillets wild Alaskan halibut (or another white fish like cod)**

1. Preheat the oven to 400°F and line a large baking sheet with parchment paper.

2. *For the aioli:* Whisk together all the ingredients in a small bowl and place in the fridge until ready to serve.

3. *For the halibut and Brussels:* Toss the Brussels sprouts with the avocado oil, half of the garlic, the salt, and black pepper and spread on the prepared baking sheet. Slide in the oven and roast for 15 minutes.

4. Meanwhile, combine the remaining garlic, the pistachios, parsley, lemon zest, and ½ teaspoon salt in a food processor and pulse until the mixture has the consistency of breadcrumbs, 5 to 10 pulses. Smother each halibut piece generously with Dijon mustard and press on a layer of the pistachio coating.

5. Once the Brussels sprouts have roasted for 15 minutes, remove the pan from the oven and push the sprouts to one side. Using a spatula, carefully transfer the coated halibut pieces to the other side of the pan. Return the baking sheet to the oven and roast for about 10 minutes, until the crust is crispy, and the fish reaches an internal temperature of 145°F.

6. Serve immediately, drizzling the fish and Brussels sprouts with the aioli.

NOTE: Cooking time for the fish will vary based on thickness: the thicker the fillet, the longer it will have to cook. Having a meat thermometer on hand will help you cook the fish to perfection!

LUTEAL PHASE BENEFITS

Rich in fiber • High in B vitamins • Anti-inflammatory • Rich in magnesium

Crispy Chicken Tenders and Root Veggie Fries + Honey Mustard

PREP: 15 MINUTES   COOK: 30 MINUTES   SERVES 4–6

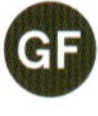
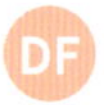
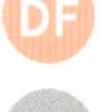

I tend to crave carbohydrate-rich comfort meals right before my period, and this nostalgic recipe hits the spot every time. The chicken is rich in protein and progesterone-boosting B vitamins, not to mention that it is seriously crispy and delicious. But I'm also partial to the fries, which contain those slow-burning, mood-boosting complex carbs, and are oh-so-satisfying when dipped in the homemade honey mustard sauce. This one is *fun* to eat and a family favorite.

Chicken Tenders and Fries

- **2 large Japanese sweet potatoes, cut into ½-inch-thick matchsticks (resembling a fry shape), or use yams, parsnips, carrots, orange-fleshed sweet potatoes, or a combo**
- **Avocado oil spray**
- **1 teaspoon garlic powder**
- **Sea salt**
- **2 cups finely crushed gluten-free crackers (or 2 cups additional almond flour)**
- **¼ cup almond flour**
- **1 tablespoon smoked paprika**
- **1 tablespoon garlic powder**
- **1 tablespoon onion powder**
- **1 pound organic chicken breasts, pounded to a ¼- to ½-inch thickness**
- **2 to 4 tablespoons avocado oil mayonnaise**

Honey Mustard Dipping Sauce

- **½ cup avocado oil mayonnaise**
- **3 tablespoons raw honey**
- **2 tablespoons Dijon mustard**
- **1 tablespoon yellow mustard**
- **1 tablespoon apple cider vinegar or white vinegar**
- **1 teaspoon smoked paprika**
- **½ teaspoon garlic powder**
- **½ teaspoon onion powder**
- **½ teaspoon sea salt**

1. Preheat the oven to 400°F. Line one large baking sheet (or two smaller baking sheets) with parchment paper.

2. *For the chicken and fries:* Add the sliced sweet potato fries to a medium mixing bowl and spray with avocado oil spray, then sprinkle with the garlic powder and ½ teaspoon salt. Use your hands to mix everything together until the fries are evenly coated. Arrange evenly on half of the baking sheet and bake for 15 minutes.

3. Meanwhile, in a large mixing bowl, combine the crushed crackers (or almond flour), almond flour, paprika, garlic powder, and onion powder. Add ½ teaspoon salt (or 1 teaspoon if you're not using crackers). Whisk until well combined.

4. Cut the flattened chicken breasts in half or thirds, until each resembles a chicken tender shape and size. Use a brush to coat each piece with a thin layer of mayonnaise, then dip in the crumb mixture until well coated.

5. Once the fries have baked for 15 minutes, remove the baking sheet from the oven and turn each fry. Add the chicken tenders to the empty side of the sheet. Return to the oven and bake for 12 to 15 more minutes, flipping the tenders halfway through, until the fries are cooked through and the chicken reaches an internal temperature of 165°F.

6. *For the honey mustard sauce:* While the chicken and fries cook, whisk together all the honey mustard ingredients in a small mixing bowl and set aside.

7. Serve the fries and chicken with the honey mustard for dipping.

NOTE: If you prefer nuggets over tenders, cut the chicken into smaller pieces before coating in the spices and keep an eye on cooking time, as they may be done closer to 12 minutes.

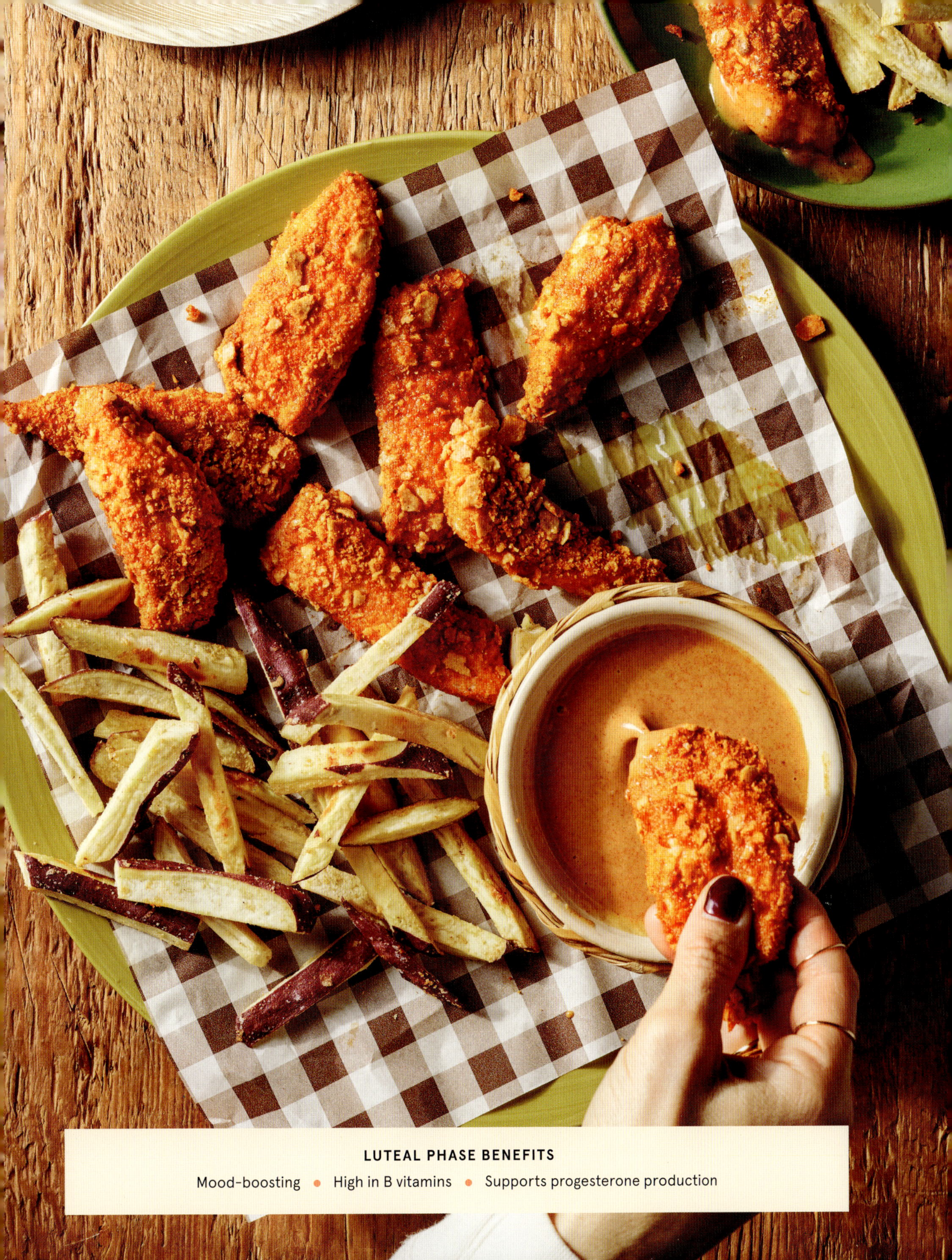

LUTEAL PHASE BENEFITS

Mood-boosting • High in B vitamins • Supports progesterone production

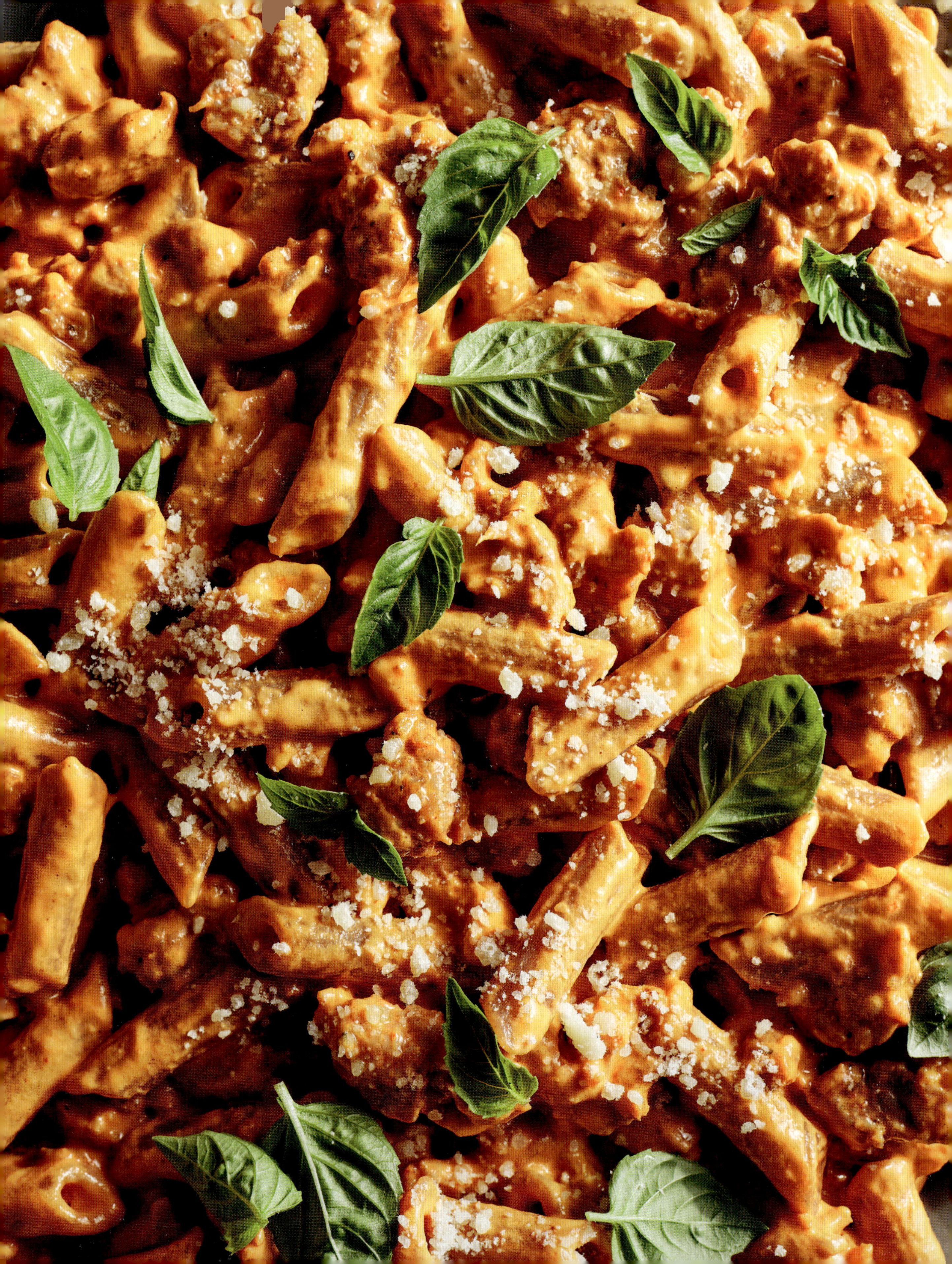

Better-for-You Pasta alla Vodka + Italian Sausage

PREP: 5 MINUTES COOK: 25 MINUTES SERVES 4

This is *the* recipe to make when a pasta craving strikes. While the title might imply a gut bomb (alcohol and carbs and dairy, oh my!), this recipe is naturally gluten-free and dairy-free-friendly (just leave out the Parm). It's also loaded with protein, thanks to the addition of Italian sausage, and the alcohol actually burns off when cooking. Despite all of these things, it's still incredibly rich, creamy, and flavorful—*and* it comes together in 30 minutes! Trust me, it's a luteal phase winner and everyone else will love it too.

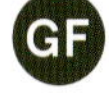

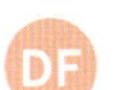

BF

- **1 (12-ounce) box gluten-free penne pasta (try lentil, chickpea, or brown rice pasta)**
- **4 tablespoons grass-fed ghee or avocado oil, divided**
- **1 pound ground Italian chicken sausage, casings removed**
- **1 yellow onion, diced**
- **4 cloves garlic, minced**
- **¼ cup tomato paste**
- **½ to 1 teaspoon Calabrian chili paste (depending on spice tolerance)**
- **¼ cup vodka**
- **1 teaspoon sea salt**
- **1 cup full-fat unsweetened coconut cream (for a very mild sweetness; if you prefer more savory, try another unsweetened nondairy milk like cashew or an organic dairy heavy cream)**
- **1 cup shaved Parmesan, plus more for serving (optional)**
- **¼ cup torn or thinly sliced fresh basil leaves, for serving**

1. Cook the pasta in a large pot of salted boiling water according to package instructions. Drain, *making sure to reserve ½ cup of the pasta water to add to the sauce later.*

2. Heat 1 tablespoon of the ghee or avocado oil in a skillet over medium heat. Add the ground sausage and cook, using a spatula to break up any large chunks and stirring occasionally, until the meat is cooked through, about 15 minutes. Remove from the heat and set aside.

3. Heat 2 tablespoons of the ghee or avocado oil in another skillet over medium heat. Once the pan is coated, add the onion and cook, stirring, for 3 minutes. Add the garlic and cook and stir for about 2 minutes more, until the onion is translucent and the garlic is fragrant. Add the tomato paste and chili paste and stir until everything is mixed. Pour in the vodka and stir for 2 to 3 minutes, scraping bits from the bottom of the skillet. Sprinkle in the salt, then stir in the coconut cream, Parmesan or nondairy substitute (if using), and reserved pasta water. When everything is fully incorporated, transfer to a blender (reserving the skillet) and blend until creamy and smooth.

4. Toss the cooked pasta with the remaining 1 tablespoon ghee or avocado oil to keep it from sticking, then add to the reserved skillet. Use a slotted spoon to scoop the Italian sausage from its pan, tapping off any excess grease or liquid, and add to the pasta. Pour the vodka sauce over the pasta and sausage and toss well to coat. Taste and add additional salt or pepper as needed. Add fresh basil leaves and more Parmesan if desired.

LUTEAL PHASE BENEFITS

High in B vitamins • Rich in fiber • Rich in magnesium • Supports progesterone production

Cozy Autumn Harvest Bowls

PREP: 15 MINUTES   COOK: 45 MINUTES   SERVES 4

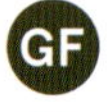

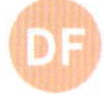

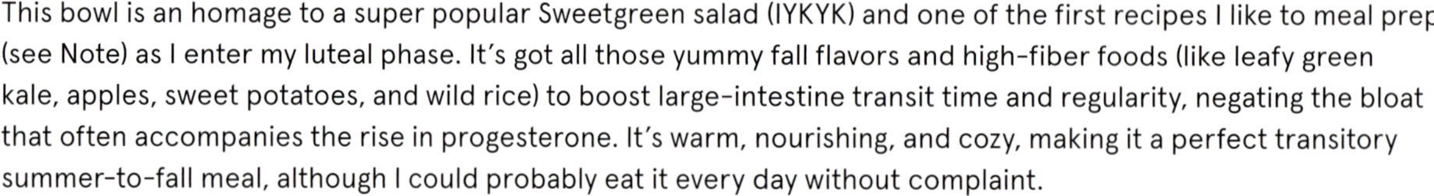

This bowl is an homage to a super popular Sweetgreen salad (IYKYK) and one of the first recipes I like to meal prep (see Note) as I enter my luteal phase. It's got all those yummy fall flavors and high-fiber foods (like leafy green kale, apples, sweet potatoes, and wild rice) to boost large-intestine transit time and regularity, negating the bloat that often accompanies the rise in progesterone. It's warm, nourishing, and cozy, making it a perfect transitory summer-to-fall meal, although I could probably eat it every day without complaint.

Wild Rice

- **1 cup uncooked wild rice**
- **About 1½ cups bone broth (try using the Super Simple Homemade Bone Broth on page 109)**

Sweet Potatoes

- **2 medium sweet potatoes, cut into half-moons**
- **2 tablespoons avocado oil**
- **4 cloves garlic, minced**
- **Sea salt and black pepper to taste**

Maple Pecans

- **1 cup pecans**
- **2 tablespoons pure maple syrup**
- **½ teaspoon sea salt**

Balsamic Dressing

- **¼ cup high-quality aged balsamic vinegar (this really elevates the taste)**
- **2 tablespoons raw honey**
- **2 teaspoons Dijon mustard**
- **2 cloves garlic, minced**
- **½ teaspoon dried thyme**
- **½ teaspoon sea salt**
- **⅓ cup extra virgin olive oil**

- **2 large bunches curly green kale, stemmed, rinsed, and chopped (about 8 cups)**
- **2 large organic chicken breasts, cooked and chopped (or 4 cups cooked rotisserie chicken or leftover Crispy Chicken Tenders, page 252, for crispy chicken)**
- **1 large apple (I like Fuji, Pink Lady, or Honeycrisp), cored and chopped**
- **Crumbled goat cheese, chopped fresh chives, and pomegranate seeds, for topping (optional)**

1. *For the rice:* Cook the wild rice according to package instructions using bone broth (typically 1½ cups) for the liquid. This typically takes 35 to 45 minutes to cook.

2. *For the sweet potatoes:* Preheat the oven to 425°F and line a baking sheet with parchment paper. Place the sweet potatoes on the sheet and toss with the avocado oil, garlic, salt, and pepper. Roast for 25 to 30 minutes, flipping the half-moons halfway through, until soft.

3. *For the pecans:* Heat a small skillet over medium heat. Add the pecans and toast, stirring every so often, for 5 to 10 minutes, until warm and toasted. Pour in the maple syrup and stir quickly, which keeps the syrup from burning and helps the pecans soak up the liquid. Sprinkle with the salt and cook until the mixture becomes sticky, 1 to 2 minutes, then remove from the heat. Use a spatula to transfer the pecans to a sheet of parchment paper to cool.

4. *For the balsamic dressing:* Combine all the ingredients except the olive oil in a small bowl. Whisk until smooth, then slowly drizzle in the olive oil and continue to whisk until well combined.

5. To assemble, massage the kale leaves with your hands to help them tenderize. Layer the kale in serving bowls with the wild rice, sweet potatoes, maple pecans, chicken, and apple. Add any other toppings of choice. Drizzle the balsamic dressing over the tops and toss to combine.

NOTE: This bowl takes a bit of time to prepare because of all the components, but it makes a huge batch. I prefer to meal prep the wild rice, sweet potatoes, maple pecans, balsamic dressing, and massaged kale at the beginning of my luteal phase and store each individually in airtight containers in the fridge for up to 5 days, enabling me to put together a delicious lunch in 5 minutes or less.

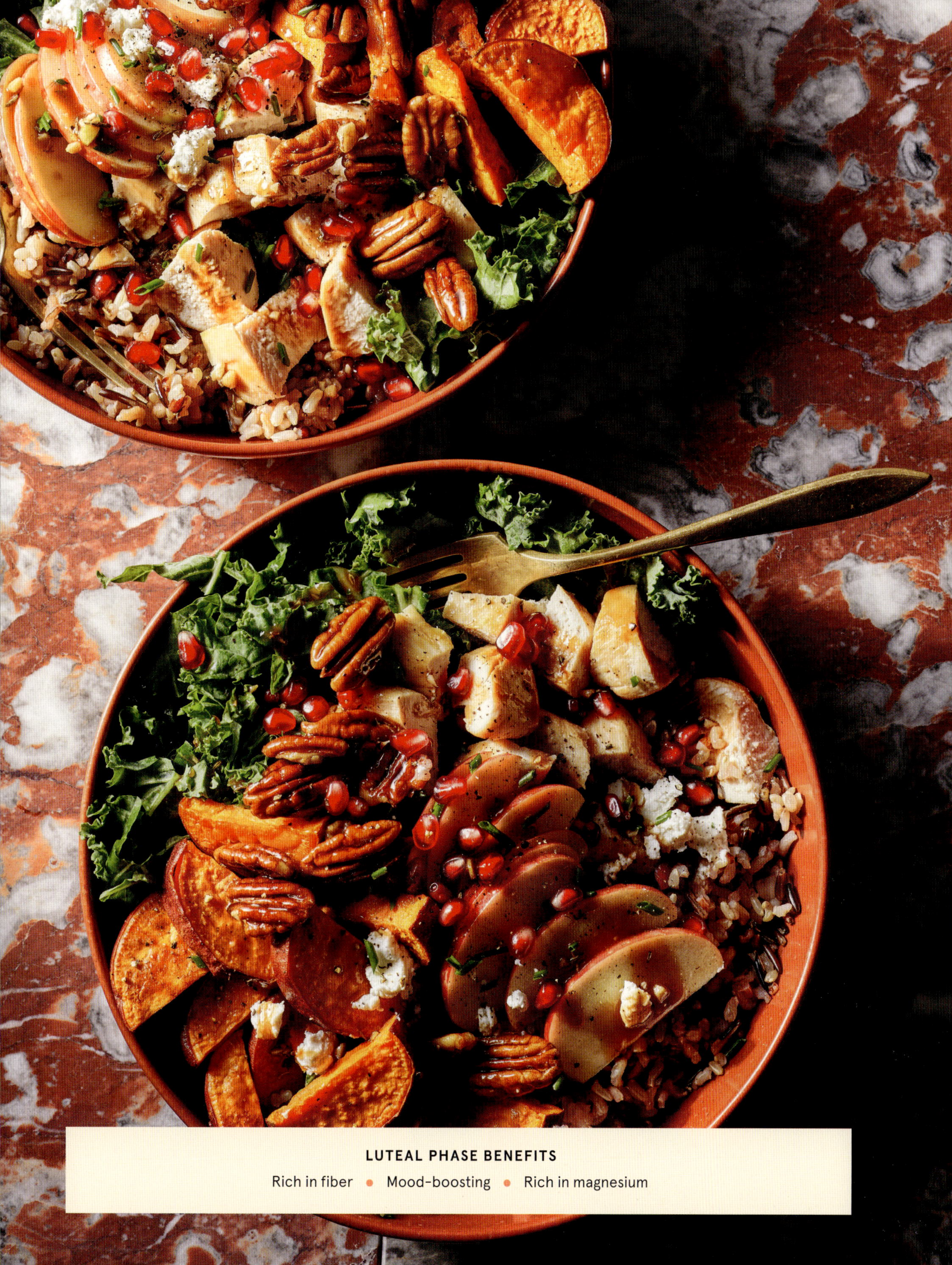
LUTEAL PHASE BENEFITS
Rich in fiber • Mood-boosting • Rich in magnesium

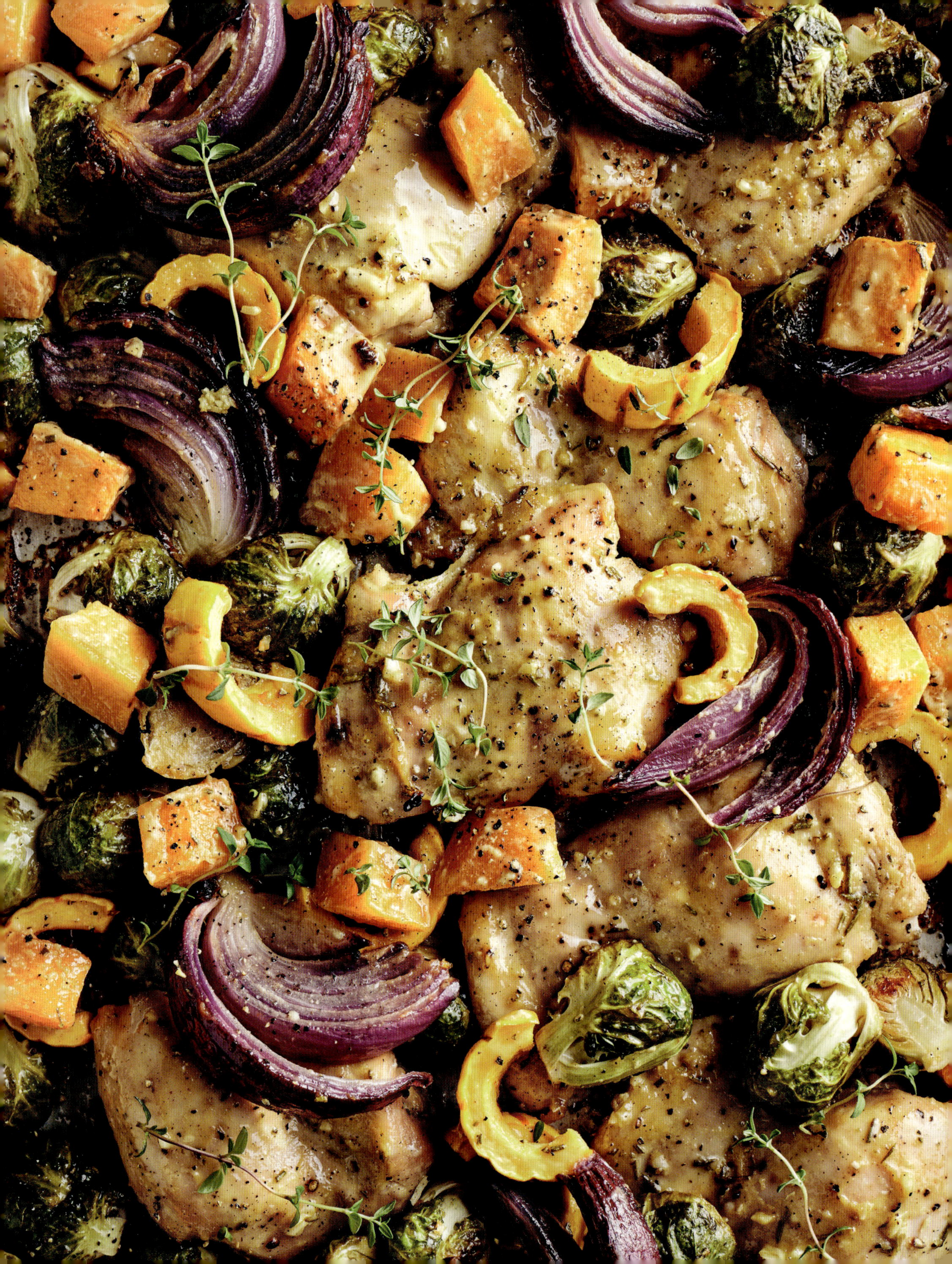

Sheet-Pan Honey-Dijon Chicken + Veggies

PREP: 15 MINUTES COOK: 30 MINUTES SERVES 4–6

This sheet-pan meal packs in a ton of flavor thanks to the honey Dijon sauce and fresh rosemary. I tend to favor fall vegetables, especially when roasted on a baking sheet, as they caramelize and become extra tender on the inside, crispy on the outside, and overall delicious. They're also perfect for the luteal phase, as they're rich in fiber and complex carbohydrates to help curb cravings and give us a little feel-good, mood-regulating boost. Serve as is or over bowls of a hearty gluten-free grain such as brown rice, quinoa, or millet.

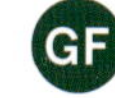

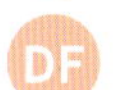

BF

- ⅓ cup Dijon mustard
- ¼ cup avocado oil (or other non-flavored cooking oil)
- ¼ cup raw honey (or pure maple syrup)
- 1 tablespoon apple cider vinegar
- 6 cloves garlic, minced
- 2 tablespoons fresh rosemary needles, chopped
- 1 delicata squash, seeded and cut into half-moons
- 1 small butternut squash, peeled, seeded, and chopped
- 1 small red onion, cut into thick slices
- 1 pound (about 2 cups) Brussels sprouts, ends trimmed and cut in half
- 2 pounds (about 8) skinless boneless organic chicken thighs
- Sea salt and black pepper to taste

1. Preheat the oven to 425°F and line a large baking sheet with parchment paper.
2. In a small bowl, whisk together the Dijon, avocado oil, honey, apple cider vinegar, garlic, and rosemary.
3. Spread the delicata squash, butternut squash, onion, and Brussels sprouts on the pan, then place the chicken thighs in between the vegetables, making sure everything is evenly spaced. Sprinkle the chicken and veggies with salt and pepper, then pour the honey Dijon sauce over everything. Use your hands to evenly spread the mixture all over the chicken and veggies, then sprinkle with additional salt and pepper (you want all sides coated in seasoning and sauce for maximum flavor).
4. Roast for 15 to 20 minutes. Flip the vegetables and chicken and roast for an additional 15 to 20 minutes, until the veggies are fully cooked and tender and the chicken reaches an internal temperature of 165°F.

NOTE: Feel free to swap in other fall seasonal vegetables like cauliflower, kabocha or acorn squash, and yams or Japanese sweet potatoes.

LUTEAL PHASE BENEFITS

Rich in fiber • Mood-boosting • High in B vitamins • Slow cooked for maximum nutrient absorption and digestion

One-Pot Thai Chicken Curry and Rice

PREP: 15 MINUTES COOK: 30 MINUTES SERVES 6–8

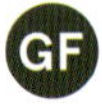
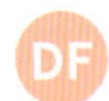

This dish is a crowd pleaser, with a creamy, almost risotto-like texture and good, hearty ingredients. I like to incorporate lots of warming spices into meals during my luteal phase, as they've been used for thousands of years in ancient medicine to combat common PMS symptoms ranging from cramping to indigestion and bloat, and this one-pot meal packs them in thanks to the garlic, ginger, and curry paste. I like using yellow curry paste, which is mild, but if you prefer it spicier try a green or red paste instead.

- 2 tablespoons unrefined organic coconut oil
- 1½ pounds skinless boneless organic chicken thighs, rinsed and patted dry (or use breasts)
- Sea salt and black pepper to taste
- 1 onion, diced
- 4 cloves garlic, minced
- 1 tablespoon minced fresh ginger
- 2 carrots, peeled and sliced into rounds
- 2 red bell peppers, seeded and thinly sliced
- 1 small head broccoli, chopped into florets
- ¼ cup yellow curry paste
- 1 (13.5-ounce) can full-fat organic coconut milk
- 2 cups chicken bone broth (try using the Super Simple Homemade Bone Broth on page 109)
- 2 tablespoons fish sauce
- 2 tablespoons coconut aminos
- 1 tablespoon coconut sugar
- Juice of 1 lime
- 1½ cups jasmine rice, rinsed three times and drained
- Fresh cilantro, coconut yogurt, chopped peanuts, and lime wedges, for topping

1. Heat the coconut oil in a large stockpot or Dutch oven over medium-high heat. Add the chicken thighs, sprinkle generously with salt and pepper, and sear for 3 to 5 minutes, until browned on both sides. Transfer to a plate and set aside.

2. Reduce the heat to medium and add the onion to the pot, cooking until translucent, about 3 minutes. Stir in the garlic, ginger, carrots, bell peppers, and broccoli and season with salt. Cook for 3 minutes, until the veggies become bright and tender. Stir in the curry paste and cook for a minute.

3. Add the coconut milk and bone broth to deglaze the pot, scraping up any bits that have stuck to the bottom. Stir in the fish sauce, coconut aminos, coconut sugar, lime juice, and jasmine rice. Bring the mixture to a boil, then reduce to a simmer. Return the seared chicken thighs to the pot, submerging them halfway. Cover the pot and cook for 20 minutes, or until the chicken reaches an internal temperature of 165°F and the rice is creamy and cooked through.

4. Remove the pot from the heat and let the curry rest for 10 minutes. Serve in a large bowl or individual bowls, topped with cilantro, coconut yogurt, peanuts, and squeezes of lime juice.

LUTEAL PHASE BENEFITS

High in B vitamins • Anti-inflammatory • Slow cooked for maximum nutrient absorption and digestion

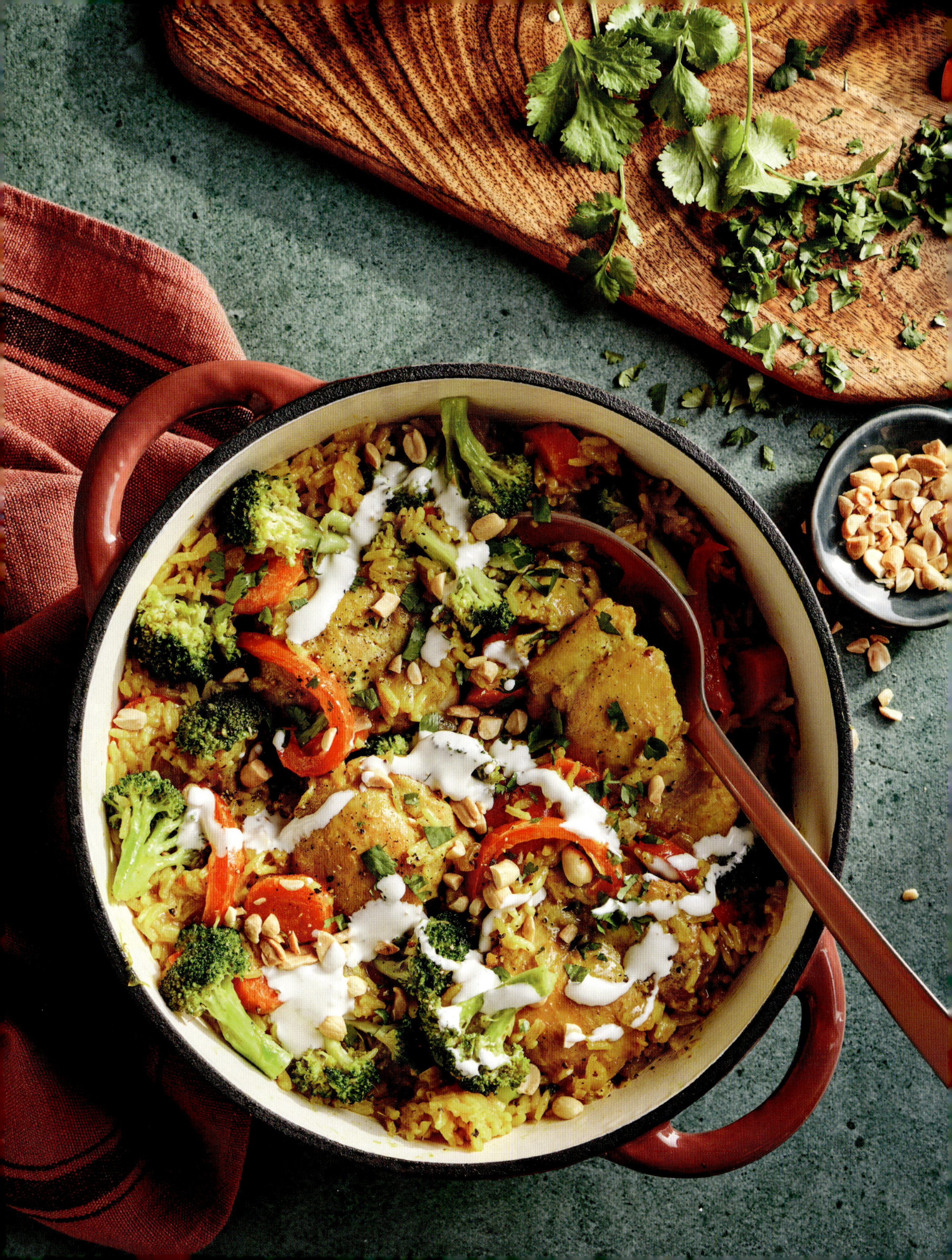

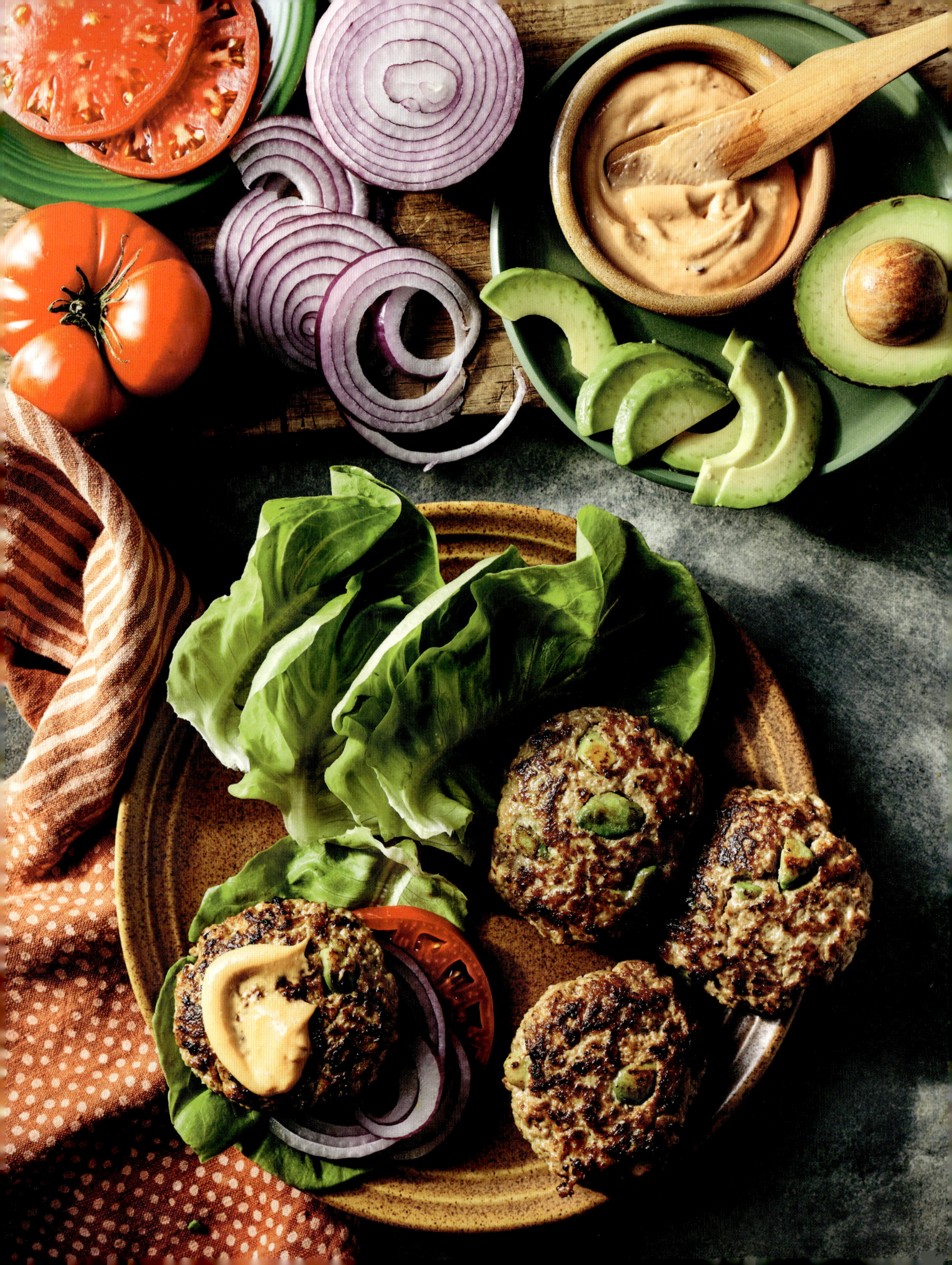

Juicy Avocado Turkey Burgers

PREP: 20 MINUTES COOK: 10 MINUTES SERVES 4–6

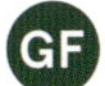

While turkey patties might sound basic, these are anything but, filled with flavor and seriously *so* juicy, thanks in part to the fiber-rich avocado. Ground turkey is also an excellent source of protein, B vitamins, and minerals like selenium that support cell energy and thyroid hormone production, all of which work to mitigate PMS. Try serving these with the Root Veggie Fries (page 252) for a feel-good complex-carb boost and ultra satisfying meal.

Turkey Burgers

- **1½ pounds organic ground turkey**
- **½ large avocado, pitted, peeled, and chopped**
- **3 tablespoons avocado oil mayonnaise**
- **2 teaspoons gluten-free Worcestershire sauce**
- **2 teaspoons sriracha**
- **1 teaspoon cumin**
- **1 teaspoon garlic powder**
- **1 teaspoon sea salt**
- **2 tablespoons avocado oil**

Chipotle Aioli

- **½ cup avocado oil mayonnaise**
- **2 teaspoons chipotle adobo sauce (make sure to use only the sauce in the jar, not the chipotle pepper itself, which might lend too much heat)**
- **½ teaspoon garlic powder**
- **½ teaspoon sea salt**

To Serve

- **Whole bibb or iceberg lettuce leaves, for wrapping**
- **Sliced avocado, sliced tomato, and sliced red onion, for topping**

1. *For the turkey burgers:* Mix the turkey, chopped avocado, mayo, Worcestershire, sriracha, cumin, garlic powder, and salt together in a medium mixing bowl, then form into six to eight medium patties.

2. Heat a large skillet over medium heat and spread the avocado oil evenly in the pan. When the oil is hot, add the patties (you may have to do this in batches depending on the size of the skillet). Cook undisturbed for about 5 minutes, until the patties are halfway cooked through and the bottom sides have browned. Use a spatula to carefully flip each patty and cook undisturbed for another 3 to 5 minutes, until the meat is cooked through and registers an internal temperature of 165°F.

3. *For the chipotle aioli:* While the burgers are cooking, mix all the aioli ingredients together in a small bowl and set aside.

4. *To serve:* Place each patty on a whole lettuce leaf, generously smear with chipotle aioli, and top with avocado slices, tomato, onion, and another lettuce leaf.

NOTE: I prefer ground turkey with dark meat rather than just breast, as the fat helps to keep the burgers intact and the texture less crumbly.

LUTEAL PHASE BENEFITS

Rich in fiber • High in B vitamins • Rich in magnesium

Loaded Spiced-Lamb Hummus Bowls + Pita Chips

PREP: 15 MINUTES COOK: 10 MINUTES SERVES 4

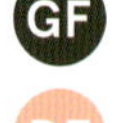
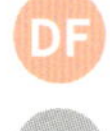
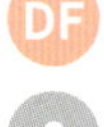
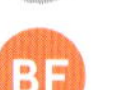

When I first made this dish, my husband exclaimed, "There is no way this is healthy. It's too good," and while his palate was partially correct (it *is* next-level good), the bowls are loaded with fresh ingredients and hormone-healthy nutrients like high-quality protein, amino acids, B vitamins, minerals, and fiber. The homemade hummus is super creamy, and so good you may never go back to store-bought again.

Hummus

- **1 (15-ounce) can organic chickpeas, rinsed and drained**
- **⅓ cup creamy tahini**
- **Juice of 1 large lemon (about 3 tablespoons)**
- **4 cloves garlic, minced**
- **1 teaspoon sea salt**
- **Black pepper to taste**
- **½ to ¾ cup high-quality extra virgin olive oil (this makes a difference with the taste!)**

Spiced Lamb

- **1 tablespoon avocado oil**
- **½ yellow onion, diced**
- **1 pound grass-fed ground lamb (or ground beef or bison)**
- **2 cloves garlic, minced**
- **½ teaspoon smoked paprika**
- **½ teaspoon coriander**
- **½ teaspoon cumin**
- **¼ teaspoon cinnamon**
- **½ teaspoon sea salt**
- **Black pepper to taste**

Cucumber-Tomato Salad

- **1 cup cherry tomatoes, halved**
- **2 Persian cucumbers, chopped**
- **Juice of ½ lemon (1 tablespoon)**
- **¼ cup chopped fresh flat-leaf parsley**
- **2 tablespoons extra virgin olive oil**
- **Sea salt and black pepper to taste**

- **Feta cheese, pine nuts, a drizzle of olive oil, and flaky sea salt, for topping (optional)**
- **Gluten-free pita chips for serving**

1. *For the hummus:* Combine all the ingredients except the olive oil in a food processor and cover. Pulse, drizzling in the olive oil from the top opening and stopping to use a spatula to scrape the sides a couple of times if needed, until the hummus is well mixed, ultra creamy, and smooth. Set aside.

2. *For the lamb:* Heat the avocado oil in a large skillet over medium heat. Add the onion and cook, stirring occasionally, until translucent, 3 to 5 minutes. Stir in the lamb, garlic, paprika, coriander, cumin, cinnamon, salt, and pepper and cook, using a spatula or wooden spoon to break up any large chunks. Turn the heat up to medium-high and continue cooking and stirring until the lamb is cooked through, about 5 minutes.

3. *For the salad:* While the lamb is cooking, combine the tomatoes and cucumbers in a small bowl and mix in the lemon juice, parsley, olive oil, salt, and pepper.

4. *To serve:* Spread the hummus on a large platter (or in individual bowls) and top with the spiced lamb. Spoon the cucumber-tomato salad evenly over the top and sprinkle with optional feta cheese, pine nuts, olive oil, and flaky sea salt. Serve with gluten-free pita chips for scooping.

NOTE: Try swapping out the pita chips for crudités or a gluten-free pita or wrap!

LUTEAL PHASE BENEFITS

Rich in fiber • High in B vitamins • Anti-inflammatory • Rich in magnesium

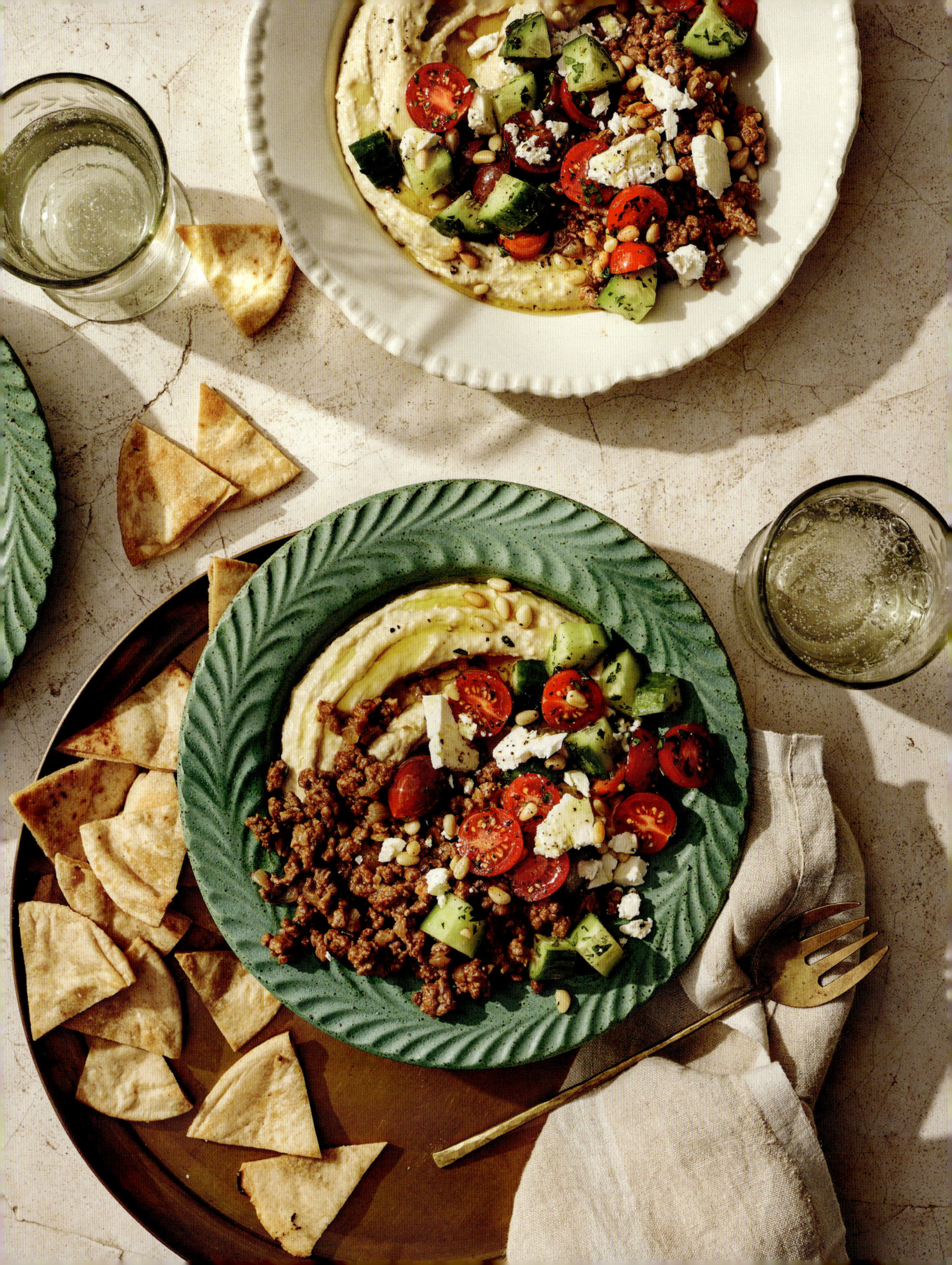

Spaghetti Squash Boats with Meatballs and Marinara

PREP: 10 MINUTES COOK: 45 MINUTES SERVES 4

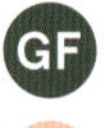
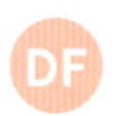
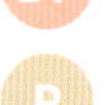
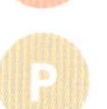

This dish is a repeat offender in our household (my husband is Italian and adores any red sauce and meatball situation). I love to make it right before my period, as grass-fed beef adds plenty of bioavailable, iron-rich protein to help prevent depletion during the upcoming menstrual phase. The spaghetti squash also adds lots of flavor and a noodle-like texture, making it the perfect fiber-rich substitute for pasta without sacrificing taste. This one gives all the cozy feels and is especially fun to eat right outta the "boat."

Spaghetti Squash Boats

- 1 to 2 tablespoons avocado oil
- Sea salt and black pepper to taste
- 2 small to medium spaghetti squash, sliced in half lengthwise and seeded (to create "boats")

Marinara

- 2 tablespoons avocado oil
- 1 small white onion, diced
- 4 cloves garlic, minced
- 1 (28-ounce) can whole peeled tomatoes (or about 4 cups fresh tomatoes cut into large chunks)
- 1 (6-ounce) can tomato paste (about ½ cup)
- 2 tablespoons apple cider vinegar
- 1 tablespoon pure maple syrup
- 2 tablespoons Italian seasoning
- 1 teaspoon sea salt

Meatballs

- 1 pound lean ground grass-fed beef
- 1 large pasture-raised egg
- 3 tablespoons almond flour
- 1 tablespoon Italian seasoning
- 1 tablespoon minced fresh parsley
- 2 teaspoons onion powder
- 1 teaspoon sea salt
- Black pepper to taste
- 2 tablespoons grass-fed ghee or butter

- Fresh basil, grated pecorino, Parmesan, or a vegan Parmesan, for topping (optional)

1. *For the squash boats:* Preheat the oven to 400°F and line a large baking sheet with parchment paper.

2. Drizzle the avocado oil and sprinkle salt and pepper on the spaghetti squash halves. Place them cut side down on the lined baking sheet and roast for 45 to 60 minutes, until a fork scraped over the flesh easily pulls it apart. The insides should have a spaghetti noodle-like consistency.

3. *For the marinara:* Meanwhile, heat the avocado oil in a large pot or Dutch oven over medium heat. Stir in the onion and cook for 3 to 5 minutes, until translucent. Add the garlic and cook for another minute. Add the tomatoes, tomato paste, vinegar, maple syrup, Italian seasoning, and salt. Bring the mixture to a boil, then reduce the heat to low and simmer for about 10 minutes, until well cooked and fragrant. Transfer the sauce to a blender and blend until thick and creamy. (Or use an immersion blender directly in the pot.) Return the sauce to the pot (if necessary) and continue simmering until you add the meatballs to the pot, about 10 minutes. (If using store-bought marinara, warm it in a pot over medium heat.)

4. *For the meatballs:* Combine the ground beef, egg, almond flour, Italian seasoning, parsley, onion powder, and salt and pepper in a medium mixing bowl and mix well with your hands.

5. Roll the meat mixture into balls (about 1½ inches in diameter, the size of a golf ball) and place on a plate until all of the meat is used up. Melt the ghee or butter in a large pot or skillet over medium-high heat. Add the meatballs and cook until the bottoms are browned, 2 to 3 minutes, then turn the meatballs and brown on another side. Repeat until all sides of the meatballs are browned, 8 to 10 minutes total.

6. Transfer the meatballs to the pot with the marinara. Bring everything to a boil, then reduce to a simmer, allowing the meatballs to cook completely through, about 10 minutes. Immediately remove from the heat and set aside.

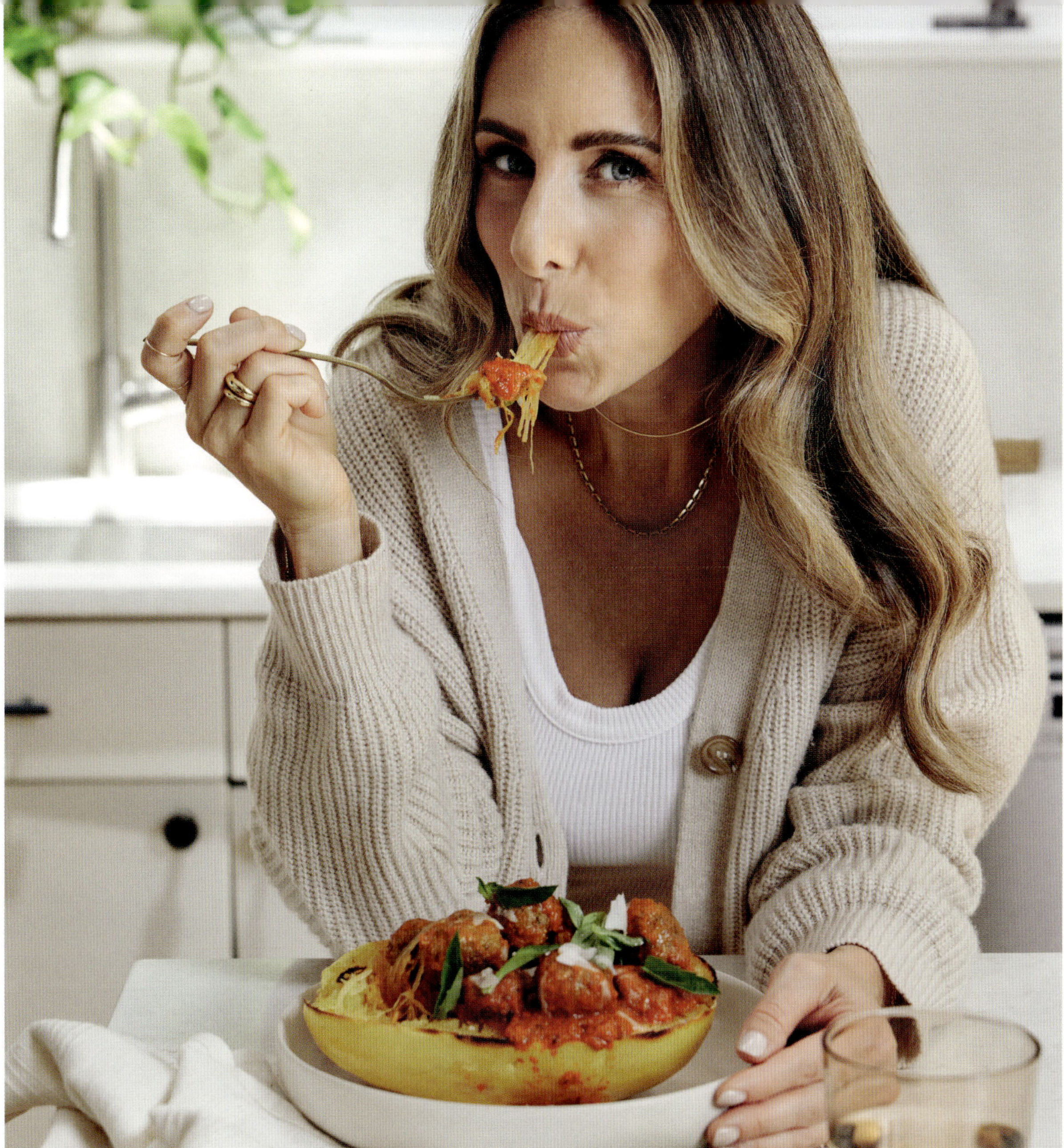

7. Place the spaghetti squash boats flesh side up on a plate and top generously with marinara, meatballs, and optional basil and grated cheese. (If you're not into the stuffed squash, you can use a fork to remove the flesh of the squash from the skin and add it to a bowl, topping with the marinara and meatballs.)

NOTES: The marinara sauce in this dish is super delish, but if you're looking to save time there are plenty of good store-bought options. Additionally, if making meatballs seems tedious, you can skip that step and simply sauté the beef in a skillet over medium heat until cooked through, then add it to the marinara and use the meaty marinara mixture as the topping.

LUTEAL PHASE BENEFITS

Mood-boosting • High in B vitamins • Supports progesterone production

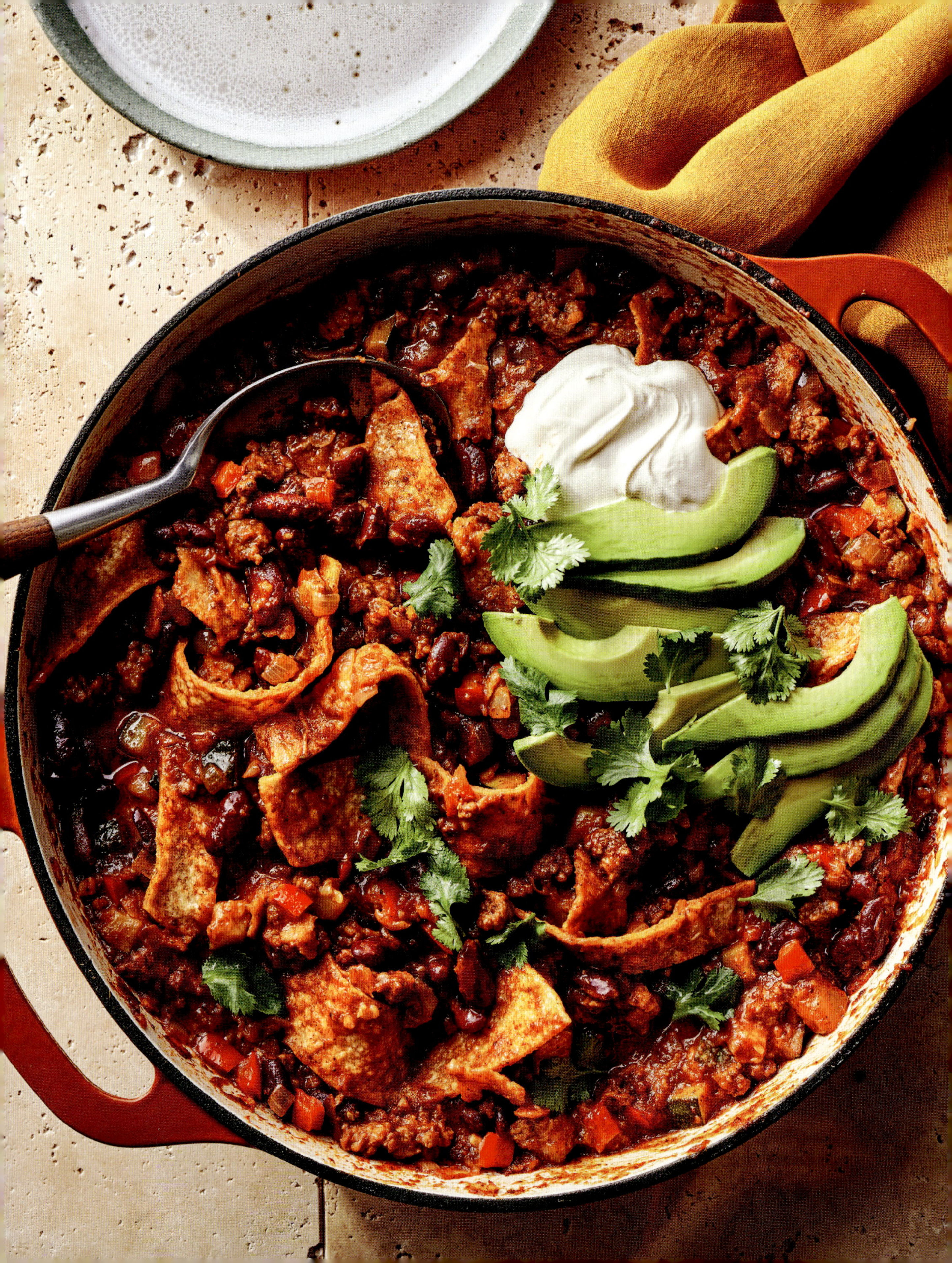

Saucy Enchilada Skillet Casserole

PREP: 10 MINUTES COOK: 25 MINUTES SERVES 4

This casserole is a warm, comforting one-pot situation with minimal dishes to wash and maximum flavor. It's also incredibly protein- and nutrient-rich, with grass-fed beef providing plenty of B vitamins to keep energy and blood sugar stable and beans and veggies contributing fiber to aid digestion and decrease bloat. I come back to this meal repeatedly, but I especially crave it right before my period. For an extra hearty option, serve over rice.

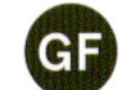

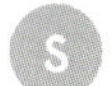

- 2 tablespoons avocado oil
- 1 medium white onion, diced
- 4 cloves garlic, minced
- 2 small zucchini, diced
- 1 red bell pepper, seeded and diced
- 1 pound ground lean grass-fed beef (or ground chicken or turkey)
- 1 teaspoon chili powder
- 1 teaspoon paprika
- 1 teaspoon cumin
- 1 teaspoon sea salt
- 1 (15-ounce) can organic kidney or pinto beans, rinsed and drained
- 1 (15-ounce) jar red enchilada sauce (I like the Siete brand)
- 1 cup shredded raw organic cheddar cheese or nondairy substitute, plus more for topping
- 4 (6-inch) corn or other grain-free tortillas, cut into 1-inch strips
- Cilantro leaves, sliced avocado, and optional sour cream, for topping

1. Warm the avocado oil in a large skillet over medium heat. Add the diced onion and sauté until translucent, 3 to 5 minutes. Add the garlic, zucchini, and bell pepper and sauté for another 2 to 3 minutes, until softened. Add the ground beef, chili powder, paprika, cumin, and salt, stirring and breaking up large chunks, until the beef is browned, 3 to 5 minutes. Add the beans, enchilada sauce, cheese, and tortilla strips and stir until everything is well mixed and the sauce is bubbling.

2. Cover the skillet, reduce the heat to medium-low, and simmer for 10 minutes, stirring once or twice to keep it from sticking to the bottom of the pan. Remove from the heat and let cool for 1 to 2 minutes.

3. Scoop into big bowls and top with cilantro and avocado, plus sour cream and additional shredded cheese if desired.

LUTEAL PHASE BENEFITS

Rich in fiber • High in B vitamins • Rich in magnesium • Anti-inflammatory

Chocolate Chip Cookie Dough Protein Bars

PREP: 20 MINUTES, PLUS 2 HOURS CHILLING   COOK: NONE   SERVES 8–12

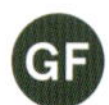
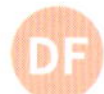

With your body naturally burning 10 to 20 percent more calories during your luteal phase, you can likely expect an uptick in your appetite. Not eating enough actually prevents your body from producing the hormones it needs to keep your metabolism burning effectively, which can lead to an increase in fat storage and destabilized blood sugar. Savoring a nutrient-dense snack is a great way to supply your body with the extra fuel it needs. These cookie dough protein bars are truly such a satisfying treat, I haven't touched a packaged protein bar since! **BONUS:** Dark chocolate is rich in magnesium, which has been shown to help reduce cramping, a common symptom during this phase.

- **¾ cup unsweetened creamy organic peanut butter (or almond or cashew butter)**
- **¼ cup pure maple syrup**
- **1 teaspoon pure vanilla extract**
- **2 tablespoons melted unrefined organic coconut oil, plus more if needed**
- **½ cup vanilla protein powder**
- **½ cup almond or coconut flour, plus more if needed**
- **½ teaspoon sea salt, plus more for topping**
- **1½ cups dark chocolate chips, divided**
- **¼ cup coconut cream**
- **Flaky sea salt, for topping**

1. In a medium bowl, whisk together the peanut butter, maple syrup, vanilla, and melted coconut oil. Add the protein powder and stir well with a mixing spoon. Add the almond or coconut flour and salt and stir until the mixture is well combined. The texture should be thick and slightly dry, mimicking that of a cookie dough. If it's too sticky or wet, add more flour. If it's too dry and crumbly, add more melted coconut oil. Stir in ½ cup of the chocolate chips. Press the dough evenly into a 4 by 8-inch baking pan lined with parchment paper.

2. Melt the remaining 1 cup chocolate chips in a microwave-safe bowl in 30-second increments, stirring after each time, until just melted. Stir in the coconut cream until smooth and creamy. Pour evenly over the peanut butter layer. Top with flaky sea salt and store in the fridge for 2 to 3 hours before slicing into squares and serving.

NOTE: You'll want to keep these bars cool (i.e., store in the fridge or in your bag with a freezer pack when on the go) as they'll start to get a bit melty at room temperature thanks to the coconut oil.

LUTEAL PHASE BENEFITS

Rich in magnesium • Supports progesterone production

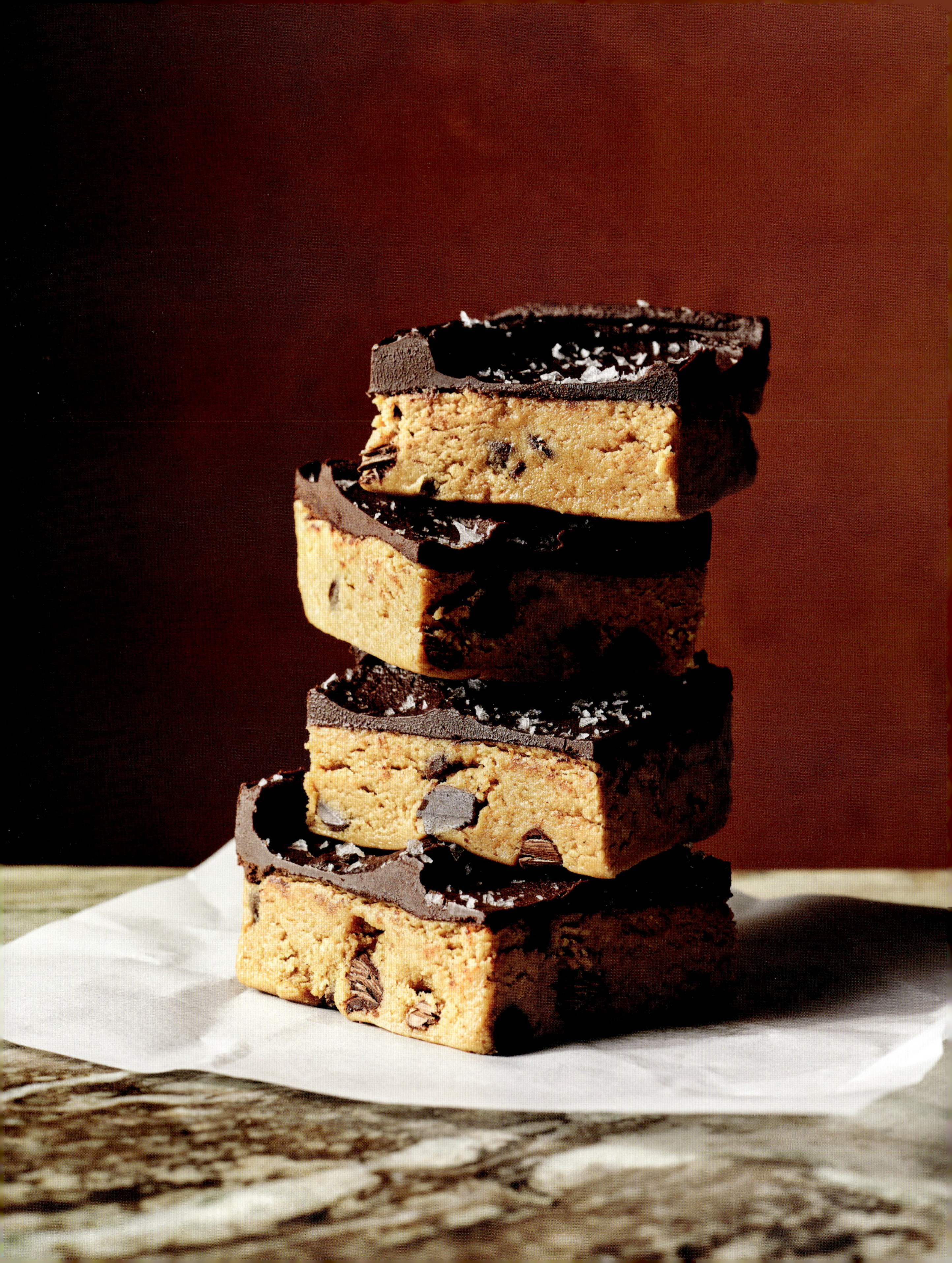

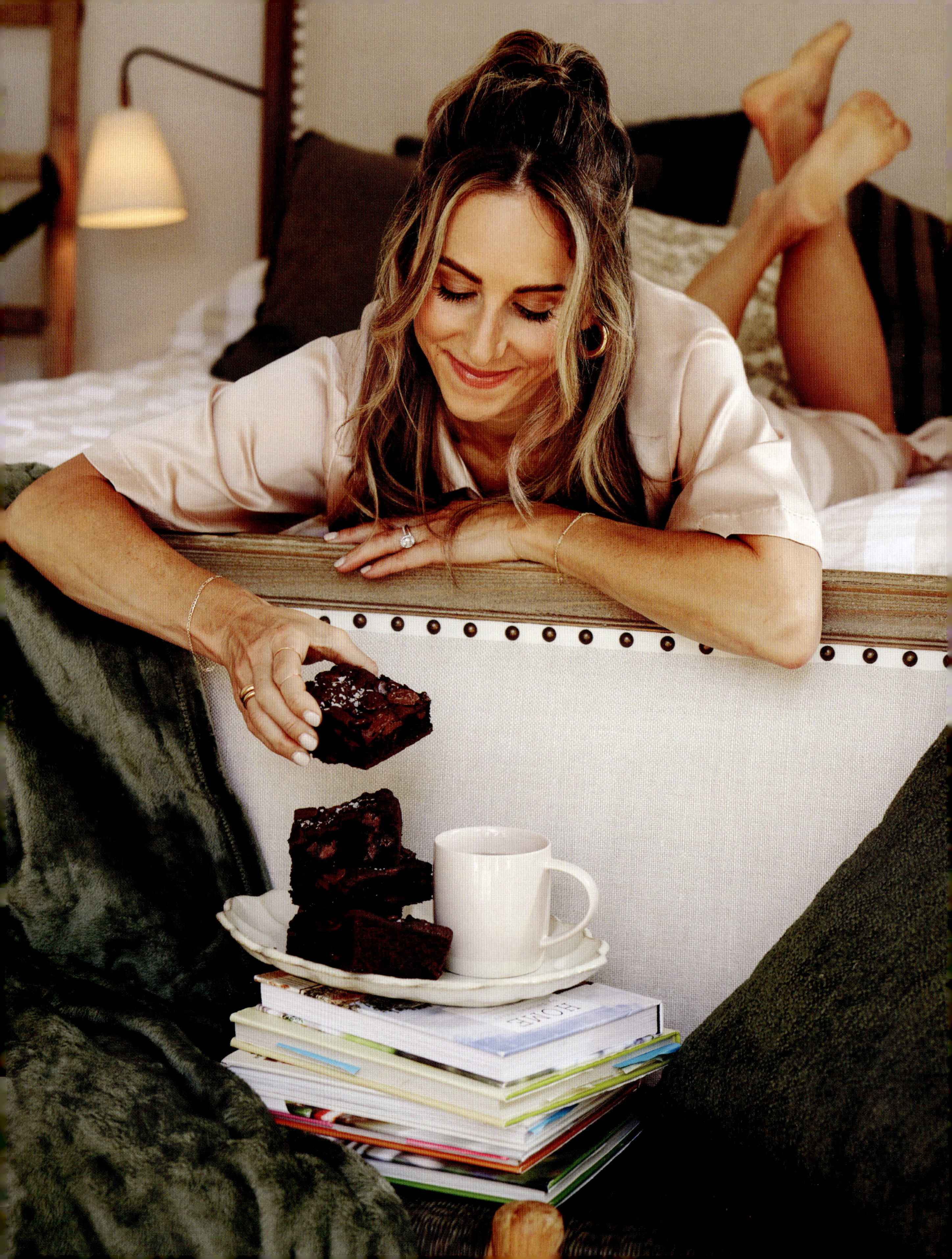
HOME

Flourless Chocolate–Peanut Butter PMS Brownies

PREP: 10 MINUTES COOK: 25 MINUTES SERVES 16

Trust me when I say you only need *one* brownie recipe in your life, and this is it! I have yet to meet a single person on this earth who doesn't *love* this dessert—it's so fudgy, dense, rich, and chocolatey no one ever guesses it's naturally grain-free, gluten-free—and dairy-free to boot. It's also loaded with magnesium, which has been shown to lower prostaglandins, the hormone-like substances that can cause cramping in the days leading up to your period, while the peanut butter provides fat to curb a blood sugar spike, along with minerals and a creamy texture. I'm not saying they're a necessity for healthy hormones...but my luteal phase is just so much better when I have a batch of these to look forward to.

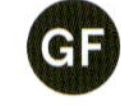

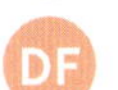

- **2 cups unsweetened organic creamy peanut butter (or almond or cashew butter)**
- **1¼ cups pure maple syrup**
- **2 pasture-raised organic eggs**
- **1 teaspoon pure vanilla extract**
- **½ cup cacao powder**
- **1 teaspoon baking soda**
- **½ teaspoon sea salt**
- **1 tablespoon instant espresso powder (can use decaf), optional**
- **2¼ cups dark chocolate chips or chunks, divided**
- **Flaky sea salt for topping**

1. Preheat the oven to 350°F and line a 9 by 13-inch baking pan with parchment paper.

2. In a large mixing bowl with a hand mixer or stand mixer, beat the peanut butter and maple syrup together until well combined. Slowly add the eggs and vanilla, continuing to mix. Add the cacao, baking soda, salt, and optional espresso powder and combine until smooth and creamy.

3. Using a large spoon or spatula, stir in 2 cups of the chocolate chunks or chips. Pour the batter evenly into the pan and top with the remaining ¼ cup chocolate. Bake for 25 minutes, until the brownies have risen and are almost crispy around the edges, but still a bit soft and gooey in the center. Sprinkle with flaky sea salt and let cool for 30 minutes before serving. Store in an airtight container at room temperature for up to 5 days.

LUTEAL PHASE BENEFITS

Rich in magnesium

Dreamy Golden Milk Latte with Coconut Cashew Milk

PREP: 30 MINUTES   COOK: 5 MINUTES   SERVES 1

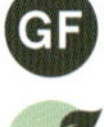

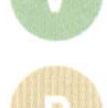

This cozy golden latte tastes good and leaves you feeling good too. It's creamy and bright, slightly sweet, slightly spiced, and filled with anti-inflammatory nutrients that have been shown to help reduce cramping, headaches, and period pain. If you don't feel like making the coconut cashew milk, you don't *have* to, but it does make this latte extra dreamy. (If you do, make sure to give yourself at least 30 minutes to soak the cashews in boiling-hot water; this increases bioavailability and softens the nuts for an ideal creamy texture.)

Coconut Cashew Milk (Optional)

- **1 cup raw organic cashews**
- **4 cups filtered water**
- **1 cup unsweetened coconut flakes**
- **2 dates, pitted**
- **½ teaspoon Himalayan pink salt or sea salt**

Golden Milk Latte

- **1 tablespoon unrefined organic coconut oil**
- **1 teaspoon ground turmeric**
- **½ teaspoon cinnamon, plus more for garnish**
- **½ teaspoon ground ginger**
- **¼ teaspoon sea salt**
- **Pinch of black pepper (increases turmeric's bioavailability)**
- **1½ cups coconut cashew milk (or organic whole milk or a nondairy milk with minimal ingredients)**
- **1 tablespoon raw honey (or pure maple syrup or 1 large medjool date)**
- **1 teaspoon pure vanilla extract**
- **1 serving collagen peptides (optional)**

1. *For the optional cashew milk:* Bring about 2 cups water to a boil. Remove from the heat, add the cashews, and soak for 30 minutes. Drain and rinse.

2. Combine the cashews, 4 cups filtered water, coconut flakes, dates, and pink salt in a high-speed blender and blend on high until smooth. If you like, strain through a nut milk bag or fine-mesh strainer for a super smooth texture, or leave as is for a thicker texture. Set aside.

3. *For the latte:* Melt the coconut oil in a small pot over medium heat. Stir in the turmeric, cinnamon, ginger, salt, and pepper and continue to stir for 1 minute, until you have a fragrant paste. Add the coconut cashew milk (or other milk of choice) along with the honey and vanilla. Let heat through, continuously stirring, for 3 to 5 minutes, until the milk begins to steam (do not boil).

4. Pour into a blender and add the collagen peptides if you like. Blend until well mixed and frothy. Pour into a 12-ounce mug and top with extra cinnamon.

LUTEAL PHASE BENEFIT

Anti-inflammatory

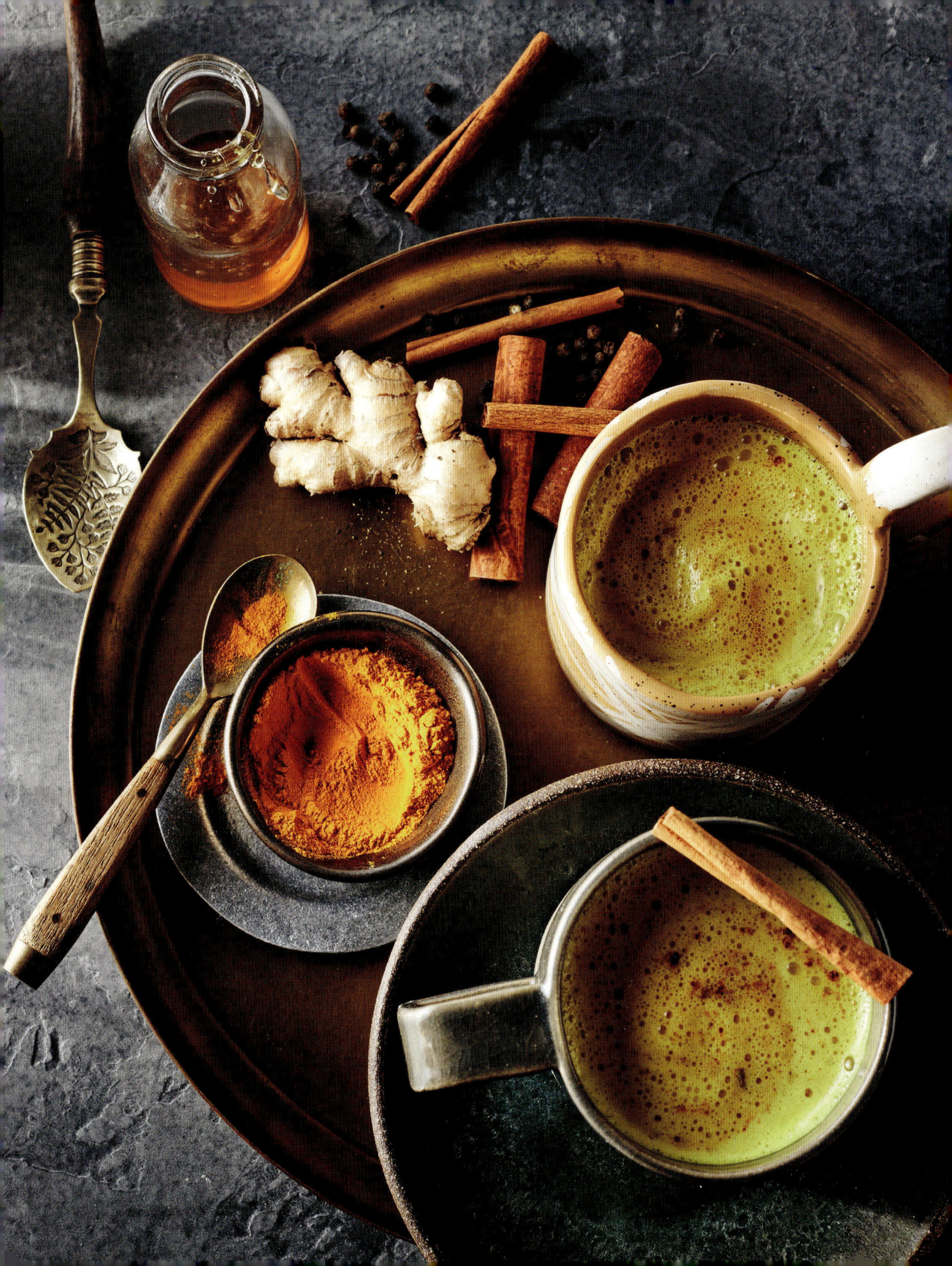

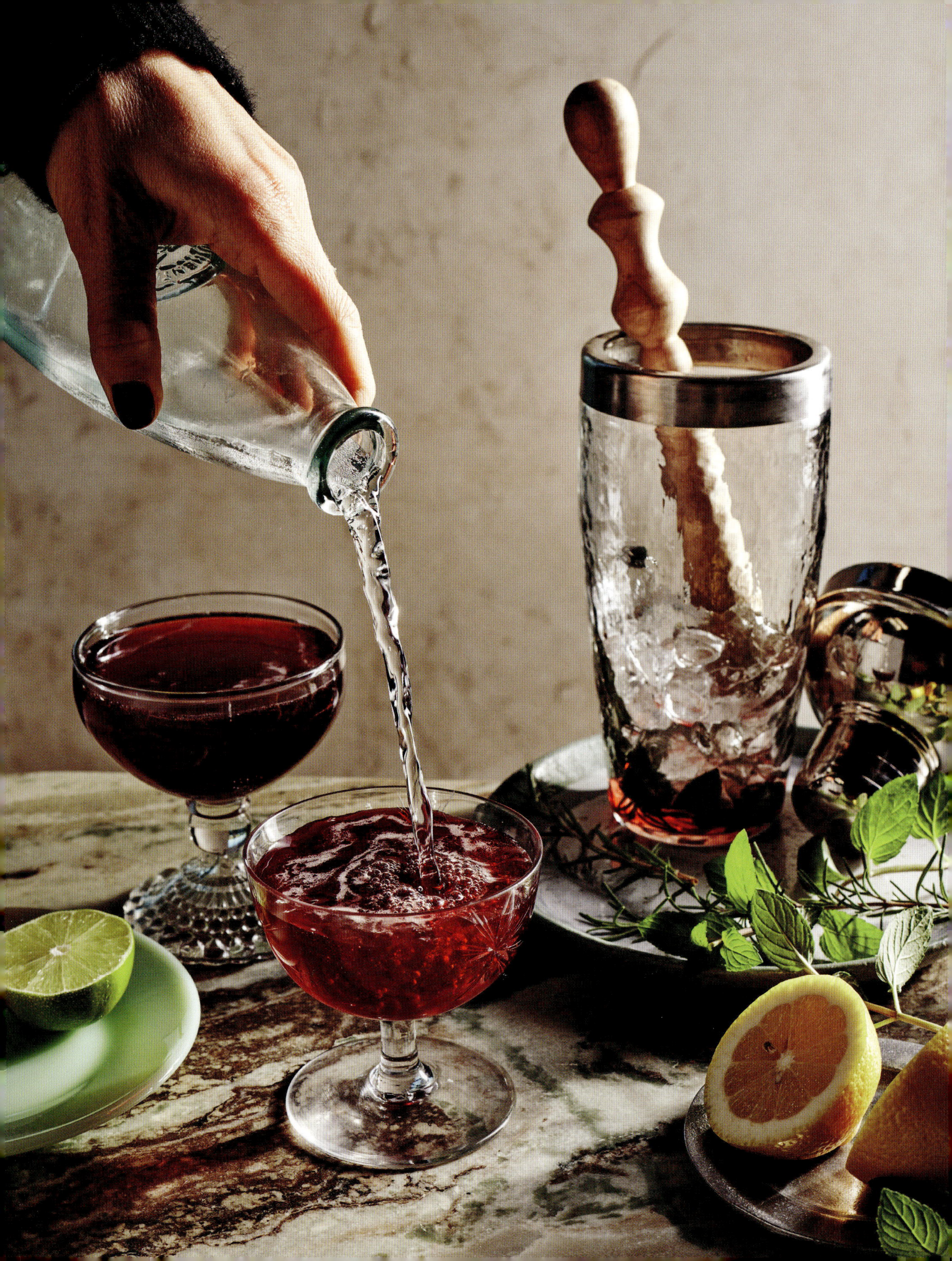

Sleepy Girl Tart-Cherry Mocktail

PREP: 5 MINUTES   COOK: NONE   SERVES 1

The sleepy girl mocktail has become a cherished part of my nighttime routine, as it's super tasty and *super* functional, especially during the luteal phase, when sleep disturbances often crop up due to hormonal imbalances related to the ratio of estrogen to progesterone. Scientific research shows that tart cherries contain a high concentration of melatonin, a hormone that guides your sleep/wake cycle and induces drowsiness at nighttime. The addition of magnesium powder also works to regulate stress hormone cortisol production and promote muscle relaxation, which (bonus!) can help with cramping.

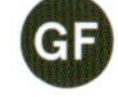

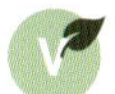

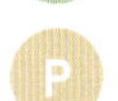

1 sprig fresh rosemary

3 sprigs fresh mint

1 to 3 teaspoons pure maple syrup

Juice of 1 small lemon (about 2 tablespoons)

Juice of 1 large lime (about 2 tablespoons)

1 cup pure tart cherry juice, unsweetened

1 serving magnesium glycinate powder

Ice cubes

¼ cup sparkling water

In a tall glass or cocktail shaker, muddle the rosemary and mint with 1 teaspoon of the maple syrup. Stir in the lemon and lime juice, then add the cherry juice. Taste and add up to 2 teaspoons maple syrup if it needs more sweetness. Stir in the magnesium powder. Add ice cubes (or if using a shaker, strain into a glass with ice). Top off with sparkling water and serve. Enjoy immediately!

NOTE: I prefer a higher ratio of sparkling water (about ¼ cup) to mellow out a bit of the tartness from the cherry juice, but feel free to experiment with the amount you like best. You can also use a little less cherry juice.

LUTEAL PHASE BENEFITS

Anti-inflammatory • Rich in magnesium

ACKNOWLEDGMENTS

To my friends, family, clients, and beloved online (and OG SFNSG) community: Thank you for the love, support, and encouragement you have shown me over the past (ten!!) years. So many of you have read my content, made my recipes, and shared with me the ripple effect it's had—whether it's positively impacted your health and quality of life, brought you and your partner closer together, or helped you feel good about feeding your family and friends. You've been the wind in my sails when times have been tough, and have brought so much meaning, purpose, and fulfillment to my life. I wouldn't be able to do what I do if it weren't for you, and this book is my way of saying thank you. I hope you love it as much as I have loved creating it for you.

To my daughters, Eloise, Amelia, and Frances: Being your mother is the greatest role and honor of my life, and being able to share this book with you just sweetens the deal! You three inspire me in countless ways—and it means so much to me knowing I get to create work that will help you learn about, honor, and nourish your beautiful bodies.

To my husband, my OG taste tester (formerly the meat-lovin' husband—MLH): You've been there since day 1 (circa 2016) when I pursued my passion in health and supported me through all of its ebbs and flows (even my raw/vegan phase!). Thank you for always believing in me, encouraging me to chase my dreams (even when they seemed *so* scary), and helping me get out of my own way. And a special shout-out to your spot-on palate and candid feedback, which ensured that only the most delicious of recipes made their way into this book.

To my parents: Thank you for always believing in me. Since I was little you instilled in me the confidence that I could do or be anything, and although there were times I questioned myself, you never once wavered. Also, Mom: Thank you for teaching me the value of home-cooked meals. You are one of the best cooks I've ever known, and I credit my love of food (especially dessert) to you.

To my mother-in-law, Lori: Thank you for the many flights you've taken to come all the way out here and help with the girls so I could work on this book, not to mention your sheer interest, excitement, and encouragement around it all. You are the ultimate cheerleader, and I'm lucky to have you in my corner.

To my agent, Anna Worrall: Working with you has simply been the BEST. Since the day we first connected I knew it was kismet, and you have made this entire process utterly seamless, supportive, and so *fun*. I only hope we can continue doing it together for many more years to come.

To Eva Kolenko, Emily Caneer, Genesis Vallejo, and Allison Fellion: My *dream* team! Your vision, attention to detail, creativity, and pure talent brought this book to life in ways I wasn't even able to fully articulate, but somehow you just knew. Working with you has been a highlight of my career, not only because of how beautiful the book turned out, but because of your friendship and the fun we had doing it.

To Cara Bedick, my editor: Thank you for your guidance, support, patience, and humor throughout this process! It's truly been a joy working with you, and I'm so grateful for everything you've done to make this book the best it could possibly be.

To the Little, Brown and Company team: Thank you for all of your hard work, expertise, and dedication to this book. You've supported me in my mission to get *Hormone Healthy Eats* out into the world and in the hands of every woman who needs it, and I appreciate you all so much!

To Thea: The champion of this book, which would have never happened if it weren't for you. I'm eternally grateful.

NOTES

HORMONES 101

1 Gudipally, Pratyusha R., and G.K. Sharma. "Premenstrual Syndrome." *StatPearls* (updated July 7, 2023). https://www.ncbi.nlm.nih.gov/books/NBK560698/.

2 Sutton, P., et al. "Toxic environmental chemicals: The role of reproductive health professionals in preventing harmful exposures." *American Journal of Obstetrics and Gynecology* S207(3) (2012): 164–173. doi: 10.1016/j.ajog.2012.01.034. Epub 2012 Mar 8. PMID: 22405527; PMCID: PMC4682569.

3 Sadeghi, H.M., et al. "Polycystic ovary syndrome: A comprehensive review of pathogenesis, management, and drug repurposing." *International Journal of Molecular Sciences* 23(2) (2022): 583. https://doi.org/10.3390/ijms23020583.

4 González-Rodríguez, L.A., M.E. Felici-Giovanni, and L. Haddock. "Thyroid dysfunction in an adult female population: A population-based study of Latin American Vertebral Osteoporosis Study (LAVOS)—Puerto Rico site." *Puerto Rico Health Sciences Journal* 32(2) (2013), 57–62. https://pmc.ncbi.nlm.nih.gov/articles/PMC3804108/.

5 Thoma, M.E., et al. "Prevalence of infertility in the United States as estimated by the current duration approach and a traditional constructed approach." *Fertility and Sterility* 99(5) (2013): 1324–1331.

6 Looijer-van Langen, M., et al. "Estrogen receptor-β signaling modulates epithelial barrier function." *American Journal of Physiology: Gastrointestinal and Liver Physiology* 300(4) (2011): G621–G626.

7 Lee, J.-J., et al. "Oral contraception and female sexual dysfunction in reproductive women." *Sexual Medicine Reviews* 5(1) (2017): 31–44.

8 Deb, S., et al. "Quantifying effect of combined oral contraceptive pill on functional ovarian reserve as measured by serum anti-Müllerian hormone and small antral follicle count using three-dimensional ultrasound." *Ultrasound in Obstetrics & Gynecology* 39(5) (2012): 574–580.

9 Basciani, S., and G. Porcaro. "Counteracting side effects of combined oral contraceptives through the administration of specific micronutrients." *European Review for Medical & Pharmacological Sciences* 26(13) (2022): 4846–4862.

10 Wang, X., et al. "Use of oral contraceptives and risk of ulcerative colitis: A systematic review and meta-analysis." *Pharmacological Research* 139 (2019): 367–374.

11 Schliep, K.C., et al. "Alcohol intake, reproductive hormones, and menstrual cycle function: A prospective cohort study." *American Journal of Clinical Nutrition* 102(4) (2015): 933–942.

12 Gill, J. "Effects of moderate alcohol consumption on female hormone levels and reproductive function." *Alcohol and Alcoholism* 35(5) (2000): 417–423.

THE HORMONE HEALTHY EATS PHILOSOPHY

1 Loucks, A.B., and J.R. Suma. "Luteinizing hormone pulsatility is disrupted at a threshold of energy availability in regularly menstruating women." *Journal of Clinical Endocrinology and Metabolism* 88(1) (2003): 297–311.

2 Pirke, K.M., et al. "Dieting causes menstrual irregularities in normal weight young women through impairment of episodic luteinizing hormone secretion." *Fertility and Sterility* 51(2) (1989): 263–268.

3 Williams, N.I., et al. "Estrogen and progesterone exposure is reduced in response to energy deficiency in women aged 25–40 years." *Human Reproduction* 25(9) (2010): 2328–2339.

4 Koebnick, C., et al. "Consequences of a long-term raw food diet on body weight and menstruation: Results of a questionnaire survey." *Annals of Nutrition and Metabolism* 43(2) (1999): 69–79.

5 Kazemi, A., et al. "Effect of calorie restriction or protein intake on circulating levels of insulin like growth factor I in humans: A systematic review and meta-analysis." *Clinical Nutrition* 39(6) (2020): 1705–1716.

6 Chavarro, J.E., et al. "Dietary fatty acid intakes and the risk of ovulatory infertility." *American Journal of Clinical Nutrition* 85(1) (2007): 231–237.

7 Rasheed, P., and L.S. Al-Sowielem. "Prevalence and predictors of premenstrual syndrome among college-aged women in Saudi Arabia." *Annals of Saudi Medicine* (2003) 3(6) (2003): 381–387.

8 Loy, S.L., et al. "Plasma glycemic measures and fecundability in a Singapore preconception cohort study." *Fertility and Sterility* 115(1) (2021): 138–147.

9 Phillips, S.M. "Current concepts and unresolved questions in dietary protein requirements and supplements in adults." *Frontiers in Nutrition* 4 (2017): 13.

10 Xiao, K., et al. "Effect of a high protein diet at breakfast on postprandial glucose level at dinner time in healthy adults." *Nutrients* 15(1) (2022): 85. https://doi.org/10.3390/nu15010085.

11 Kane, K.K., et al. "Effects of varying levels of undegradable intake protein on endocrine and metabolic function of young post-partum beef cows." *Theriogenology* 57(9) (2002): 2179–2191.

12 Schutt, A.K., et al. "Preovulatory exposure to a protein-restricted diet disrupts amino acid kinetics and alters mitochondrial structure and function in the rat oocyte and is partially rescued by folic acid." *Reproductive Biology and Endocrinology* 17(1) (2019): 1–13.

13 Gold, E.B., et al. "Diet and lifestyle factors associated with premenstrual symptoms in a racially diverse community sample: Study of Women's Health Across the Nation (SWAN)." *Journal of Women's Health* 16(5) (2007): 641–656.

14 Chavarro. "Dietary fatty acid intakes and the risk of ovulatory infertility."

15 Houghton, S.C., et al. "Protein intake and the risk of premenstrual syndrome." *Public Health Nutrition* 22(10) (2019): 1762.

16 Nichols, L., and L. Hendrickson-Jack. "Fertility Nutrition Fundamentals" in *Real Food for Fertility*. Fertility Food Publishing, 2024, p. 44.

17 Houghton, S.C., et al. "Intake of dietary fat and fat subtypes and risk of premenstrual syndrome in the Nurses' Health Study II." *British Journal of Nutrition* 118(10) (2017): 849–857.

18 Fayezi, S., et al. "Oleic acid in the modulation of oocyte and preimplantation embryo development." *Zygote* 26(1) (2018): 1–13.

19 López-Gómez, C., et al. "Oleic acid protects against insulin resistance by regulating the genes related to the PI3K signaling pathway." *Journal of Clinical Medicine* 9(18) (2020): 2615. https://doi.org/10.3390/jcm9082615.

20 Fayezi. "Oleic acid in the modulation of oocyte and preimplantation embryo development"; Karayiannis, D., et al. "Adherence to the Mediterranean diet and IVF success rate among non-obese women attempting fertility." *Human Reproduction* 33(3) (2018): 494–502.

21 Jandacek, R.J. "Linoleic acid: A nutritional quandary." *Healthcare* 5(2) (2017): 25; Fontana, R., and S. Della Torre. "The deep correlation between energy metabolism and reproduction: A view on the effects of nutrition for women fertility." *Nutrients* 8(2) (2016): 87.

22 "New WHA Resolution to Accelerate Efforts on Food Micronutrient Fortification." 2023. https://www.who.int/news/item/29-05-2023-new-wha-resolution-to-accelerate-efforts-on-food-micronutrient-fortification.

23 Institute of Medicine. "Dietary Reference Intakes for Vitamin A, Vitamin K, Arsenic, Boron, Chromium, Copper, Iodine, Iron, Manganese, Molybdenum, Nickel, Silicon, Vanadium, and Zinc." Washington, DC: National Academy Press, 2001; Hurrell, R., and I. Egli. "Iron bioavailability and dietary reference values." *American Journal of Clinical Nutrition* 91(5) (2010): 1461S–1467S.

24 Kim, K., et al. "Dietary minerals, reproductive hormone levels and sporadic anovulation: Associations in healthy women with regular menstrual cycles." *British Journal of Nutrition* 120(1) (2018): 81–89.

25 Gold. "Diet and lifestyle factors"; Janowsky, D.S., et al. "Correlations between mood, weight, and electrolytes during the menstrual cycle: A renin-angiotensin-aldosterone hypothesis of premenstrual tension." *Psychosomatic Medicine* (1973) 35(2) (1973): 143–154.

26 Fathizadeh, N., et al. "Evaluating the effect of magnesium and magnesium plus vitamin B6 supplement on the severity of premenstrual syndrome." *Iranian Journal of Nursing and Midwifery Research* 15(suppl1) (2010): 401; Fis-Jacobs, S. "Micronutrients and the premenstrual syndrome: The case for calcium." *Journal of the American College of Nutrition* 19(2) (2000): 220–227.

27 Lord, T., et al. "Accumulation of electrophilic aldehydes during postovulatory aging of mouse oocytes causes reduced fertility, oxidative stress, and apoptosis." *Biology of Reproduction* 92(2) (2015): 33–1; Hansen, S.O., and U.B. Knudsen. "Endometriosis, dysmenorrhoea and diet." *European Journal of Obstetrics & Gynecology and Reproductive Biology* 169(2) (2013): 162–171; McDougall, M., et al. "Lethal dysregulation of energy metabolism during embryonic vitamin E deficiency." *Free Radical Biology and Medicine* 104 (2017): 324–332.

28 Chavarro. "Dietary fatty acid intakes and the risk of ovulatory infertility."

29 Fontana and Della Torre. "The deep correlation between energy metabolism and reproduction."

30 Abou-Donia, M.B., et al. "Splenda alters gut microflora and increases intestinal p-glycoprotein and cytochrome p-450 in male rats." *Journal of Toxicology and Environmental Health, Part A*, 71(21) (2008): 1415–1429.

31 Pałkowska-Goździk, E., et al. "Type of sweet flavour carrier affects thyroid axis activity in male rats." *European Journal of Nutrition* (2016): 1–10.

32 Schliep, K.C., et al. "Alcohol intake, reproductive hormones, and menstrual cycle function: A prospective cohort study." *American Journal of Clinical Nutrition* 102(4) (2015): 933–942.

33 Perry, E.D., et al. "Genetically engineered crops and pesticide use in U.S. maize and soybeans." *Science Advances* 2(8) (2016): e1600850. https://doi.org/10.1126/sciadv.1600850.

PHASE 1: MENSTRUAL PHASE (INNER WINTER)

1 Kulkarni, S.A., et al. "Beneficial effect of iron pot cooking on iron status." *Indian Journal of Pediatrics* 80 (12) (2013): 985–989. https://doi.org/10.1007/s12098-013-1066-z.

PHASE 4: LUTEAL PHASE (INNER FALL)

1 Cross, G.B., et al. "Changes in nutrient intake during the menstrual cycle of overweight women with premenstrual syndrome." *British Journal of Nutrition* 85(4) (2001): 475–482; Dalvit-McPhillips, S.P. "The effect of the human menstrual cycle on nutrient intake." *Physiology and Behavior* 31(2) (1983): 209–212.

INDEX

NOTE: Page references in *italics* indicate photographs.

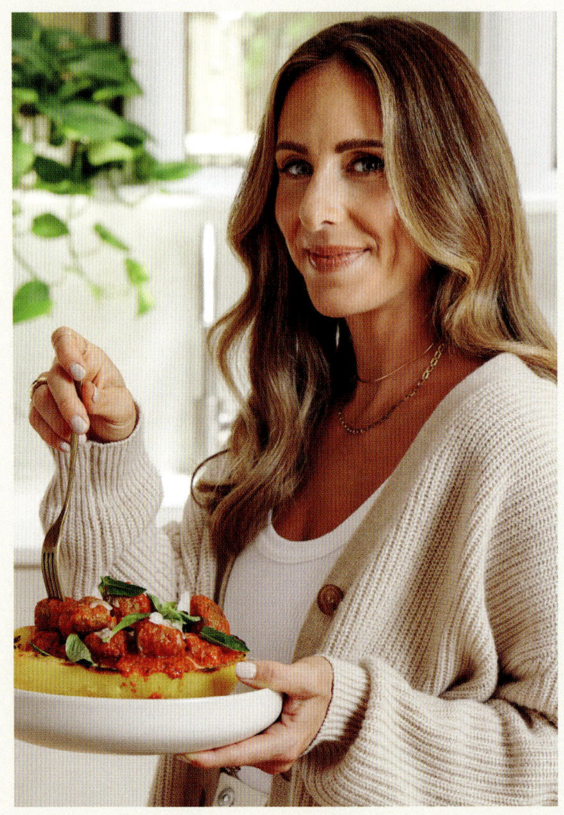

ABOUT THE AUTHOR

Lauren Chambers is an author and nutrition and hormone health coach on a mission to help women balance their hormones and reduce symptoms to feel their best through delicious, nutrient-dense recipes. At any time, you'll probably find her sipping on a beverage of sorts (coffee, mocktail, smoothie, tea, hot cocoa—she doesn't discriminate) and dreaming up her next recipe. She's married to her best friend and is a mom to three girls, who are the loves of her life and also keep her *very* busy. Chambers lives in the Pacific Northwest and enjoys hiking, camping (especially if it involves s'mores), and spending time in nature. To learn more, visit her website at sofreshnsogreen.com or Substack at hormonehealthyeats.substack.com.

"Whether you're struggling with PMS, PCOS, or perimenopause, or just want to feel more like yourself again, *Hormone Healthy Eats* is your invitation to eat your way to vibrant health. With practical tips, empowering education, and flavors you'll crave, Lauren Chambers makes it easy."

—DR. JOLENE BRIGHTEN, FABNE,
author of *Is This Normal?* and *Beyond the Pill*

"This book is a beautiful crash course on the female endocrine system and will help every reader ditch diet culture, support a healthy menstrual cycle, and eat incredibly deliciously while doing so."

—JENNA RADOMSKI, MScN,
coauthor of *The Moon Cycle Cookbook*

"*Hormone Healthy Eats* is more than a cookbook—it's a guide to living in harmony with your body. With 100 delicious, hormone-supportive recipes designed around the four phases of the menstrual cycle, Lauren Chambers shows you how to nourish yourself in sync with your biology. Part education, part empowerment, and entirely practical, this book will change the way you think about food, your period, and your health—inviting you to ditch deprivation and embrace a way of eating that feels aligned, intuitive, and deeply nourishing."

—NICOLE JARDIM,
certified women's health coach
and author of *Fix Your Period*